Uncertain Bioethics

"Stephen Napier argues with verve and subtlety for a cautious and restrained approach to acts of killing in bioethics; central to his argument is the difficulty of being sure that active interventions are permissible. This book intriguingly combines insights from a wide variety of different recent philosophical literatures to offer an important and interesting contribution to numerous current debates."

Sophie-Grace Chappell, Professor of
Philosophy at Open University, UK

Bioethics is a field of inquiry and as such is fundamentally an epistemic discipline. Knowing how we make moral judgments can bring into relief why certain arguments on various bioethical issues appear plausible to one side and obviously false to the other. *Uncertain Bioethics* makes a significant and distinctive contribution to the bioethics literature by culling the insights from contemporary moral psychology to highlight the epistemic pitfalls and distorting influences on our apprehension of value. Stephen Napier also incorporates research from epistemology addressing pragmatic encroachment and the significance of peer disagreement to justify what he refers to as *epistemic diffidence* when one is considering harming or killing human beings. Napier extends these developments to the traditional bioethical notion of dignity and argues that beliefs subject to *epistemic diffidence* should not be acted upon. He proceeds to apply this framework to traditional and developing issues in bioethics including abortion, stem cell research, euthanasia, decision-making for patients in a minimally conscious state, and risky research on competent human subjects.

Stephen Napier is an associate professor of philosophy at Villanova University. His previous publications include *Virtue Epistemology: Motivation and Knowledge*, and he edited *Persons, Moral Worth, and Embryos*. His interests include epistemology, bioethics, and the metaphysics of persons.

Routledge Annals of Bioethics

Series Editors:
Mark J. Cherry
St. Edward's University, USA
Ana Smith Iltis
Saint Louis University, USA

Uncertain Bioethics
Moral Risk and Human Dignity

Stephen Napier

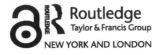
Routledge
Taylor & Francis Group
NEW YORK AND LONDON

First published 2020
by Routledge
605 Third Avenue, New York, NY 10017

and by Routledge
2 Park Square, Milton Park, Abingdon, Oxon, OX14 4RN

First issued in paperback 2021

Routledge is an imprint of the Taylor & Francis Group, an informa business

Publisher's Note
The publisher has gone to great lengths to ensure the quality of this reprint but
points out that some imperfections in the original copies may be apparent.

Library of Congress Cataloging-in-Publication Data
Names: Napier, Stephen E., author.
Title: Uncertain bioethics : human dignity and moral risk / by Stephen Napier.
Description: New York : Taylor & Francis, 2020. | Series: Routledge annals
     of bioethics ; 19 | Includes bibliographical references and index.
Identifiers: LCCN 2019012772| ISBN 9780815372981 (hbk : alk. paper) |
     ISBN 9781351244510 (ebk)
Subjects: LCSH: Bioethics. | Dignity.
Classification: LCC QH332 .N35 2020 | DDC 174.2—dc23
LC record available at https://lccn.loc.gov/2019012772

ISBN 13: 978-1-03-209099-3 (pbk)
ISBN 13: 978-0-8153-7298-1 (hbk)

Typeset in Sabon
by Swales & Willis Ltd, Exeter, Devon, UK

To Katherine,
lux quia lucet

Contents

Acknowledgments

The following individuals contributed to the present project in various ways. David Benrimoh, Joe Butera, John Carvalho, Dan Cheely, Rev. Alfred Cioffi, Michael Degnan, Mark Doorley, Jason Eberl, Karl Hahn, Stephen Heaney, Rev. James McCartney, Matthew O'Brien, David Prentice, Benjamin Richards, Mike Rota, John Travaline, Helen Watt, Peter Wicks, and Brett Wilmot commented on some of the material present here. Edmund Howe and Matthew Braddock wrote separate essays in reply to some of the material herein (Howe's is published). Sarah-Vaughan Brakman and Peter Koch formed a writing group that involved sharing comments on our respective work. This proved immensely helpful. David Hershenov reviewed, in exquisite detail, two penultimate chapters. I sent him 8,000+ word count documents, and received 5,000+ ones in return. I have no excuse for any errors except that philosophy is difficult. I'd like to thank two anonymous reviewers and the editors at Routledge, namely, Mark Cherry, Andrew Weckenmann, Allie Simmons, and freelance editor Judith Harvey for their very helpful guidance and feedback on this project.

In writing this book I have made use of previously published material. Chapter 3 includes some material from my article, "The Justification of Killing and Psychological Accounts of the Person," *American Catholic Philosophical Quarterly* 89(4) (2015): 651–680. Chapter 6 includes paragraphs from "Vulnerable Embryos: A Critical Analysis of Twinning, Rescue, and Natural-Loss Arguments," *American Catholic Philosophical Quarterly* 84(4) (2010): 783–812. Chapter 8 includes paragraphs from "Perception of Value and the Minimally Conscious State," *HEC Forum* 27(3) (2015): 265–286; and "The Minimally Conscious State, the Disability Bias and the Moral Authority of Advance Directives," *International Journal of Law and Psychiatry* (2018), doi: 10.1016/j.ijlp.2018.03.001. Chapter 9 derives mostly from "When Should We Not Respect a Patient's Wish?" *Journal of Clinical Ethics* 25(3) (2014): 196–206. And Chapter 10 derives mostly from "Challenging Research on Human Subjects: Justice and Uncompensated Harms," *Theoretical Medicine and Bioethics* 34(1) (2013): 29–51. I wish to thank the editors

and the anonymous reviewers of these journals for their significant contributions to my thinking. Finally, I wish to thank the Office of the Provost
at Villanova University for funding the Veritas Award which helped me
write significant portions of the manuscript.

1 Introduction

An informative introduction should frame the content that follows such that the reader is better able to understand the author's intent and fundamental concerns. It should suggest how the work may be looked *along* as well as looked *at*. The change in preposition is important. *This book should be understood as an essay on what the intellectual virtues of humility and justice look like in discrete areas of bioethical inquiry.* Looking at it, one will find arguments for and against various claims. Looking along it, one should glean why one should take a more epistemically humble stance when arguing for permissible killing or harming. By looking *along* this essay, one catches a glimpse of *how* one should weigh the evidence and measure one's credulity on certain bioethical positions. For any inquiry, there is the object of inquiry, and the inquirer; both receive attention in this book.

Bioethics is a field of inquiry and as such is fundamentally an epistemic discipline. It aims to know what the right/wrong action or policy is. The locus of attention for this project is on the epistemic significance of various developments in moral psychology and contemporary epistemology applied to bioethical inquiry. Specifically, this book aims to answer the following question: under what conditions is an agent S justified in believing that P [an act of killing a human being] is permissible when S is the agent of that action? Or more simply, under what conditions is an agent justified in believing a proposition 'it is permissible to kill x' when one is acting on that belief?

The idea of moral risk referenced in my title can be understood in relation to our typical way of using risk in healthcare delivery. Typically, risk is understood as roughly parasitic on cause–effect relations as when we say, "there is a risk of nausea and vomiting if you take this drug." Here, risk is understood as a probability that a disvaluable state of affairs might occur. The notion of moral risk with which I am concerned pertains rather to the very judgment of disvalue (or value). Moral risk is a function of acting on what might very well be an erroneous moral judgment. Hence, the first step in this project is to articulate how our moral judgments might err.

Knowing how we make moral judgments can bring into relief why certain arguments on various bioethical issues appear plausible to one side and obviously false to the other. This is the first feature of my project that aims to make a significant contribution: namely, to cull the insights from contemporary moral psychology to highlight the epistemic pitfalls and distorting influences on our apprehension of value.

A second contribution of my project is to collate the lessons learned from the epistemological literature addressing moral risk (cf. Fantl & McGrath, 2009), the nature of presumptions in argument (Freeman, 2005), and the epistemic significance of peer disagreement (Christensen, 2011; Elga, 2007) to justify what I refer to as *epistemic diffidence* on numerous bioethical issues. The notion of moral risk and the significance of peer disagreement are simple to understand and that they exert epistemic effects is clear in many cases (consider the stronger standard of evidence for criminal cases versus civil cases). The difficult project is explaining why risk and disagreement exert epistemic effects at all.

The first two contributions together justify epistemic diffidence when one is considering harming or killing human beings. The cost of being wrong that 'killing a human being is permissible' is high; it is subject to peer disagreement, and it is doubtful that, given the evidence from the cognitive sciences, we should be so trustful of our moral intuitions (or the post-hoc reasoning justifying those intuitions (Haidt, 2001)). Beliefs subject to epistemic diffidence should not be acted upon.

The argument I wish to defend in this book may be understood in outline as follows:

1   The belief B that 'x is permissible,' where x is an act of intentional killing or harming of a human being, is subject to *epistemic diffidence*. (Hereafter, 'x' is a variable only for the issues I discuss in this work.)
    A belief B is subject to epistemic diffidence if and only if:[1]

    i   B suffers from an undercutting defeater or is unstable (both notions explained below),
    ii The justification for B does not offset the cost of being wrong, and
    iii The justification for B does not discharge the effects of peer disagreement.[2]

2   If B is subject to epistemic diffidence, it would be impermissible to *act* on that belief.
3   Therefore, it is impermissible to act on 'x is permissible' where x includes the specific actions that I address in this book.

A few points are worth noting about this argument. First, the belief B is restricted to those acts of intentional killing or harming that I address in this book. I remain neutral as to whether this argument is sound for *any* case of intentional killing or harming either of a human being, or non-human animal. Second, the dialectical work of the chapters is to justify that the epistemic standards or degree of justification needed to permit acting on the belief that 'x is permissible' are not met. Third, the dialectical work of this book is *not* to argue that all things considered the beliefs that 'x is permissible' are false. My argument requires a lower horizon of acceptability while also arguing that one should be epistemically diffident towards *acting* on such beliefs. This is probably the most distinctive aspect of my project. Lowering the dialectical horizon is not done best by defending one's favored theory, and then applying it to specific cases. The horizon is lowered partly by focusing on how we form our theoretical commitments in the first place. Fourth, the notion of epistemic diffidence is, in this work, an epistemological notion. The moral implications of it are made explicit in premise 2. As such, Chapters 2 and 3 (summarized below) aim to justify premise 2. The remainder of the chapters aim to justify premise 1, substituting in for 'x' each issue – whether it is abortion, euthanasia, etc.

The project aims to frame both traditional and novel bioethical problems in light of the epistemological lessons I highlight. In doing so, I argue that a dialectical shift occurs to the advantage of those who take a prohibitive stance on the issues discussed.

Chapter 2 aims to answer the question, "How do we typically think on moral issues?" The chapter explicates what is called Moral Foundations Theory (Graham et al., 2013), which includes four theses: nativism, cultural influences, intuitionism, and pluralism. There are two pericopes of the theory I wish to highlight in this chapter. The first is that intuitions come first, and moral reasoning comes second. The second aspect of the theory that I draw attention to is the explanation for why we have the intuitions we do. On this point Graham et al. (2013) highlight the importance of cultural influences and more subjective motivational influences (Kunda, 1990).

Knowing that our intuitions are subject to such influences may *undercut* our confidence in them. An undercutting defeater is a reason for thinking that things might not be as they appear (Pollock & Cruz, 1999). I see widgets on an assembly line that look red. The foreman informs me that they look red because they are illuminated by red incandescent bulbs such that they look red whether or not they really are. What the foreman tells me is an undercutting defeater to my belief that the widgets are red. That something looks red is still a reason for thinking that it is red, but an undercutting defeater renders that appearance inert *to justify* believing that x is red. Discovering how we morally think and process moral information functions in a similar way. Whether or not an action really is permissible, my moral intuitions might apprehend it as permissible anyway given certain facts about how we think morally. The non-alethic influences on our moral perception function like the red incandescent light bulbs; they give me reason for thinking that the moral world might not be as it appears to be.

Another conclusion that follows from Chapter 2 is slightly weaker but still sufficient for my purposes. One could say that upon taking seriously the empirical evidence outlined in Chapter 2 one's noetic system suffers no defeater at all, undercutting or otherwise. The evidence does, however, render one's noetic system more easily *destabilized* by defeaters highlighted in later chapters. Consider an analogy with an unruptured brain aneurysm (BA). An unruptured BA does not cause any deleterious health effects, but the health situation of the person who has one is more easily destabilized. Something as simple as elevated blood pressure can rupture the BA. Likewise, the evidence canvassed in Chapter 2 might not cause any deleterious epistemic effects, but the justification one has for her beliefs is more easily destabilized – even by somewhat weak defeaters such as peer disagreement.

So Chapter 2 does not argue for moral skepticism. Chapter 3, however, acuminates our reasons for epistemic diffidence based on concrete dialectical engagements. I argue for a local skepticism based on two features of these engagements: the cost of being wrong in one's judgment that a particular action is permissible to perform, and the epistemic pressure that peer disagreement exerts on my moral beliefs. Why there is such 'pressure' is explained with reference to intellectual virtues.

The previous two chapters present an argument for epistemic diffidence in high-stakes cases based on how we typically think on moral issues, and the justifiable doubt we should have for our own views in the setting of peer disagreement. In contemporary bioethics, however, it is far from innocuous and picayune to suppose that the cost of being wrong that, for example, 'abortion is permissible' is a high-stakes belief that justifies epistemic diffidence. To that end, the next two chapters argue that the costs in being wrong about the permissibility of killing any human being are asymmetrical – the costs are on the side of thinking that such actions are permissible. Specifically, the costs of being *wrong* that abortion, or any other act of killing a human being, is *permissible* are sufficient to justify epistemic diffidence.

Chapter 4 argues that you and I are individual human substances that come into existence at conception. But do we have intrinsic dignity? Are we valuable at every point in our existence? More to the point, is it permissible to kill us intentionally? – pollarding away complications such as capital punishment and just war. In Chapter 5 I argue that human beings do have intrinsic dignity. If you and I have intrinsic dignity at every point in which we exist, then a lot is at stake when one considers intentionally killing or harming you or me.

The first part of the book argues for epistemic diffidence in relation to actions intended to kill or harm human beings. Epistemic diffidence, if justified, means that there are insufficient reasons for acting on a belief that x is permissible, where x is an act of killing/harming a human being. The reason: the cost of being wrong is irrecusable.

The dialectical goal of Chapter 6 is to defend premise 1 substituting in for 'x' the act of direct abortion. To this end I outline two principal arguments in support of direct abortion. I consider in detail the argument from bodily rights (Thomson, 1971; Boonin, 2002). Arguments based on personhood (Warren, 1973; McMahan, 2002) are addressed in Chapter 4. I argue that none of the arguments exceed a threshold of justification that would override the epistemic diffidence we should have towards killing human life.

The goals of Chapter 7 are to address the four principal arguments used in support of human destructive stem cell research. The four arguments are the argument from twinning (Persson, 2009; and DeGrazia, 2006), totipotency (Smith and Brogaard, 2003), rescue cases (Sandel, 2005), and natural loss (Ord, 2008; McMahan, 2007). The conclusion in this chapter is the same as in the previous one. I argue that none of the arguments exceed a threshold of justification that would override the epistemic diffidence we should have towards killing human life.

Pro-euthanasia arguments fall into two broad camps: those that argue for the normativity of personal or subjective features of a patient – i.e., arguments from autonomy (Brock, 1992; Jackson & Keown, 2012); and those that argue for the normativity of objective features – such as the avoidance of unnecessary suffering (Rachels, 1986; Jackson & Keown, 2012). As in the previous chapter, I argue that premises 1 and 2 are true when substituting in for x, "euthanasia is permissible."

In the third part of the book, I turn to address more specific clinical scenarios wherein the values of dignity and autonomy can encounter axiological friction. I focus on clinical and research ethics cases where the same themes of moral risk arise. The first clinical scenario concerns end-of-life decision-making for those patients who suffer suppressed consciousness, for example, patients in a minimally conscious state.

My thesis in this chapter is that there exists a disability bias against those who may be severely disabled. This is a bias because those who become severely disabled rate their own quality of life (QoL) at or just slightly below the QoL assessments of normal controls. This is a source of skepticism regarding third-person QoL judgments of the disabled. I argue that this skepticism applies as well to those who are in the minimally conscious state (MCS). For rather simple means of sustaining an MCS patient's life (for example, tube feeding), the cost of being wrong that the patient would not want further support is high. Pair this cost with the reason to be skeptical of third-person judgments, and my argument suggests not withholding food and water from MCS patients.

The prevailing orthodoxy in terms of competency assessment is to test for the presence of certain abilities. Chapter 10 argues that the presence of certain abilities is not enough in cases where the patient refuses a life-sustaining/saving measure that promises to work and does not present obviously onerous burdens. In such cases, the push and pull between dignity and autonomy is most palpable. I argue, however, that we need to know whether the patient has rendered a *competent refusal* of such measures. Whereas the former refers us to test for certain abilities, the latter refers us to assess the quality of one's judgment. I argue that, for competent adults (i.e., intact abilities), who refuse means of saving or sustaining their lives with manageable burdens, a higher degree of justification is needed to honor such refusals. Unless such justification is present, we should have epistemic diffidence for the belief that their refusals represent the patient's stable self.

There are few challenges to research when the subjects are competent and the research presents more than minimal risk with no promise of direct benefit. The principal reason for allowing such research is that we should respect the autonomy of competent subjects. In the final chapter I argue that we have additional moral intuitions stemming from commutative justice. I argue that concerns generated by commutative justice serve as an additional criterion for assessing permissible research. My argument aims to justify having epistemic diffidence for the claim that "risky research is permissible because the subjects consented to it." To this end, I highlight our intuitions informing this notion of commutative justice and conclude that all human subjects who are exposed to more than minimal-risk research should enjoy the same protections as those given subjects who cannot consent (e.g., children).

A concluding chapter summarizes the dialectical territory covered. The advance this project makes is to mine findings in recent moral psychology and epistemology to the effect that even if one achieves widely coherent views on an issue that involves moral risk, that is *still* tenuous epistemic comfort. That strikes me as a bold conclusion, but I offer what I see as plausible reasons for it. The feature that makes it bold, however, is also the feature that makes it ecumenical. I resist placing too many theoretical demands on my interlocutors. To take one example, my readers need not subscribe to a substance view of the person vis-à-vis the abortion issue to appreciate the force of my argument. It is enough for my purposes to argue that such a view is plausible enough to set the presumptions of that dialectical exchange, and that those who hold such a view can function as epistemic *peers* with whom one may disagree. This is enough, I argue, to motivate diffidence in the setting of moral risk.

Notes

1 In making these jointly sufficient and necessary conditions, I am raising the bar for my argument. It is plausible that there are weaker conditions such that (2) remains plausible as well. The Radiology case (Chapter 3) might illustrate how satisfying condition (iii) and (ii) is sufficient to make (1) and (2) true. Conditions (i) and (ii) might be sufficient for diffidence if one thinks that her beliefs might suffer from one of the biases explained in Chapter 2.

2 If peer disagreement is evidence for one having made a performance error, which provides an undercutting defeater, condition (i) is redundant given (iii). In some circumstances I would agree. But my virtue interpretation of disagreement's effects does not *entail* that disagreement is an undercutting defeater. No doubt, (i)–(iii) are related, but my task does not require disaggregating them. It is enough to argue that such epistemic features are present for my substitution instances of B.

Part I
Foundational Matters
The Perception of Value, Persons, and Human Worth

2 Moral Inquiry and the Apprehension of Value

When we think about moral issues and what is right and wrong, we have to address how we apprehend moral values. As such, in the first section I discuss the idea of moral perception, particularly how that perception is motivated. Moral perception is a cognitive faculty in that it is oriented towards generating beliefs, or cognitive contact with moral values.[1] As with any cognitive faculty, a question in epistemology is whether that faculty is reliable. Does it function well? Does it put our minds in contact with the reality it is meant to apprehend? Answering these questions meets what's called the problem of epistemic circularity. The basic idea, explained in more detail below, is that we cannot prove the reliability of a faculty without using the very outputs of that faculty. We can *take* our faculties to be reliable but we can never prove them to be so. This by itself does not justify skepticism, but it does if we have reason for thinking that our faculties are in what Bergmann (2004) refers to as a questioned-source context. The empirical research on moral cognition reveals that our moral perception is prey to a number of influences that would render them unreliable. Thus, in the second section, I discuss the problem of epistemic circularity and in the third section I discuss the evidence for distrusting our moral perception. The conclusion reached at the end of this chapter is that we have reasons for questioning the reliability of our moral perception in certain contexts. The next chapter argues that the scope of epistemic diffidence includes judgments on controversial issues with high costs in being wrong. One could understand this chapter as arguing for diffidence in regard to our moral *faculties*; and the next as imputing diffidence to specific *justifications* for our moral beliefs.

Motivated Cognition, Attention, and Moral Perception

Cognitive processing is a motivated activity in the sense that it is a goal-directed activity. This is true for perceptual judgments as well as other more extended processing such as scientific inquiry. The evidence of inattentional blindness (Mack & Rock, 2000; Pashlar, 1999) and change blindness

(Rensink, O'Reagan, & Clark, 1997) suggests that perceptual knowledge cannot be obtained apart from attention. Attention is the directed allocation of cognitive resources to process *fully* a stimulus, and attentional processes are motivated. "The idea that attention is motivated . . . is not new in psychology, nor is the view that limbic and subcortical emotional processes play a role in directing attention" (Ellis, 2001, 299). Conversely, inattentional blindness is the phenomenon of agents not seeing (or hearing) what is clearly within one's visual (or auditory) field and this is because one is not motivated to process the stimuli – attention is not directed to process the visual/auditory information. Change blindness refers to one's inability to detect rather obvious changes in scenes suggesting that memorial encoding requires attention as well. And, attention is a motivated activity even if it is not a *consciously* motivated activity (Chartrand & Bargh, 2002). I defended this view in Napier (2008)[2] and it is summarized as follows. Attention is an act in the sense that there is an allocation of cognitive resources, and such an allocation is goal directed. Attention is motivated (Ellis, 2001, 2005) and perception depends on attentional resources. Thus attention is required for perceptual knowledge. Attention is a function of an agent's motivations. Therefore perceptual knowledge is a function of one's motivations. This view is compatible with and relies on the empirical fact that much of perceptual processing takes place without conscious awareness. Information that 'makes it' to consciousness is a function of the motivational goals of the agent.

It is, of course, not necessary to grant that all perceptual processing is motivated to grant that moral perception is. Moral perception is subject to attentional effects and is thereby a motivated activity as illustrated by Lawrence Blum (1994).

> John and Joan are riding in a subway train, seated. There are no empty seats and some people are standing; yet the subway car is not packed so tightly as to be uncomfortable for everyone. One of the passengers standing is a woman in her thirties holding two relatively full shopping bags. John is not particularly paying attention to the woman, but he is cognizant of her. Joan, by contrast, is distinctly aware that the woman is uncomfortable.
>
> (Blum, 1994, 31–32)

Here are two people who have the same visual abilities, are situated alike in the same environment, but only for Joan are the moral aspects of the situation salient because she attends to them. Blum remarks that what is salient for John is simply that there is a woman who is standing holding two bags; what is salient for Joan is that she is standing holding two bags, *and* is uncomfortable. "John misses something of the moral reality confronting him" (Blum, 1994, 33) whereas Joan discerns what is morally salient in her environment. Blum's basic point is that there is such a thing as moral perception,[3] according to which one is able to have an apprehension of value and disvalue in the world. Joan sees what is morally salient in her environment, John does not and the difference is likely traceable to differences in motivational and emotional dispositions. John suffers an inattentional moral blindness if you will. Margaret Olivia Little is explicit on this point. She states, "The extent to which one actually cares about and is responsive to moral ends . . . has enormous impact on how accurately and reliably one sees the moral landscape . . ." (Little, 1995, 123). Of course, the apparatus of attention for moral stimuli is different than perceptual stimuli. For perceptual stimuli it may involve eye gaze, whereas for moral content, one may need emotional sensitivity (Blair & James, 1995; and Lacewing, 2015) and motivations which may be a function of one's overall ideological orientation (Haidt, 2012; Gilovich, 1991). Consequently, what we attend to is a function of what value commitments we already have; and conversely, what we may miss is a function of what we do not value.

I emphasize the idea of moral perception being motivated because most of our moral judgments begin with a basic perception of value. Moral perception is the faculty that disposes one to apprehend values/disvalues in one's environment. There is a priority to moral perception in generating our moral judgments. On this point there seems to be much agreement. Describing the epistemic deficiencies of a Vulcan (a fictional character from *Star Trek* who reasons well, but has sublimated their emotional capacities) David Pizarro writes that "while the Vulcan might be capable of making accurate moral judgments based on the application of principles, the Vulcan may not always know when a moral event is taking place" (Pizarro, 2000, 371). Ishtiyaque Haji recapitulates the same idea while commenting on Aristotle's virtue-theoretic account of moral perception. For Aristotle, discernment of moral values in discrete circumstances rests with perception (1109b23). Haji explains,

> We cannot, for instance, decide whether to help someone unless we notice that she is in need, and we perceive that because she is in need, she ought to be helped. In this manner, in practical reasoning how we perceive the situation has priority over what we decide or what choices we make.
>
> (2010, 138)

Nancy Sherman, also commenting on Aristotle, makes a general point about the conditions for making moral judgments, and endorses the priority of moral perception as well. She notes that "an ethical theory that begins with the justification of a decision to act begins too far down the road. Preliminary to deciding *how* to act, one must acknowledge that the situation requires action" (Sherman, 1991, 29). And recognizing that the situation requires action cannot be but the work of perception. One may extend the same point to the recognition of a moral principle as being *moral*. Noticing the difference in content between the principles 'do no harm' and 'never conclude the consequent when denying the antecedent' is a function of moral recognition.[4]

My understanding of moral perception shares features with Charles Starkey (2006) but departs in instructive ways. Starkey is correct to reject definitions of moral perception that focus on the specific contents of one's moral judgments. He eventually defines moral perception as "morally appraisable perceptual apprehension" (Starkey, 2006, 88). Where I depart from Starkey is that he is still trying to define moral perception with reference to discrete instances of it, namely, instances of perceptual apprehension and not with reference to a cognitive *faculty* or *ability*. Moral perception on my view is a cognitive faculty, an ability to apprehend moral values in one's environment – it can be reliable or unreliable. Starkey's definition leads him to say, "failing to perceive can be morally appraisable and is thus a form of moral perception" (Starkey 2006, 90). It seems clear to me, however, that not having a moral perception cannot be a form of moral perception. One might criticize *another* agent for not having a moral perception in response to a discrete morally charged circumstance – and that criticism itself may be a function of the critic's moral perception. But if we keep straight which agent is having (or not having) the perception, not perceiving values in one's environment when one should is still not an instance where moral perception is *functioning*. Not perceiving a real rabbit out in my yard is not a form of visual perception, it is an absence of it.

The Problem of Epistemic Circularity

The reason it is important to highlight the priority of perception is because moral perception is a basic source of knowledge. It is a cognitive faculty that is basic insofar as moral reasoning depends on it, but moral perception does not depend on some other faculty.[5] This is not to say that in order to apprehend battery on a street corner late one evening I do not need functional visual capacities. Of course I do. What it means is that for the *moral* judgment, I need functional moral perception. The point is simply that we have numerous cognitive faculties, such as reasoning, visual perception, auditory perception, memory, etc.[6] When we form beliefs, we do so as a function of the cognitive faculty that produces that belief type. Without, for example, a visual system like humans have, we could not form visual beliefs. Some synesthesiacs can be said to have acquired anomalous sensory capacities that dispose them to have beliefs about geometrical designs in a nature scene. Without such a capacity, no such beliefs could be formed without some additional technical apparatus. So, moral perception is a basic faculty that disposes one to have cognitive contact with moral reality.

How could one prove that one's moral perception is reliable except by appeal to the very outputs of that faculty? Any track-record-type argument would involve circularity. To illustrate, we would not rely on a person's say-so that she is telling the truth if it is an open question whether she is or not. As Baron Reed (2006, 186) notes succinctly, "no customer would ever ask a used car salesman if he is honest." Taking him at his word, when whether he is telling the truth is in question, is clearly circular – it begs the very question at stake. The same idea can be applied to one's own justification that her cognitive faculties are reliable. One *may* just assume that they are reliable. My question is what would be the justification for their reliability? Take a particular faculty labelled F1. Again, Reed explains,

> In order to know that F1 is a reliable source of knowledge, S will have to use either F1, or another faculty. But if S uses F1 his belief that F1 is reliable will be epistemically circular. So, S must instead use (say) F2. But S should not use F2 unless she knows that it is a reliable source of knowledge itself. In order to come to know this, S will have to use F2, or some other faculty. But S cannot use F2 on pain of epistemic circularity. And S cannot use F1, without first knowing that it is a reliable source of knowledge, which is still in question.
>
> (Reed, 2006, 187)

One can see here three options looming: there is either an infinite regress, a circular justification, or we embrace externalism according to which what matters is that the faculty is *actually* reliable, not whether I can provide noncircular justification that it is reliable. Though I harbor sympathies with externalism, none of these options is fully attractive. For externalism, my beliefs arising from a faculty F are justified if F is actually reliable. But as Alston observes, externalism cannot tell us whether or not a practice like crystal ball gazing is reliable (Alston, 1991, 148). When we are interested in discriminating which epistemic faculties or practices are reliable, externalism cannot give an answer. The argument from epistemic circularity means only to show that we cannot have any noncircular reason for thinking that our moral perception is rightly attuned. Wholesale skepticism does not necessarily follow, but it makes it easier to mount an argument for local skepticism since we have no justification *for* reliability.

Our epistemic diffidence in trusting our faculties/practices becomes live when one is in what Bergmann (2004) refers to as a *questioned-source context*. "A context in which epistemic circularity is a bad thing is one in which the subject begins by doubting or being unsure of [a faculty's] trustworthiness" (Bergmann, 2004, 717). Notice, it is not difficult to find oneself in a questioned-source context. The reason is that epistemic circularity has shown that a person must simply trust her faculties. There is no noncircular argument *for* their reliability. They are viewed as innocent, but not for any reason. Of course the deliverances of our basic faculties seem correct, but the very seeming that it is correct is based on and is entirely a function of the seeming itself.[7] Reasons for challenging the reliability of one's faculty, then, are easy to come by since they need not offset any reasons for their reliability.

"Questioned-Source Contexts"

A key idea for motivating epistemic diffidence with regard to our faculties is that I cannot look back upon that by which I look.[8] I have to trust. The outputs of our moral faculties may look unproblematic to us; but of course they would even if they were unreliable. Leibniz gives the example of the Caribs – who made their children fat so that they could eat them – to illustrate that heinous actions can look unproblematic to the one who thinks such actions are permissible (Leibniz, 1996, 92). He also relates a story of Honorius, an Emperor of Rome, according to which, "when he was brought the news of the loss of Rome, [he] thought they meant his hen which was also called 'Rome'; and that distressed him more than the truth did when he learned it" (Leibniz, 1996, 512). Leibniz offers Honorius as an example of someone whose moral conscience is obtuse. With rare hyperbole, he observes that "[i]f geometry conflicted with our passions and our present concerns as much as morality does, we would dispute it and transgress it almost as much – in spite of Euclid's and Archimedes' demonstrations" (Leibniz, 1996, 96). Leibniz goes on to diagnose correctly that the causes of becoming morally purblind are rooted in our passions, prejudices, and cultural customs (1996, 93).

It is tempting to think that someone else's moral faculties are purblind if they disagree with us, but the lesson I wish to draw here is to consider what things might look like from the one whose conscience is obtuse. Again, because we cannot look back upon that by which we look, the Caribs' moral beliefs look fine when viewed through their corrupt moral faculties. Any explanation for such corruption that does not refer to the will, one's self-interests, one's motivations, and one's culture are likely deficient explanations. In the sections that follow I discuss in more detail sources of distortion of one's moral perception in three broad categories: ill-motivations (internal), ill-influences (external), and deficient resources (defects).

Ill-Motivations

Moral Foundations Theory (hereafter MFT; Graham et al., 2013) confirms several important points I wish to highlight in the material that follows. MFT includes four theses: (1) nativism is the view that human development enables one to have a sensitivity to value and disvalue. (2) Intuitionism is the view that most of our moral judgments result from quick and seemingly automatic processing. (3) Cultural learning refers to the fact that our initial native template for moral processing is malleable.

Just as we are born with a certain set of taste receptors that become more sensitive or insensitive to certain flavors depending upon sets of cuisine, so too our moral perception can become more sensitive or insensitive depending upon culture. For example, our native moral perception may not see anything good about loving one's enemies. Those who do must have attuned themselves partly as a function of a moral culture in which such a value is recognized. (4) Pluralism is the view that there are numerous values to which we can be attuned.

I emphasize two pericopes of the theory, namely, 2 and 3. MFT holds that intuitions come first and moral reasoning comes second.[9] Haidt (2001 and 2012) provides evidence to the effect that, on moral issues, people have an initial intuition on whether an action, event, or person is right or wrong. On my view, this intuition is the specific output of the moral perceptual faculty. Moral reasoning is typically hired out like a lawyer to defend the initial intuition or preconception; we typically do not reason as judges (Haidt's analogy (2001)). What is important is that our sensitivity to certain moral values is basic (though malleable). The empirical evidence for the basicality of moral perception comes from what Haidt refers to as moral dumbfounding. When subjects are asked to defend their moral position when confronted with a putative case of harmless wrongdoing (e.g., masturbating with a chicken carcass) subjects are unable to provide justification beyond appeals to autonomy (in the case of permissive judgments) or impurity (in the case of non-permissive judgments).

Can our moral perception be subject to something analogous to inattentional blindness? To the extent that one's moral perception is a function of non-alethic motives, the answer is yes. In what follows, I both canvass what motives may function to direct our moral attention to non-alethic features, and illustrate their furtive nature. The discussion of certain motives and how they can distort one's moral perception is important for justifying that one can be in a questioned source context and not know it.

Coherence Motives

A putatively admirable epistemic motive might be the desire for one's beliefs to cohere with one another. In certain epistemic settings, however, the motive to maintain coherence among one's beliefs is a vicious motive.

Roberts and Wood (2008) discuss numerous epistemic vices many of which can be traced back to a motive to maintain one's own beliefs and ideas when it would be rational to reconsider those beliefs and ideas. For example, they discuss failures of "concern to know" as being vices opposed to the virtue of love for knowledge. They describe failures of the concern to know as an "insufficient concern for truth . . . that when such people are given an opportunity to test their more cherished beliefs, they . . . offer defenses of the beliefs that are weaker than any that these people would accept in other contexts" (Roberts & Wood, 2008, 170). Epistemic rigidity, which is a vice opposed to intellectual firmness, is defined with reference to motives to maintain one's beliefs when it is rational to reconsider them. For example, dogmatism (which is a subspecies of rigidity) is not "just strong adherence to a belief for inadequate reasons. It is a disposition to *respond* irrationally to *oppositions* to the belief" (Roberts & Wood, 2008, 195, emphasis original). Under the same heading of rigidity, they describe comprehensional rigidity as an,

> inability to grasp theoretical alternatives to one's own; it is the tendency for the views from other vantage points to look stupid or infantile or uninteresting or just opaque. Comprehensionally inflexible is the Freudian who can see no value in cognitive behavioral psychology.
>
> (Roberts & Wood, 2008, 204–205)

Motives to maintain one's own views in the face of rational challenge account for a number of epistemic vices. I refer to these motives simply as coherence motives following Haidt (2001). I begin the discussion of motives with a discussion of cognitive dissonance since dissonance typically occurs in the setting of a challenge to one's beliefs.

We generally desire consistency; consistency between each of our beliefs, and between our beliefs and actions. When we discern inconsistency between our beliefs or between our behavior and beliefs, we may experience what psychologists call cognitive dissonance (CD). Cognitive dissonance refers to the *discomfort* one feels if either (i) she is presented with new information that conflicts with previously held beliefs, expectations, or assumptions; or (ii) she discovers an inconsistency between a belief and her behavior (Festinger, 1962).[10] Because CD involves discomfort leading to certain motivational goals – discussed below – it does not occur unless the subject sees the dissonant information as meaningful; for example, the subject is told that her score on an IQ exam is lower than the person had previously believed and it matters to her that she think of herself as smart. We have a basic psychological drive for consistency – which is a good thing. What is concerning is how we handle the perceived inconsistency.

There are three basic responses to such dissonance: (1) *ignore* the dissonant information, (2) find a way to *reject* the dissonant information, or (3) *modify* one's beliefs in light of the new information. Psychological evidence has shown that in the case where an agent senses dissonance between her current beliefs and new information (scenario (i)), the typical preference is to maintain the current belief.[11] Why? Some of our current beliefs have a lot of support going for them, we have lived with them, we have acted on them, and we have held them for some time. Fastidiously subjecting each new piece of information that apparently conflicts with our current beliefs is not feasible. It is not obviously rational either. I am well within my epistemic rights not to consider putative 'scientific proof' that there is life on Mars or conspiracy theories about the Moon landing. However, there are features of our beliefs that make them resistant to change. Some of these features are epistemically deleterious.

Beliefs with the following properties are typically more resistant to change than beliefs without these properties.

a   Clear-cut empirical beliefs such as that the sun is shining.
    This first category is worthy of some additional comments. Immediate empirical beliefs are likely the only type of belief resistant to change that is resistant *because* it is likely *true*. Empirical beliefs acquired through extended scientific study may be less resistant to change than ones acquired without extended investigation but they may also be subject to more biases.[12] The properties that follow are likely resistant to change not because they are true.

b   Beliefs that are *fundamental* to our worldview or belief system – since changing one or several of them would involve changing a constellation of other beliefs (Roberts & Wood, 2008, 157; and MacNair, 2009, 39). Furthermore, fundamental beliefs typically implicate the person's self-identity (Steele & Liu, 1983).

c   Beliefs that are acquired more recently (MacNair, 2009, 39).

d   Publicly announced beliefs, whether shared with friends, family, or classmates.

e   Beliefs held by one's peer group (Chaiken, 1987).

f   Beliefs which we acted upon.[13]

g   Beliefs that contribute to one's self-esteem, self-concept, or self-identity (Aronson, 1968).[14] If we consider ourselves liberal (or conservative), we would be more inclined to hold positions that we associate with liberal (or conservative) views.

Ignoring dissonant new information is either benign, as in the case of claims that there is life on Mars, or it is clearly close-minded, as in the case of ignoring evidence that pharmaceutical companies bring to market inferior drugs that can harm numerous patients (Garattini & Bertele, 2007; and Light, Lexchin, & Darrow, 2013). If a person ignores plausible contrary new information, she may do so to protect her beliefs from dissonant new information.

How may we come to reject dissonant new information? Gilovich thinks that there are usually three means by which our preconceptions exert their epistemic effects on dissonant or preference-inconsistent new information. We either "subject inconsistent information to more *critical scrutiny* than consistent information; . . . we seek out *additional information* only when the initial outcomes are inconsistent with our expectations" (Gilovich, 1991, 52), or we *weigh* or assign meanings to new information depending on whether it is inconsistent or consistent with our preconceptions.

To illustrate critical scrutiny, Gilovich relates a study on participants who were either proponents or opponents of the death penalty (Lord, Ross, & Lepper, 1979). Subjects were presented with (fictitious) studies showing that there is a deterrent effect on homicide rates in states with the death penalty, and studies showing that there is not a deterrent effect. Additionally, they read criticisms of both sets of studies. Both groups read both types of studies, critiques, and responses to those studies. For the study that presented evidence consistent with the participant's view, the participant noted that it was a well-conducted and important study. For the study that presented evidence inconsistent with the participant's view, the participants spent more time considering the critiques, and they remembered more of the facts presented in preference-inconsistent studies. Both features indicate that more cognitive resources were devoted to reviewing the opposing view (Edwards & Smith, 1996). Because participants accepted agreeable views without too much critical assessment and rejected disagreeable views after extensive reflection, participants became *more* convinced that their view was right. And this was so even after having been presented with empirical evidence that in its entirety is ambiguous. The culprit is a cognitive motivation aimed not at getting the truth, but at preserving one's preconceptions.[15]

The final result of the critical scrutiny is to diminish the evidential force of the new dissonant information. This is called disconfirmation bias (Edwards & Smith, 1996). What is important to note is that the motivation informing this end is to preserve one's preconceptions. And viewed from the inside, subjects thought that they were being objective and rational – they reviewed the critiques and responses to each study and had a very coherent set of reasons for their position. As Lord, Ross, and Lepper point out, however, their cognitive sin "lay in their readiness to use evidence already processed in a biased manner to bolster the very theory or belief that initially 'justified' the processing bias" (Lord, Ross, & Lepper, 1979, 2107).

Similar results can be seen in studies on divorce and child care.[16] Divorced couples viewed the harm that divorce may have on children as significantly less than never-divorced couples. A similar difference was noted between divorcees who initiated the divorce and those who did not (Moon, 2011). Bastardi, Uhlmann, and Ross (2011) enrolled couples all of whom initially viewed daycare as inferior to at-home childcare. There were two groups according to whether they planned on using daycare or did not plan on it. Those who planned on using daycare were referred to as the conflicted group since they viewed it as inferior. Couples were exposed to ambiguous evidence according to which one study suggested the superiority of daycare, and another study suggested the superiority of home care. All subjects read both studies. On a nine-point Likert scale (1 = daycare far superior, 9 = home care far superior) the conflicted group dramatically changed their attitudes from a mean of 7.72 to 4.89. Across 18 subjects this is a dramatic change in attitude and this after only reading one study in favor of daycare! There was virtually no change in attitude among the unconflicted group (7.89 to 7.17). Clearly, coherence with one's desires and planned behavior heavily influenced the beliefs one would hold.

The second means does not require further explanation; the third, however, does. What does "weighing" new information look like? To illustrate, Rachel MacNair relates a story of a nurse who is describing her first experience with a late-term abortion.

> I was watching the doctor struggle with the cannula, trying to pull it out . . . I didn't understand what the resistance was all about. And I was very alarmed and all of a sudden the doctor pulled the cannula out and there, as I was at the woman's side, I looked down at the cannula and there was a foot sticking out. I will never forget the feeling I had in my chest as the doctor pulled the cannula out . . . This sounds terribly cavalier, I suppose, but within about a month, like everything else we do after a while, it just becomes pretty routine and it has never bothered me since then.
>
> (MacNair, 2009, 60)[17]

The new information here is the experience of abortion as the dismemberment of a human being or, more simply, a destructive act.[18] The experience appeared to be weighed less than the belief that abortion is part of one's work or that it is a necessary evil. Whatever evidential force the experience should have had was discharged by a preferential weighing of one's beliefs against the experience. This preferential weighing is common. Abortion doctor Don Sloan notes, "I don't think there's anyone doing abortions who hasn't wished at some point that the situations creating the demand for them wouldn't just go away" (MacNair, 2009, 73).[19] With the settled preconception that abortion is permissible, the nurse and Dr. Sloan weighed the dissonant information of dismembering a human being less than the weight of being employed, or doing a perceived necessary evil.

The motivation for coherence is usually a good epistemic motivation. It can lead us away from the truth, however, if we take our starting beliefs as infallible data that are recalcitrant to revision. Of course, some beliefs should be immune to revision (e.g., torturing children for fun is wrong), and some should not be. Deciding which ones to put on the exam table requires the intellectual virtue of justice (and *phronesis*), discussed in the next chapter.

Self-Identity/Self-Interest Motives

Robin Hanson asks us to consider the reliability of our moral intuitions informed as they might be by one's self interests.

> Consider, for example, the moral intuition that slaveholders should protect slaves from freedom because slaves are incapable of managing such freedom well. Or consider the related intuition that the upper class in a given society should rule due to its superior education and intelligence. Such intuitions are widely suspected of being mere fronts for self- and group-interest, even when they seem to be quite sincerely felt.
>
> (Hanson, 2002, 160)

Can Hanson's worries be broadened beyond the obvious example of a slaveholder? The answer is yes and, in explaining why, I wish to illustrate two key points: the first is to argue that our self-interests can distort our perception of moral reality, and, more importantly, I wish to illustrate how these motives function furtively. It is hard to get 'out of ourselves' to reflect on the epistemic effects of our self-interests.

One important category of beliefs that are under the aegis of our self-interested motivations are beliefs about ourselves. "One of the most documented findings in psychology is that the average person purports to believe extremely flattering things about him or herself – beliefs that do not stand up to objective analysis" (Gilovich, 1991, 77). I shall refer to this as a self-esteem bias, but it is a broader category than the more familiar self-attribution bias. One important self-esteem bias is the belief that one is objective and open-minded. Kunda remarks that "people motivated to arrive at a particular conclusion attempt to be rational and to construct a justification of their desired conclusion that would persuade a dispassionate observer" (Kunda, 1990, 482–483). But, she continues, the construction of a justification is done by selecting only confirming evidence for their preconceived view. The person who creates such constructions thinks she is being objective and thorough.

One of the more important points to note is that these biases are not moderated by IQ. Numerous studies confirm that the esteem bias operates even for those who think they may be 'above' such influences. The first type of study concerns the my-side bias. My-side bias is the evaluation or generation of evidence aimed to confirm one's prior opinions or assumptions.[20] The basic experimental paradigm asks subjects of varying degrees of education (high school to graduate) or IQ (low to high) to generate or evaluate arguments on both sides of an issue. For generating arguments, their initial opinions on the issue were recorded and their arguments were scored for the number of points made and what conclusion the arguments were meant to support. The researchers discovered that higher

IQ students were able to think of slightly more arguments than lower IQ students on belief-consistent arguments, but the higher IQ group did not differ from the lower IQ group in terms of offering counter-arguments to their own opinion. That is, all of the subjects were dismal in generating counter-arguments to their own opinions. "Although IQ correlated significantly with my-side arguments produced without prompting . . ., its correlation with other-side arguments was nonsignificant and negative" (Perkins, Farady, & Bushey, 1991, 95). Perkins, Farady, and Bushey conclude, "in effect, people invest their IQ in buttressing their own case rather than in exploring the entire issue more fully and evenhandedly" (Perkins, Farady, & Bushey, 1991, 95). Stanovich, West, and Toplak replicated these experiments and concluded that the "magnitude of the my-side bias shows very little relation to intelligence" (2013, 259).

Self-identity biases are a preference for positions that are identity-consistent, and a strong antipathy for identity-inconsistent positions. Evidence of self-identity biases comes from automatic activation of stereotypes and/or negative heuristics. Iyengar and Westwood (2015) found that negative attitudes across ideological convictions (liberal v. conservative) far exceeded other negative stereotypes on the basis of race (see also Brandt et al., 2014). That is, liberals viewed conservatives and vice versa far more negatively than how, for example, Caucasians view African-Americans and vice versa. Although the researchers did not measure response times, it is well known that emotions facilitate early selective attention and subsequent processing (Vuilleumier, 2005). It is also well known that the stronger the negative association, the easier it is to adopt additional negative associations, and the more motivated one is to avoid the stereotyped person (Kunda, 1999). Likewise, negative associations of an ideological *position* makes it easier to disagree with it (Iyengar and Westwood, 2015) in an uncharitable and simplistic manner (Graham, Nosek, & Haidt, 2012). Graham, Nosek, and Haidt conducted a study where they asked liberals (and conservatives) to answer a moral questionnaire in two conditions: (a) authentically and (b) *as if* they were answering as a member of the out-group would answer. The subjects were instructed to be as accurate as possible. The evidence was clear though surprising to some. They note that the "largest inaccuracies were in liberals' underestimations of conservatives' Harm and Fairness concerns, and liberals further exaggerated the political differences by overestimating their own such concerns" (2012, 10). For example, liberals believed (falsely) that conservatives do not believe that justice is an important feature of society or that defenseless animals should not be hurt. This evidence is consistent with most in-group/out-group studies in that negative stereotypes and false heuristics cloud one's perception of the out-group.

The conclusion to draw from these studies and from the Caribs is that our moral perception may be unreliable and that, if it were unreliable, *we would not know it*. Our moral perception can see everything except the 'eye' by which it sees. Biases are equal opportunity inhabitants and are probably more dangerous for higher IQ people who can generate more arguments on 'their side' of an issue.

Ill-Influences

The motives previously mentioned have adaptive purposes but *can* be epistemically devastating. There are other external factors that influence one's moral perception.[21] I have divided the discussion here into influences from close associates and influences from culture.

Friendship and identification with a community are good things, and our cognitive apparatus has and should conform to these more social goals. Imagine how unpleasant a person would be if she or he had no motivation to fit in or to agree with at least a subset of one's community. Haidt (2001) summarizes, however, the studies on belief formation as showing that our desire for agreement with others exerts strong effects on which beliefs we adopt. Haidt mentions several examples. The basic experimental paradigm is that subjects are told that they will interact with another person and what that other person's views are on an issue; or they are given a description of that person's personality. When they are expected to discuss a certain moral issue with that person, the subjects' beliefs on the issue become more homogenous with those of the interacting person with *no* effect for non-interacting persons (Chen & Chaiken, 1999). When they are expected to interact with the other person, they rate the personality description corresponding to the interacting person as better than descriptions of non-interacting persons (Darley & Berscheid, 1967). More generally, Haidt notes that the desire to harmonize with those close to us is so strong that the "mere fact that your friend expresses a moral judgment against X, is often sufficient to cause in you a critical attitude toward X" (Haidt, 2001, 821).

What is particularly worrisome about this latter fact is that such uptake of beliefs from others can happen automatically and without conscious deliberation (Bargh & Chartrand, 1999; and Ditto, Pizarro, & Tannenbaum, 2009, 311–312). For example, rude versus polite behavior can be induced unconsciously by exposing subjects either to words related to rudeness, such as 'impolite' or 'obnoxious,' or to words related to politeness such as 'respect' or 'considerate.' The subjects were told this was a semantic test. After that portion of the test was done, subjects were placed in a situation in which they could either behave in a rude fashion or a polite fashion. "Results show that significantly more participants in the rude priming condition (67%) interrupted the conversation than did those . . . in the polite condition (16%)" (Bargh & Chartrand, 1999, 894). The evidence from unconscious priming paired with the evidence that our opinions typically follow those with whom we associate, suggests that our moral judgments can be a function of belonging and not the cold hard truth of the matter.

Regarding the influence of culture, we can return to MFT. Graham et al. note that "the moral foundations [of an individual] are not the finished moralities, although they constrain the kinds of moral orders that can be built" (Graham et al., 2013, 65). The idea is that we can acquire modules according to which one gains a sensitivity to other values or, conversely, a culture can restrain what sensitivities one may develop.

Graham et al. give the example of Hindu children who are taught to bow to elders and in religious worship. The Hindu greeting *namaste* means something like, "I bow to the divinity in you." By the time Hindu children enter adulthood, these salutary gesticulations translate into beliefs about who one honors and respects in the community. Graham et al. observe that "this knowledge is not just factual knowledge—it includes feelings and motor schemas for bowing and otherwise showing deference" (2013, 64). A child raised in secular America will have no such experiences, and consequently no sensitivity to respect or honor certain people in society. Haidt relates how after immersing himself in such a culture – specifically the Orrisans – he came to apprehend better the values that his hosts apprehended. He states,

> I had read about Shweder's ethic of community and had understood it intellectually. But now, for the first time in my life, I began to feel it. I could see beauty in a moral code that emphasizes duty, respect for one's elders, service to the group, and negation of the self's desires.
> (Haidt, 2012, 102)

Haidt's conversion illustrates nicely both the foundational aspect of one's intuitions and the malleability of our moral modules in light of the surrounding culture. One can acquire a sensitivity (or insensitivity) to other sets of values.[22] Haidt's is a case of acquiring a moral sensitivity by participation in practices indigenous to a moral culture that emphasizes community and human dignity ("preciousness," as Raimond Gaita notes, discussed further in Chapter 5).

Vetlesen (1994) discusses at length how one's moral perception can become insensitive by analyzing the moral psychology of moral failings. Vetlesen is concerned with limning the epistemic state of the perpetrators of the Holocaust. His analysis centers on the idea of psychic numbing, which is characterized by a lack of empathy and emotional insight to the woe of one's victims. Numbing is achieved, according to Vetlesen, through ideology, technology, and bureaucracy, all of which were a function of National Socialist culture. I focus on ideology as that is the feature indicative of cultural influences on one's moral perception.

Nazi ideology aimed to undercut empathy. Nazi doctors could adore and love their children and at the same time be numb to the suffering and destruction of Jewish children. A necessary condition for such a contradiction is a culturally accepted ideology in the background that engaged in what Vetlesen calls boundary drawing. The boundary drawing characteristic of eugenic and utilitarian ideologies was able to distinguish what is in truth indistinguishable. In general, through the educational system, laws, and customs, all societies prescribe

> a particular way of drawing boundaries between moral and nonmoral objects to its members . . . Against the background of this most general feature, a given society will encourage its members to observe that the desired and thus allegedly "correct" way of drawing boundaries is this one particular way.
>
> (Vetlesen, 1994, 193)

Importantly, when a society draws such lines, perception is affected.

> Perception – *here* a boundary exists, and *this* is what it contains – is not a spontaneous making of the individual. Far from arising *de novo* . . . perception is taught to individuals . . . Accordingly, society awaits and readily rewards or condemns individuals' displayed ability to adopt society's way of seeing as *their* way of seeing.
>
> (Vetlesen, 1994, 194)

What our moral attention is directed to, and thus what values we can apprehend, is a function of the cultural and, importantly, ideological assumptions we may have.

Empirical evidence for Vetlesen's reflections comes from cross-cultural studies on perception. Park and Kitayama (2011) summarize studies on East Asian and American subjects (representing cultures that emphasize interdependent relations and independence respectively). Both cohorts were presented with visual scenes involving focal objects (e.g., airplanes) and a background (e.g., sky). Tracking eye saccades, both groups focused on the objects, but around 400ms after presentation Asian subjects divided their saccades between background and object, whereas American subjects continued exclusively on the objects. In a comparison task, a scene with object-background was presented and then a second exposure was done with the background changed. American subjects were dismal at detecting the background changes but Asian subjects were exceptional at it. Conversely, Asian subjects did not perform as well as American subjects in identifying changes in the focal objects between scenes. Consequently, culture affects *what* we perceive, by directing our attention to different aspects of our environment. If it can do this for emotionally neutral and morally irrelevant stimuli, moral stimuli requiring various emotional and attentional sensitivities would seem much more dictated by culture and background ideology.

The effect of boundary drawing on one's perception cannot be overstated given its effects and its subtlety. It is tempting but incorrect, however, to understand Vetlesen or Park and Kitiyama as calling for wholesale moral skepticism. We are not like victims of *The Matrix* regarding our moral beliefs. We are, however, challenged by these comments to at least consider our moral beliefs with *hesitation* – especially our moral beliefs that rely on boundary drawing.

Defects

Perceptual knowledge requires categorization. When I correctly perceive a chair, I have the concept chair. If I am to recognize a moral situation correctly and comprehensively, I need to have the conceptual and emotional resources necessary for understanding the issue. I say emotional resources as well, as illustrated in cases like John and Joan above. John may understand what being compassionate involves, but he does not see the suffering in the discrete circumstances – or if he does, he does not see the suffering as bad. One needs what Joan has, both to see the discomfort and to see it as bad. Conversely, the psychopath will not see suffering as bad due to a deficiency in her emotional resources. So, even if psychopaths have the concept of suffering, and can discern correctly that a person is suffering, they will not see it *as* bad. Psychopaths have a defect in their faculty of moral perception.

The kind of defect I have in mind here is like the notion of perceptual rigidity discussed by Roberts and Wood (2008, 202ff). Perceptual rigidity "is a defective perceptual disposition, but it is compatible with 20–20 vision and perfect hearing. The deficit of versatility is categorial or conceptual . . . one's perceptual acuity is stuck within certain categories, outside of which one is 'blind' or 'deaf'" (2008, 202). Roberts and Wood relate the research by Bruner and Postman (1949) according to which subjects were asked to identify playing cards, some of which were normal and others anomalous (e.g., red seven of spades, black ten of diamonds). After very short exposures (28 ms), normal cards were correctly identified, but anomalous cards were also identified as normal with no hesitation (e.g., the red six of spades was seen as black, or the spades was seen as a heart/diamond). Bruner and Postman call this perceptual process "domination," according to which a percept is made to fit the agent's established perceptual categories. As I will explain immediately below, something like this happens in moral perception as well. Whereas the causes of perceptual rigidity on moral issues likely include motivational sources and/or emotional deprivations, I wish to emphasize the possible linguistic sources of this defect here.

William Brennan begins his book *Dehumanizing the Vulnerable: When Word Games Take Lives* with the following observation,

> The power of language to color one's view of reality is profound. In many instances, the most significant factor determining how an object will be perceived is not the nature of the object itself, but the words employed to characterize it.
>
> (Brennan, 1995, 1)

Brennan spends the remainder of his book empirically supporting the importance of language. In the field of bioethics where the ethical treatment of human beings is a principal concern, the question with language is whether it is being used to distort moral reality through marginalization or boundary drawing. Important for the argument at present is that when perception draws boundaries, that perception itself is a function of the very schemas/categories which constitute the boundary-drawing ideology.

An interesting display of how descriptions draw boundaries comes from the libel case of Dr. Carolyn Brown. Dr. Brown was a doctor who performed abortions in Anchorage, Alaska, and she was suing pro-life protesters for libel. The reason: they noted that the procedures she used were so "horrible"[23] that her own nurses refused to cooperate. She took the stand in court and was questioned by one of the attorneys for the protestors. She noted that she refers to the unborn human being as a baby when the mother wants the baby; but she refers to it as a fetus if the mother indicates an interest in abortion (see Brennan, 1995, 79). Brennan comments, "When the occupant in the womb is wanted, *he* or *she* is called 'a baby'; when unwanted, *it* is called 'a fetus'" (Brennan, 1995, 79). Here is an example of perceptual rigidity according to which the doctor continues to see the objects of abortion in dehumanizing concepts, but those who are wanted are seen without boundary drawing.[24] More recently Gómez-Lobo and Keown (2015) observe that, outside the context of abortion, we typically use terms such as "child" or "baby," rather than "fetus," when discussing the pre-born. "For example, we naturally say that a woman has 'conceived a child,' and we ask a pregnant woman 'how is the baby doing?' Not 'how is the fetus doing?'" (2015, 51). Not only can dehumanizing language be used to draw boundaries, but, on the abortion issue in particular, the use of dehumanizing language is discriminatory as it is not used elsewhere.

Conclusion

Because the data presented here is rather diverse, it may be helpful to end this chapter with an example that embodies the principal points made above. Michael Depaul (1993) considers a fictitious character named Jay – a young, zealous, and impressionable man who has a romantic view of warfare whereby war is good because it supplies a theater in which courage, honor, and bravery are realized. Jay has never been in a war but he watches numerous movies which glorify the valor and triumph associated with it. He converses frequently with the "old-timers" at the local American Legion listening attentively to their stories of triumph against improbable odds. Depaul observes that "Jay is rather naïve. The experience . . . that grounds his view of war is very narrow; none is first hand, and the rest is exclusively of reports, essays, novels, and films that romanticize warfare" (Depaul, 1993, 149). His experience is limited, and his motivations to identify with a soldier's courage and triumph exert enormous epistemic effects – this is due in part to his emotion of admiration (Zagzebski, 2012) and the ideology he has accepted from his elders.

Suppose Jay goes off to college and encounters arguments for very strict conditions for going to war, conditions that initially strike Jay as overly restrictive and pointless. Jay reacts somewhat like the subjects in the death penalty studies reacted. Jay reads materials that rebut these stricter conditions – an illustration of my-side bias and coherence motives in general. As a result, Jay's romantic view of warfare now takes on deeper and more philosophically sustained support. Suppose Jay encounters a moral principle that appears plausible, but it suggests that warfare is subject to strict conditions. Because Jay's starting intuition and preconception is that warfare is good, this starting intuition wins out in cases of conflict with unqualified principles.

If the professor who teaches Jay tries to dislodge Jay's commitment to his romantic views by showing him emotionally charged accounts of the collateral damage caused by war, Jay remains unmoved because his schemas representing warfare include valor and honor in the face of extreme sacrifice. He sees the sad costs of war, but not *as bad*; rather, he sees them *as necessary sacrifices*. If he feels pity, he *weighs* that evidence against the good goals of warfare – similar to how Dr. Sloan and the nurse reacted to abortion. His moral perception is such that when you show him bodies of dead children, for example, he acknowledges that this is bad, but it is a harsh reality outweighed by other goals such as defeating an evil enemy. Jay has a set of beliefs which have the following properties: (a) he has well-developed philosophical arguments against the non-romantic view of warfare, and (b) a host of positive arguments for his view. (Of course, these positive arguments rely on premises that are only plausible against the backdrop of his other beliefs.) Lastly, (c) Jay has an explanation for why his opponents arrived at the beliefs they have – he has a hermeneutic of suspicion. They have their beliefs because they have ulterior motives or are not really concerned about the real issues at hand – similar to how polarized disputants stereotype the out-group (Graham, Nosek, & Haidt, 2012). This last feature allows Jay to avoid seriously considering his opponents' view further since he thinks that they are the ones with distorting motives.

Clearly, Jay's belief system regarding the ethics of warfare is dismal. Notice, however, that he has a widely coherent set of beliefs on the issue, complete with counter-arguments and a hermeneutic of suspicion of his opponents. The principal problem with Jay's belief system is *Jay*. He conducted his inquiry as a function of coherence motives. His self-identity and schemas shape and condition his moral perception such that he does not see the moral realities of warfare in their proper light. He does not necessarily reason badly; he sees badly. So, as illustrated, there are various biases that can distort our ability to see and think clearly on ethical issues, these biases do not announce their presence, and they do not discriminate in terms of IQ.

The purpose of this chapter is to motivate the position that our moral perception suffers an undercutting defeater or that beliefs produced by it are more easily destabilized. How so? If there is a moral phenomenology – a 'what it's like' to apprehend a state of affairs as valuable (or disvaluable) – that phenomenology would be the same whether or not that state of affairs really is valuable (or disvaluable). More succinctly stated: I could be wrong about the true value of a putative human being, for example, and things would look just the same nonetheless; just as the widgets would look red even if they were not.

The conclusion reached is that we need to be skeptical of our preconceptions and our initial responses to moral argument. Why? Our moral perception is fragile in that it is susceptible to distorting influences – not all of our motivations, emotional sensitivities, and uses of language are ordered to obtain the truth. I am not suggesting that we hold with suspicion our judgment that torturing cats is wrong. Rather, the evidence suggests that we are in a questioned source context on issues involving rational disagreement. In the next chapter I discuss why the scope of epistemic diffidence is local and not ubiquitous. This localizing involves a discussion of peer disagreement and moral risks.

Notes

1 The phrase 'cognitive contact' is from Zagzebski's (1996) helpful definition of knowledge as involving cognitive contact with reality. The notion of cognitive contact remains neutral about whether this contact is mediated by propositions or experience. See Sayre (1998) for extensive discussion of the latter option.

2 My view shares features with Ellis (2005) and Noë (2004).

3 Throughout I hold that moral intuitions are specific outputs of moral perception where moral perception is understood as a faculty. See further discussion below.

4 See Chappell (2008) and Audi (2013) for further discussion. Chappell explores the boundaries of moral perception nicely and there appears to be little disagreement in the literature concerning her project.

5 This is not to say that moral perception is not multi-modal. The emotion of compassion, for instance, may be required to see the suffering of others as bad; the emotion of anger may be required to see injustices, etc. To illustrate the idea of basicality, a psychopath who has deficiencies in empathy simply does not apprehend the suffering of others as bad. And there is really no way to get her to have such an apprehension without some form of rational-emotive therapy or something else. This hardly entails, however, that all moral perception is reducible to the emotion of empathy. The point in the text is only about the basicality of moral perception.

6 The question of individuating or identifying faculties is viewed by some as a hopeless endeavor. The idea is that whether a faculty turns out to be reliable or not depends not on the faculty type per se, but on the beliefs we include in the reference class. For example, if we include only human perceptual beliefs

formed at long distances in sub-optimal conditions, we are not going to judge perception to be reliable; and vice versa for short distances under optimal conditions. So, how we carve up the perceptual faculty determines whether we would find the faculty reliable. My question in the text is logically prior to the task of individuating faculties: how could we justify reliability at all, however we carve up the faculty in question?

7 While I think that phenomenal conservativism (PC) is correct, PC does not affect what Alston or Reed or many others are saying who think that epistemic circularity is a live problem. Phenomenal conservativism tells me that my *belief* p is prima facie justified if it seems to me that p. The problem of epistemic circularity concerns the reliability of one's *faculty* that produced the belief. A crystal ball gazer could be prima facie justified in believing p (which results from ball gazing) because it seems to her that p. But this does not tell us much. If she wants to say that crystal ball gazing is a reliable method for discovering reality because it seems to her that p is true, and p is produced by ball gazing, she is using the very outputs of the faculty to justify the *reliability of that faculty.*

8 This is from an observation by E. F. Schumacher (1977, 44), "everything can be seen directly except the eye through which we see. Every thought can be scrutinized directly except the thought by which we scrutinize." His point is similar to mine in this chapter, namely, that one's moral evaluation of the world is a function of one's presuppositions, and those presuppositions are as basic as they are difficult to critically assess from the agent's own view.

9 There is not wholesale agreement on exactly what an intuition *is*. Haidt (2001) considers intuitions as a type of cognitive *process* that delivers its results immediately and automatically (without conscious effort). Sabine Roeser (2011) thinks that intuitions are *beliefs* that are not based on or justified by other beliefs – if they are justified they are non-inferentially. My belief that it is wrong to torture children does not need another belief to support it to make it rational for me to believe it. Others seem to think that intuitions, and moral intuitions in particular, are a type of perception or *apprehension* of value/disvalue (Chudnoff, 2013). As illustrated by the example from Blum (1994) in the text, I prefer to think of moral perception as a faculty that enables one to apprehend value/disvalue, and an intuition is a specific output of that faculty. Such intuitions are usually accompanied by a non-inferential belief, but not necessarily so. An abortion worker may *apprehend* certain abortion procedures as destructive bloody messes (Roe, 1989), but *judge* them as morally permissible (the example is from MacNair, 2009, discussed below).

10 Some theorists appear to describe the dissonance as possibly resulting from a perceived inconsistency between two or more beliefs that the agent already holds – call this condition (iii). I do not think this is a separate category from (i) because appreciating the inconsistency will be a new belief. Suppose p and q are contradictory propositions. Suppose I believe both p and q. I will not believe that I believe contradictory beliefs until I also believe that p *entails* not-q. The proposition 'p entails not-q' is the new information consistent with scenario (i). Of course, if I already believe all three and consider them in working memory, I have far deeper problems than mere cognitive discomfort! So (iii) is an empty category.

11 Lord et al. observe that "there is considerable evidence that people tend to interpret subsequent evidence so as to maintain their initial beliefs" (Lord, Ross, & Lepper, 1979, 2099).

12 Because scientific study is extended and involves many steps, a practitioner of science is justified in having a little intellectual humility. But this is not always so. See Staley (2004).

13 Cooper and Fazio (1984) showed that dissonance is aroused only when one engages in a dissonant behavior freely. In general, conditions b–f are sub-species of condition g – dissonance typically is not aroused unless there is a perceived incoherence within the self, and the items that are dissonant matter to the individual.

14 Aronson's observations (1968) suggest that coherence motives and self-esteem motives may overlap and may even be co-extensive since the effects of CD only appear when there is a perceived inconsistency with one's self-concept. I would still urge a third category covering cases of self-interest. Examples are not hard to find. Coffee drinkers and non-coffee drinkers were presented with evidence indicating that caffeine was associated with higher incidences of cancer or cardio-vascular disease. As expected, coffee drinkers were more critical of such studies than non-coffee drinkers. I doubt the motivation informing such reasoning had to do with self-esteem, but rather with their self-interests, particularly their interest in enjoying the pleasures of a morning drink. Self-interest motives are meant to cover motivations for power, prestige, and pleasure; see Kunda (1987).

15 The opposite effect occurs in cases of attitude alignment. Attitude alignment occurs when relatedness motives are activated – discussed below.

16 I thank Michael Rota for drawing my attention to these studies.

17 Quoted from Gianelli (1993).

18 Kathleen Roe (1989) studied abortion clinic workers' own conceptions of their work doing abortions. In open-ended interviews, 77% of the workers described abortion as a "destructive act."

19 Quoted from Sloan and Hartz (1992), 248.

20 As I have characterized it, my-side bias is a species of a coherence motive in so far as it functions in such a way as to bring about coherence (Baron, 1995). But it is also activated by self-esteem motives in so far as we have an interest in thinking we are correct, or smart. In any case, I wish not to gripe about sharp divisions between these motives because such divisions do not affect my argument and these motives are often confluent in human behavior. I make these divisions for pedagogical reasons – to order the information into some pattern.

21 Another word of caution regarding taxonomy. External influences such as that we experience from friends, associates, or the broader culture, can be a function of one's desires or motivations to fit in with or identify with a social group. So, personal social motives can make the influence of associates and culture *operational*.

22 Given Haidt's description, it appears that acquiring a sensitivity to other sets of values requires open-mindedness and participation in certain practices.

23 The procedure used was prostaglandin abortions for second and third trimester pregnancies. Infants can be born alive with this procedure, but are usually killed in utero via lethal injection.

24 This is dehumanizing because the human being at the fetal stage is clearly living. Prior to animation, Frankenstein is at most potential life, nascent human beings are at least actual life.

3 Epistemic Justification, Peer Disagreement, and Moral Risk

The previous chapter argued that given what we know about how our moral perception can function, the possibility of being morally purblind is a live option. By live option I mean to say that it is a skeptical hypothesis that needs to be addressed since there is no noncircular reason *for* the reliability of one's moral apparatus. I argued that our moral perception is subject to the visual analog of inattentional blindness insofar as it may be a function of non-alethic motives which direct our moral attention to non-salient features. On the other hand, I observed that certain moral judgments, e.g., that torturing children for fun is wrong, are not suspect. This chapter, then, acuminates the focus of epistemic diffidence regarding one's moral judgments. The punchline is that judgments that involve disagreements with one's epistemic peers and involve a high cost in being wrong, are the foci of epistemic diffidence.

To this end, I discuss first the epistemic relevance of peer disagreement. I argue that the epistemic effects of peer disagreement (if any) result from an agent's alethic motivation to conform her inquiry to certain intellectual virtues. If I moderate the credence in my belief p when I discover that a putative peer conscientiously believes ~p, it is because I want to avoid dogmatism. Conversely, if I maintain my belief in the setting of a putative peer disagreement, it is because I want to avoid being epistemically flaccid. The intellectual virtues explain whatever epistemic effects disagreement exerts on one's own beliefs.

The second section addresses the epistemic effects of practical risks. I argue that when a belief has a high cost in being wrong if one were to act as if it were true, the justification for acting on such beliefs are more sensitive to defeaters.

To appreciate the integrity of discussing both issues in one chapter consider the following example. Suppose you are a radiologist looking at a chest graph and you see localized tumescence in the lower lung lobe. You diagnose the patient with pneumonia. You have reviewed chest graphs like this before and your past record in diagnosis has been accurate. To your surprise you discover that your colleague, also an expert radiologist, reviewed the same chest graph and diagnosed the patient with pulmonary fibrosis.

The latter interpreted the tumescence as interstitial tissue. Suppose that the drugs involved in treating fibrosis versus pneumonia are significantly different and involve widely divergent risk profiles. Giving a patient drugs for pneumonia when she really has fibrosis exposes the patient to significant risk of harm or death and vice versa. The cost of making a mistake is high. On this point Richard Rudner noted long ago,

> [O]ur decision regarding the evidence and respecting how strong is 'strong enough', is going to be a function of the *importance*, in the typically ethical sense, of making a mistake in accepting or rejecting the hypothesis. . . . *How sure we need to be before we accept a hypothesis will depend on how serious a mistake would be.*
>
> (Rudner, 1953, 2)

Finding out that your colleague arrived at a different judgment should give you pause in how you treat the patient. Acting on the belief that the patient has pneumonia has a high cost in being wrong such that it is more easily threatened by defeaters – in this case, your peer's disagreement. Your belief that the patient has pneumonia should be held with epistemic diffidence. Suppose further that there is not a more fundamental way to resolve this diffidence. The basis of the diagnosis is a perceptual judgment behind which one cannot peek or get more fundamental information.[1] At this point, the disagreement appears basic and incorrigible. Amplified as such, the example illustrates how disagreement with a peer concerning a belief B can undercut one's justification for acting on B. Call this the Radiology Case.

The Epistemic Effects of Disagreement: Dogmatism and Flaccidity

Why does peer disagreement motivate epistemic caution in the Radiology Case? More generally, why is peer disagreement epistemically significant at all? How does someone else's belief affect the justification for my own beliefs?[2]

In the Radiology Case, you come to hold your own diagnosis with caution. A plausible starting point for explaining why is that you believe that your colleague has epistemic credentials like your own, e.g., similarly attuned perceptual abilities (Myles-Worsley, Johnston, & Simons, 1988). But this is not enough to justify why one should hold the diagnosis with caution. For one could just as well use one's own belief that B as an argument that one's interlocutor's epistemic abilities are not operating properly on this one issue. Prior to discovering the disagreement, you believed that your colleague had similar epistemic abilities as you. But upon realizing the disagreement you have a choice to make. You could infer from, 'she has similar epistemic credentials as me,' to, 'I should hold my diagnosis with caution.' But you could also infer from your belief that the patient has pneumonia to questioning whether your colleague's epistemic abilities are functioning properly in this one case. You are not forced by any standard of rationality to hold constant the belief that your colleague is an epistemic peer.

If we have the intuition that a peer disagreement exerts epistemic effects, a plausible explanation for why is that we want to avoid *dogmatism*. David Christensen notes that the motivation behind a conciliatory stance to disagreement is "to prevent blatantly question-begging dismissals of the evidence provided by the disagreement of others" (Christensen, 2011, 2). Using my own beliefs to argue that others are not epistemic peers can amount to an egotistical privileging of my own beliefs *simply because they are my own*.[3] Michael Huemer calls such a position "agent centeredness." Huemer notes, that "[a]gent-centeredness seems to call for a kind of epistemological egotism . . . Each agent seemingly must say, 'my experiences, considered as such, are prima facie better indicators of reality than the experiences of others'" (Huemer, 2011, 24). On this view, how things seem to other conscientious agents provides me with little to no prima facie justification. While I think Huemer is right to reject epistemic egotism, with its implicit embrace of dogmatism, the appeal is merely to our sympathies with not wanting to be dogmatic. But why is being dogmatic in this sense so wrong? Labeling a position dogmatic does not argue for why it might be wrongheaded. The next few paragraphs articulate those reasons. This is an important step in my argument since I consider epistemic diffidence to be an intellectually virtuous response to *certain contextual features of one's inquiry*; one of those features is peer disagreement.

The previous chapter argued that the problem of epistemic circularity (for proving the reliability of our cognitive faculties) entails that our inquiry and reliance on our faculties must proceed on trust. For Linda Zagzebski, however, trust is not a fallback position after seeing that no proof for the reliability of one's faculties is possible. "Before we reflect upon the justification of our beliefs or the reliability of our faculties, we already trust ourselves and our environment" (Zagzebski, 2012, 42). For Zagzebski, epistemic self-trust is a starting point for any reflective activity, including the activity of discovering that the reliability of one's faculties cannot be proven. But this fact leaves us in the epistemically precarious position of not being able to prove that our faculties are reliable. The better part of wisdom is to use them in epistemically conscientious ways. Zagzebski defines epistemic conscientiousness as "the quality of using our faculties to the best of our ability in order to get the truth" (2012, 48). Importantly, she notes that conscientiousness is required particularly in cases involving extended inquiry whereby the evidence must be interpreted or handled carefully. She notes, "she [an agent] trusts evidence in virtue of her trust in herself when she is conscientious, not conversely. Her trust in herself is more basic than her trust in evidence" (2012, 49). For Zagzebski, judging whether E counts as evidence for P requires a prior trust in myself, namely, that I am being conscientious *in assessing* whether E counts as evidence for P.

Whether a piece of data counts as evidence for P, however, requires interpretive work. States of affairs do not carry labels indicating that for which they are evidence. Borrowing an example from Longino (1979), suppose my daughter has red spots on her stomach and I come to believe that my daughter has measles based on that fact. Clearly, however, red spots alone do not indicate anything. I need background medical knowledge to infer from red spots to the presence of measles. Prior to modern medical knowledge, red spots may have been taken as evidence for any number of things other than measles.

It follows that arriving at some of our beliefs is not a function of *evidence* leading directly to a belief that P,[4] but it is a result of *us* interpreting, assessing, weighing, and/or inferring from evidence to beliefs. It is because cognitive processing can be extended over time and on a complex matrix of information that one has reason for thinking that one may make a mistake. So, when confronted with someone who I initially think is a peer and she disagrees with me, I suffer a defeater to my belief that I have handled the evidence well. Clayton Littlejohn expresses the point this way, "the fact that you disagree is a reason to think that you and Tilda [a putative peer] were out of your depths or that one of you suffered from a performance error" (Littlejohn, 2013, 170). And since you cannot provide a non-circular justification for why your faculties are functioning reliably in the dispute, a disagreement is undischarged evidence for a performance error.

This idea is confirmed by the cases used to support Conciliationism – the view that I should suspend or lower credence in beliefs about which there is known peer disagreement. Following Lackey (2010), cases motivating the steadfast position – the denial of Conciliationism – are cases where the beliefs are virtually self-evident; viz. cases of perceptual recognition under epistemically ideal circumstances (e.g., good lighting, close proximity) or well-rehearsed memorial beliefs. Cases motivating the conciliatory position are cases of extended inquiry requiring numerous inferences and/or the weighing of apparently relevant information. Lackey reflects on the bill calculation case (Christensen, 2007), which involves doing complicated mental math to determine the distribution of a restaurant bill between five people given that the bill total is a large decimal number. The hypothesis that I have made a mistake becomes live when I encounter someone for whom I conscientiously believe has similar abilities as me and comes to a different conclusion.

We are now in a place to explain why dogmatism is an intellectual vice. One cannot prove the reliability of one's faculties but must trust and use them as conscientiously as possible. Moving from evidence to belief can be a complicated matter and requires using one's faculties in the best way one knows how to satisfy the desire for truth. If there are others for whom I conscientiously believe are using their faculties in a conscientious manner, I believe well to accept their beliefs at least as prima facie justified. The reason is that I should treat like cases alike. If I trust the deliverances of my own faculties, I believe well by accepting the deliverances of others who have the same faculties and for whom I believe are using their faculties conscientiously. Zagzebski notes, "[w]hen I am believing conscientiously, I come to believe that many of them [other persons with similar cognitive endowments] are just as conscientious as I am when I am as conscientious as I can be" (Zagzebski, 2012, 57). So, if I trust the deliverances of my own inquiry because I believe that I am conscientiously using my epistemic faculties, I have no reason not to trust others when I come to believe that they too are conducting their inquiry conscientiously. "I cannot consistently trust my own faculties but not those of others" (Zagzebski, 2012, 56). Epistemic egoism is irrational, and, therefore, so is dogmatism. I cannot privilege my own beliefs simply because they are my own, since the reason I trust the deliverances of my inquiry are duplicated when I conscientiously believe that others are conscientious in their inquiry.[5] I might believe that others are not conscientious in their inquiry, but I cannot justify that position with reference to the beliefs in dispute without circularity.

Another argument against dogmatism can be generated by appealing to common-sense intuition. This might be an odd claim since our starting intuitions are typically on the side of intellectual autonomy. But I suggest that we have equally strong intuitions supporting the idea of taking seriously disagreements with putative peers. Consider a species of disagreement which occurs in *intra*-personal conflict. Suppose I believe, plausibly enough, that knowledge is true justified belief. I then discover a Gettier-type counterexample to knowledge as true justified belief. Two or more of my beliefs are now in conflict. I suspect that, among philosophers, this is a common enough occurrence to proceed without further description. Notice that when one discerns the conflict, the phenomenological grip on each belief usually lessens. We become cautious towards both beliefs.[6] We may even hold both beliefs based on plausible reasons and have exercised our faculties in equally conscientious ways in forming them. It also seems plausible that in analyzing my own inquiry certain aspects of it will be opaque to that reflection. The same lessons apply to *inter*-personal disagreement; I may not have access to every epistemically relevant feature of my interlocutor's inquiry, and yet they may provide reasons for their beliefs. In both inter- and intra-disagreement, then, the same epistemic features may be present which prompt holding one's disputed beliefs with caution or lessening one's credence in them.

So, using my own belief as a premise in an argument that my interlocutor's epistemic faculties are not reliable is dogmatic and dogmatism is inconsistent with both epistemic justice and common-sense intuition. The basic idea is that, *with respect to the belief that is in dispute*, one has reasons for thinking that she has made a mistake in cases involving extended inquiry on complex information[7] and my interlocutors appear to be using their epistemic faculties in conscientious ways. Imagine the other radiologist in the Radiology Case responding to your judgment saying, "you must be wrong because it appears *to me* that there is interstitial tissue!" While there is no disputing what the other's appearances are, inferring from them to "you must be wrong" ignores how things appear *to you*. Consider an intra-personal version of this: after discerning that there is tumescence, you entertain the possibility that it might be interstitial tissue instead of inflamed tissue. You would hold both interpretations with diffidence.

Objections

In reviewing the literature on disagreement, it appears that there are at least two ways to mollify the negative character of dogmatism. Jennifer Lackey (2010) considers what she refers to as the "modified bill calculation case." As above, you are dining with four other friends, you agree to a 20% tip and to evenly split the bill, which is a large decimal number. Suppose you do the calculation in your head. You discover the disagreement, and then proceed to do the calculation on paper *several times*. Lackey observes that as your degree of confidence goes up, the more implausible it is for you to revise your belief (by suspending or lessening your credence in it). On this modified bill case, I think Lackey is correct. Lackey is quick to note, however, that even high confidence is not enough to justify asymmetry.[8] She states that, while one's confidence may be quite high, it cannot be the only epistemic feature that justifies your remaining steadfast. If it were, "this would have the consequence that the hyper-dogmatist – who is supremely confident in all of her beliefs – is never rationally required to adjust her doxastic states in the face of ordinary [peer] disagreement" (Lackey, 2010, 317). For Lackey, the additional feature we need is that the belief is, *actually*, *very well*-justified.

For Lackey, then, one avoids dogmatism by actually being very well justified in a belief that is in dispute. Whereas I find sympathy with Lackey's intuitions on the cases she discusses, I do not think that her arguments succeed in mollifying what is bad about dogmatism. That the belief is well justified must be accessible from the agent's own point of view. For the question 'what disagreement *rationally* requires?' has typically been understood as a question to specific agents given what that agent believes.[9] Being very well justified is assessed by the agent herself. But this does not avoid the hyper-dogmatist riposte. So long as being 'very well justified' is assessed from the subject's own point of view, one can easily stipulate that she has the better justification than her interlocutor. Consider Jay, introduced at the end of Chapter 2, who upon reviewing his justification for a romantic view of warfare concludes that he is very well justified. He may be, and I described him as being so, but that hardly justifies him in setting aside the judgments of those with whom he disagrees. He has reasons in the form of peer/superior disagreement for doubting the veridicality of his inquiry.

Related to this point about subjective justification are Lackey's comments on "personal information" (Lackey, 2010, 318).[10] For Lackey, personal information can function as a symmetry breaker in putative peer disagreements. Personal information can mean either one of two things. First, it can mean that, in forming my belief, there are many tacit features, such as a phenomenological experience that cannot be adequately communicated verbally, or "massive amounts of evidence accumulated over many years that I couldn't possibly remember, or data acquired from various sources in contexts that I am unable to articulate" (Lackey, 2010, 312). Personal information could also mean the results of my self-reflection on how I thought about, for example, the calculation of the bill. That is, it can involve a meta-level monitoring of my thinking. The former notion of personal information highlights the possibility of tacit justification; the latter highlights a monitoring procedure for how I arrived at my beliefs.[11] Tacit justification would purportedly add to my justification, monitoring merely checks the genesis of my belief.[12]

Personal information understood as tacit justification would count as a symmetry breaker only if those tacit elements in fact add to one's justification for the disputed belief. But the tacit component of one's cognition could just as easily include, unbeknownst to the agent, ill motivations, non-alethic cultural influences, or other non-alethic influences canvassed in the previous chapter. I agree with Lackey that there are tacit components to human cognition (Polanyi, 1962, chs 5–7), but I do not agree that all such components are alethic in nature. So, I do not see that personal information understood as tacit elements is sufficient to count as a symmetry breaker since one cannot assume that it is veridical.

Furthermore, monitoring my procedures for arriving at my beliefs does not necessarily function as a symmetry breaker, especially when I am simply rehearsing my justification. The very agent who is doing the monitoring might be duplicating the biases that led to having just those beliefs in the first place. Consider again my-side bias discussed in Chapter 2; when we rehearse our justification for B, we typically focus only on our side of the argument. Consider also Jay who may recalculate his moral reasons for a romantic view of warfare and meta-monitors the history of his inquiry. One notable fact is that this meta-monitoring would be done from the agent's own perspective. And, as noted in the last chapter, our moral eyes can see everything except the eye by which we see. So, of course Jay's inquiry is going to look veridical to him since he is the one doing the monitoring. Recall also that the epistemic problem was not with Jay's justification, but it was with *Jay*. Thus, meta-monitoring can be just another way of maintaining an illusion of objectivity. On any plausible interpretation of what Lackey means by personal information, then, it is not sufficient to function as a symmetry breaker in cases of ordinary peer disagreement.

Adam Elga (2007) proposes that remaining steadfast could be justified if one discovers that the beliefs in dispute begin to metastasize into numerous other beliefs. Elga holds to what he refers to as the "equal weight view" (i.e., Conciliationism) according to which, in the setting of known peer disagreement, parties should suspend or lower the credence in their beliefs that are in dispute. Elga admits that acting on such a view leads to what he calls "spinelessness" since the view appears to recommend flaccidly giving up your beliefs and not sticking to your guns (notice the connotation of an intellectual vice). Since spinelessness is intuitively an intellectual vice, it looks like Conciliationism recommends being intellectually vicious. Elga thinks, however, that Conciliationism can avoid such a consequence.

He considers an example involving Ann and Beth who have opposing views on the abortion issue. They have both considered the issue for the same amount of time, they have access to the same facts, and they appear to be equal in intelligence. Elga thinks, however, that neither Ann nor Beth should lower their credence in their respective beliefs and that this is consistent with Conciliationism.

Ann (or Beth) can use reasoning independent of their disagreement about abortion to justify remaining steadfast on those very beliefs. If Ann and Beth discuss claims closely associated with the abortion issue (such as views on human nature) and find that they disagree on each one of them, Ann (or Beth) can use their respective disagreements on these other issues as an argument that the other has made a mistake *on the abortion issue*. Elga states that,

> [b]y Ann's lights, Beth has reached wrong conclusions about most of these closely related questions. As a result, even setting aside her own reasoning about the abortion claim, Ann thinks it unlikely that Beth would be right in case the two of them disagree about abortion.
> (Elga, 2007, 493)

Elga claims that Ann (or Beth) can set aside their reasoning about the abortion issue *without* setting aside their reasoning on other allied issues. And, if Ann and Beth disagree on these other allied issues, they can use these other disagreements to argue that the other is not a peer on the abortion issue.

There are two ways to understand Elga's argument in terms of what justifies Ann (or Beth) remaining steadfast while assuming Conciliationism.

The first is to understand the inference as moving from the discovery that the other person disagrees with you on *many* issues to the claim that the person must be wrong on the target issue. On this first reading, what is justifying you in remaining steadfast is the *number* of propositions about which you disagree. But this understanding entails several odd results. Presumably, Conciliationism remains intact if Ann and Beth disagree only on a few other issues. If so, then my beliefs do not suffer a defeater when I encounter someone who shares *radically* different beliefs than mine, but they do when my interlocutor shares similar beliefs as mine. This is the wrong result. Would not each of my beliefs in the numerous disagreement case suffer a defeater on Conciliationism?

To see why, consider a concrete set-up. Suppose I believe that abortion is permissible. I also hold to a psychological account of the person which is, roughly, the position that you and I do not come into existence until our mental capacities are exercisable – i.e., after most abortions take place. And I hold that account based on intuitions in response to brain transplant cases. My interlocutor thinks that abortion is impermissible and holds to an animalist account of the person – we are essentially human animals. This account is based on the too-many thinkers problem and an error-theory for our transplant intuitions (these issues are discussed in Chapter 4). Elga would have us believe that, prior to discovering that my interlocutor holds to an animalist account, my belief in abortion suffers a defeater. After discovering that my interlocutor is an animalist and can provide a coherent network of beliefs which mutually support a negative judgment on abortion, my beliefs retain their justification and escape unscathed because of the number of our disagreements. This is the wrong result since the more one faces coherent and articulate reasoning, the more one's beliefs should be challenged.

The second way to understand Elga's justification for remaining steadfast is not the number of disagreements but the *quality* of those disagreements. So, suppose Beth comes to hold not-p, and not-p is supported by Q, R, S, and together they form a coherent system which realizes wide reflective equilibrium (Daniels, 1979; Rawls, 1971); and Ann has a coherent network as well. Understood as such, there are two sets of problems. The first pertains to the development of one's widely coherent view and the second to the finished product.

In developing one's views in accordance with what reflective equilibrium recommends, I may start with an intuition on an action or case description and proceed to formulate moral principles that would explain my intuition on such actions or cases (Kelly, 2008). But suppose we are confronted with a conflicting idea: for example, I believe that abortion is permissible based on a psychological account of the person, but I may also find intuitively plausible the key premise in the too-many thinkers problem. According to D. W. Haslett (1987, 306 ff.), I have what he calls an "adjustment decision" to make. I could either modify my belief that abortion is permissible or find a way to rebut the too-many thinkers problem. How one makes these adjustment decisions, however, can be problematic. Haslett explains,

> All coherence considerations enable us to decide is that the one *or* the other must be chosen, they do not enable us to decide, definitely, *which* one. . . . Because of the lack of any clear-cut guidelines for governing these decisions, reflective equilibria are extremely "under-determined" by their starting points.
>
> (Haslett, 1987, 310)

The problem is that, when it comes to making adjustment decisions, they are surprisingly unprincipled and arbitrary. The quality of the justifica-tion, then, depends upon whether these decisions were made with alethic motivations and in light of what really are the best reasons. The point to make is that the quality of one's justification can justify 'sticking to one's guns' only if the development of an agent's wide equilibria was itself an intellectually virtuous inquiry; and assessing the latter involves looking beyond the quality of coherence one's belief may enjoy.

If we just consider a widely coherent view itself, we still do not have a good justification for sticking to one's guns. The problem is simply to point out that one can have a comprehensive and coherent network of moral beliefs that is outrageous. The neo-Nazi view might be logi-cally coherent but fails to reflect moral reality. Beauchamp and Childress (2001) give the example of the "Pirates' Creed of Ethics" (2001, 400), which is logically coherent but morally outrageous. Any coherence the-ory is subject to some species of the no-contact-with-reality objection, according to which one can have coherence but no belief in the network reflects reality. If quality justification is defined with reference to coher-ence, and coherence is subject to the no-contact-with-reality objection, we still do not have a symmetry breaker with strong enough epistemic credibility – certainly we don't if both Ann and Beth have coherent views.

A final problem with Elga's proposal is the following dilemma. If I am justified in inferring from our disagreement on other issues to the belief that my disputant is not a peer on the target issue, then the relevance of these other issues *is not independent* of the reasoning one may invoke on the target issue. If they are not independent, it appears circular to use them to break the symmetry on the target issue. For then, the jus-tification J for the target issue Ti (e.g., abortion) can now become the disputed claim. At *this* stage in the dialectic I can either use my belief that Ti to discharge the dispute about J, use J itself, or a further justifica-tion for J, J-J. The first two options are obviously circular, and nothing prevents the third (i.e., J-J) from becoming the focus of a third-tier dis-pute, and so on. For each justification, I have no non-circular reason for discharging the epistemic weight of my putative peer's belief or I transfer the axis of disagreement to further justifications. If these other issues are independent, I cannot infer from our disagreement on them to the claim that my disputant is not a peer on the target issue.

One may object to my reflections so far by arguing that, if coherence is a sufficient condition for being rational and how one responds to disagreement is a question of how that response satisfies standards of rationality, then having achieved wide equilibrium suffices to discharge the effects of disagreement. Coherence can function as a symmetry breaker for discrete beliefs within rival networks of equilibria. In response, peer disagreement is not an undercutting defeater to one's justification for B specifically, but a defeater to one's belief that she has *not* made a performance error while constructing her wide equilibrium. It is a defeater directed to the faculty or agent who has the beliefs, not the beliefs themselves. A coherent view on romantic warfare, for example, cannot itself discharge the defeater from one's peers who disagree.

Elga has not given us a good justification for mollifying what is bad about dogmatism. Metastasized disagreements do not suffice. The correct response to the spinelessness objection requires being clear about what it is to be spineless.

Spinelessness is understood in this context as a vice, a defect in one's intellectual character – as is dogmatism. In this regard, Elga is right that, if Conciliationism entails being spineless, one should reject Conciliationism. Recall, however, that the reasons for Conciliationism were that rejecting it looks like one is being dogmatic. *The values at stake in this debate make essential reference to the intellectual virtues and vices.* But being virtuous or avoiding vices is not subsumed under an exceptionless epistemic principle or position such as Conciliationism or steadfastness.[13] The elixir for spinelessness is to throw oneself in the messiness of the intellectual life and discern as best as one can – while seeking to inculcate alethic motivational patterns – the reality confronting one. Principles are not the right tool to solve the problem; aiming to inculcate the relevant virtues are. One avoids spinelessness by being intellectually courageous; one avoids dogmatism by being intellectually humble and just; and one avoids both at the same time by being practically wise, i.e., *phronesis.* This is not to parry from providing principles governing one's rational response to disagreement,[14] but are reflections concordant with the messiness and difficulty of discerning moral reality.

So the explanation for why disagreements exert epistemic effects in circumstances involving extended inquiry, or inquiry that exercises the upper limit of human cognitive capacities, is that resisting those effects is dogmatic or otherwise vicious. And I have rebutted arguments to the effect that dogmatism is tolerable in certain of these cases.

Summary

We can now appreciate the following argument for why disagreement with a peer can justify diffidence. Being dogmatic is a deficiency in treating my interlocutor justly. In the face of a putative peer disagreement, I cannot simply ignore the fact that my interlocutor believes not-P when I believe P, and I have no evidence (other than the dispute about P) to believe that my interlocutor was not conscientious in forming her belief that not-P. So did my interlocutor assess the evidence for not-P correctly? Who has the requisite epistemic credentials? Answering this question cannot use the very belief in dispute as a justification that the other does not have the credentials. Consider just how tight the circularity is: you would discharge the first-order dispute, viz., your interlocutor's belief that not-P, because she does not realize credential C. And credential C is the correct credential because P is the right belief! One could use one's *justification* for P to moderate the epistemic effects of peer disagreement. But then the same dialectical schema is iterated for each justification. Al believes P on the basis of J1, Bob believes not-p on the basis of ~J1. Now the dispute is about J1; and so on for whatever supporting beliefs J1 or ~J1 enjoy in their respective noetic networks. For each belief that is in dispute, that belief cannot itself be used to justify that you are, but your interlocutor is not, conscientious.[15] Given the problem of epistemic circularity for the reliability of our own faculties, we do not have direct access to whether our inquiry is veridical. So, disagreement with a putative peer is evidence of a performance error, and this defeater cannot be discharged by the very belief in dispute without another epicycle of circular justification.

Of course, this is only a schematic argument that is not meant to apply to every disagreement. Again, the guiding heuristics are to avoid dogmatism and flaccidity. Kelly (2013) offers an example of Moorean rejections of revisionist metaphysical reflection – e.g., those who think that tables and chairs do not exist. The arguments for the nonexistence of tables and chairs are not obviously false. But a Moorean committed to common sense says that tables and chairs clearly do exist, therefore there must be something wrong with the arguments for their non-existence. If Moorean rejections are rational and being dogmatic precludes being rational, then Moorean rejections cannot be dogmatic. But they recapitulate the basic schema noted in the previous paragraph. The lesson learned is not that the schematic argument is inert, but that dogmatism and flaccidity are intellectual vices, specifically a defect (dogmatism) and an excess (flaccidity) of intellectual justice towards my interlocutors. Intellectual justice requires giving my interlocutors their due relative to the circumstances as the virtuous person would determine.

The epistemic effects of peer disagreement are a function of being intellectually virtuous (or vicious).[16] Ignoring the epistemic credentials of my interlocutor is dogmatic in certain contexts. Conversely, revising or exchanging my beliefs every time I discover that they are in dispute is epistemically flaccid (Roberts and Wood, 2008). It would be epistemically flaccid to change my beliefs on human cannibalism simply because someone endorses, for example, the custom of the sea. Finding the mean in complicated intellectual discourse is a work of *phronesis* and epistemic justice.

Moral Risk, Presumption, and Burden of Proof

Whereas peer disagreement exerts symmetrical epistemic effects,[17] the epistemic effects of costs or risk in being wrong plays favorites. Suppose Arien and Irving enter a Starbuck's with the intention of buying some brownies. They are very hungry and could use a good dose of glucose. There are two baskets of brownies, one labeled 'made with peanut flour' and the other labeled 'no peanut flour.' Suppose Irving has a severe nut allergy and has forgotten his Epi-pen. Before making their choice, they notice that another patron who is overwhelmingly busy with children, inadvertently returns a peanut brownie into the non-peanut basket (they saw the child take it from the peanut basket, but this was unnoticed by the parent). Arien grabs a brownie from the 'no peanut' basket because he does not like the taste of peanuts. Irving, however, thinking that these are open baskets and other customers (or employees who stock them) can make the same inadvertent mistake the parent did, refuses to buy a brownie without checking further. Arien's actions seem perfectly rational, as do Irving's; even though they have the same intentions, same evidence, and are situated in the same environment. What makes Irving's refusal to buy a brownie rational is that, for him, the effects of being *wrong* in *acting* on the judgment that 'this brownie from the no-peanut basket does not have any peanut flour in it' are drastic – death or severe hypoxia. Furthermore, the risks appear asymmetrical. There are no equally drastic effects in buying a safer option, except that Irving had his heart set on a brownie.

The case illustrates the epistemic relevance of risk. But what exactly is risk *doing*? There are basically three distinct though related epistemic roles that risk might play.

1   Risk might be considered relevant in adjudicating *who* in a dialectical exchange bears the burden of proof. The basic idea is that if risks are not symmetrical, the proponent of the riskier position – the position that if one is wrong involves greater harms – bears the initial burden of proof. Suppose the position bearing the greater risk of harm in being wrong is a judgment of permissibility. The proponent of impermissibility enjoys a presumption in favor of her position and does not need to argue for it – initially. Defendants in the court of law, for example, enjoy a presumption in favor of not guilty; the plaintiffs must prove guilt. Call this the burden of proof role.

2   A risk in being wrong about P might make P more sensitive to defeaters. Quite independent of whether or not the proponent of P bears the burden of proof, one could say that a higher risk in being wrong about P renders P more easily undermined by counter considerations. Consider the Radiology Case again. In this case, the risks are symmetrical and yet the evidence for P (or not P) is epistemically destabilized simply by the say-so of another epistemic peer. Call this the sensitive to defeater role – or simply the defeater role.

3   A risk in being wrong about P renders one's action on the basis of P immoral (or insufficiently justified). On this understanding, the relevance of risk has less to do with the epistemic standing of my belief that P, and more to do with my moral responsibility to consider the potential harms in being wrong about P. But this understanding can be split into two separate positions. On the one hand, cases where we have the intuition that it would be irresponsible to act on P are used to justify the claim that risks in being wrong about P can render one's action based on P as wrong (Reed, 2012) whether the agent knows P or not. On the other hand, cases where we have the intuition that it would be wrong/unjustified to act on P justifies thinking that the agent does not know P to begin with (Fantl and McGrath, 2009). The latter position holds that knowledge is subject to pragmatic encroachment, the former holds that knowledge is immune to pragmatic considerations, but our moral responsibility is not. For both positions – discussed in more detail below – a risk in being wrong about P can render acting on P morally unjustified. In some cases, we might know that P but not enough to justify *acting* on it – acting on it may be deemed careless or negligent. Call this the bar of justification role, or simply the justification role.

In complicated dialectical exchanges where risk is relevant, there is no reason to think that only one role is functioning. It is not my task, then, to specify which role, but to argue that 1, 2, and/or 3, is functioning. I focus on the burden of proof role throughout only to streamline the presentation and to avoid cumbersome and protracted qualifiers.

For the purposes of illustration, let's consider the burden of proof role in more detail. In arguments, presumptions fix which propositions bear the burden of proof. To presume a claim means that discussants will accept the initial plausibility of that claim. There may be good reasons for the presumption: Irving's observation of the misplaced brownie is enough given the risks he would bear, even though it is statistically very unlikely he would select a peanut brownie. Irving, then, takes Mislabeled as a starting point. Nicholas Rescher comments that "a presumption is not something that certain facts *give* us by way of substantiating evidentiation: it is something that we *take* through a lack of counter evidence. A presumption is more akin to a theft than a gift" (Rescher, 2006, 6, emphasis original). Consider an analogy: I take my perceptual beliefs to be veridical and I am justified in holding my basic perceptual beliefs *unless* I have reason to doubt their reliability. By presuming the veridicality of my perceptual experiences, I create a burden of proof on those who wish to challenge that veridicality. Suppose I am informed that I have been hit with a painless blow dart that, unbeknownst to me, affects my vision. Notice that, even if it were true, I would need some evidence before I just suspend my perceptual beliefs – to do otherwise strikes me as epistemically flaccid. I would need to believe my informant after she cites a few examples of error, for example. The point is that presumptions stand so long as there are no positive reasons against them. This explains how presumptions function, but what are they?

James Freeman (2005) claims that in normal discourse between two interlocutors, a proponent and a challenger, what gets presumed is going to depend upon the stage of the dialectical exchange. For example, prior to seeing that the parent misplaced the brownie, neither Arien nor Irving had a reason to presume Mislabeled. Add the evidence of misplacement and the stage of the dialectic advances to a point where, for Irving, Mislabeled is presumed and not-Mislabeled incurs a burden of proof.[18] The notion of presumption, then, should consider the development of a discussion and the crucial interchanges that can occur. As such, Freeman (2005, 29–30), defines presumption relative to a challenger, a proponent, and a dialectical interchange.

> There is a presumption in favor of a statement S at a point p in the dialectical exchange for the *challenger* C of that exchange if and only if C is obliged to concede S at p.
>   There is a presumption in favor of a statement S at a point p in a dialectical exchange for the *proponent* P of that exchange if and only if P has answered all the challenges against S at p.
>
> (2005, 29–30)

If a *challenger* has no reason to object to S, given certain assumptions about our intellectual obligations, it is plausible to suppose that the challenger ought to presume S at p. Conversely, if a *proponent* has answered all the objections to S at p, nothing stands in the way of presuming S at p. The key idea is that presumptions are statements for which it is broadly rational to accept without explicit argument or positive reasons for them – relative to an interchange of a dialectic.

Notice that for Irving (after seeing the misplacement) the inquiry into the proposition non-Mislabeled is aimed at rather high epistemic goals. Irving is not concerned merely with whether non-Mislabeled is plausible enough to justify further inquiry. His goals are to discern whether it is certainly true; he should not eat a brownie unless he has done so. When we speak of a burden of proof, what counts as proof depends on the goal. If the goal is to justify *further inquiry* on an idea that initially strikes one's interlocutors as implausible, my burden is lighter than, for example, justifying that the idea is *true*. In this book, meeting the burden of proof must give one reasons for thinking that the proposition in question is true.

What justifies distributing presumptions unequally between a proposition and its denial is the cost in being wrong in settings where the costs are asymmetrical – a possible exception is noted below. Whether the ladder I am about to climb on is safe (to do some trivial work on my house) inherits a burden of proof. Aijaz, McKeown-Green, and Webster note that,

> [i]nsofar as we are interested in how sensible it would be to climb my ladder, there is an attitudinal burden on anybody who takes it that my ladder is safe, but no burden on anybody who takes it that it is unsafe.
>
> (Aijaz, McKeown-Green, & Webster, 2013, 269)

Prior to seeing the misplacement, Arien and Irving would distribute the burden of proof equally between Mislabeled and not-Mislabeled. Upon seeing the misplacement, the cost in being wrong about non-Mislabeled[19] becomes immense for Irving, the effect of which is that Mislabled is presumed and the burden of proof is on not-Mislabeled. Thus, the costs in being wrong about P are relevant for indexing the burden of proof. It is not my view that the cost in being wrong changes the amount or strength of one's justification for or against P. For example, suppose Irving's evidence for non-Mislabeled includes the barista telling him that he just stocked the baskets and that the parent's inadvertent misplacement is very likely the only one. These are still reasons, maybe even good enough reasons, for thinking that eating a brownie from the no-peanut basket is safe. The moral risk does not change their *status* as reasons.

How might the three roles function together? Because of the cost in being wrong, the burden of proving non-Mislabeled raises the strength of justification (role 3) *required to justifiably act on it*. And the burden of proving non-Mislabeled is incurred because Mislabled is more sensitive to defeat (role 2) given Irving's health status.[20]

A burden of proof may exist even in cases where the costs in being wrong are high and symmetrical – i.e., no matter what belief you act upon (P or not-P) there are serious costs to being wrong. The Radiology Case might be an example of this but I prefer to understand that case as a case where risk is functioning as 2 or 3. Nonetheless, it is possible that the burden of proof be evenly distributed in cases of high, symmetrical cost. However, I do not consider in this book actions for which there are symmetrical costs between action A and not-A, *and* doing one or the other is morally required.[21]

It is important to note how my view differs from both the precautionary principle (PP) and uncertainty arguments based on risk, and how it relates to pragmatic encroachment. To count as a PP, several conditions are necessary (Kramer, Zaaijer, & Verweij, 2017): (i) a harm condition according to which there is a possible harm to doing an action; (ii) an epistemic condition according to which there is a probability that the harm will occur; (iii) an action plan that guides actions in light of (i) and (ii); and finally (iv) a judgment about the force of the action plan. It is often assumed that the harm and epistemic conditions are met, disagreements concern the shape and scope of what condition (iii) outlines. That is, the precautionary principle tells us that *when* there is a relevant probability of harm in doing action A, one needs to think about other harm-reducing actions or choose not to do A. On the issues I discuss, however, it is not obvious that the harm condition is met – that is the argumentative role of the chapters that follow. Furthermore, the specific content of the epistemic condition I endorse is not identical to typical formulations of the PP. Typical formulations will emphasize a quantifiable threshold of probability for x (a harm) happening. My view is much more parsimonious in that epistemic diffidence is a function of (i) taking seriously our moral processing apparatus (Chapter 2), (ii) in discrete dialectical contexts involving peer disagreement on issues that tax the upper limit of human capabilities, (iii) with serious injustices that would result in being wrong when acting on 'it is permissible to intentionally harm or kill Y.' The third feature allocates who has the burden of proof; thus, the justification for acting on such judgments requires meeting a higher threshold of justification. Epistemic diffidence does not follow simply from observing that there are moral risks to being wrong about A, one must assess the respective justifications for and against A.

Likewise, my view differs slightly from uncertainty arguments. Dan Moller (2011) rightly supposes that there are three vectors by which we assess whether the risk in being wrong in P would render acting on P wrong. Those vectors are: the reasons for being wrong about P; the gravity of the wrongdoing in acting as if P (if P were false); and the cost in not acting on P. David Boonin's (2002) criticism of uncertainty arguments in defending abortion is that, in assessing the risk of being wrong about P, one is being asked to set aside all of one's reasons for P.[22] Of course there is a probability that the pro-choice position, for example, could be wrong. But the probability of being wrong applies to any other moral claim such as that the grass in my lawn does not have moral status. "Numerous arguments . . . have been offered in defense of the claim that nonhuman animals, and even plants or ecosystems, have the same right to life that you and I have" (Boonin, 2002, 314). Given the arguments, Boonin supposes that one cannot honestly be certain that such claims are false. If they were true and we acted as if they were false, we would do serious wrong. So, Boonin understands uncertainty arguments to entail the following advice: when one is not certain that P is morally permissible, one should act as if it is morally impermissible; one should not mow her lawn (2002, 315), eat meat, or even drive (since driving causes a high incidence of roadkill).

Boonin is right that, on a probabilistic understanding of moral risk, uncertainty arguments "must insist that the mere fact that an argument for one conclusion convinces you while arguments for a contrary conclusion do not, is not in itself a good reason for you to act on that conclusion" (2002, 323). On this understanding of uncertainty arguments, they appear to require an agent to give equal weight to another's view if there is a high cost to being wrong about your own, even if you do not find the other's view remotely plausible. Giving equal weight seems to violate epistemic integrity, and it fails to acknowledge that a person might have good reasons for his belief even if being mistaken about that belief would have drastic moral consequences.

It should be clear that, on my view, the epistemic effects of moral risk are not co-extensive with how uncertainty arguments understand them to be. Suppose I act on P believing it to be true and I know that being mistaken about P would involve killing an innocent person unjustly. Assume that I'm deeply concerned about not killing people. Uncertainty arguments would tell me that I should not act because of the grave consequences of being wrong about P. My position is that it may be permissible for me to act, but the *burden of proving* that it is permissible to act is on me. Not-P enjoys a presumption in its favor. So, my view is more parsimonious in this sense: I do not look simply at the lack of certainty paired with the drastic consequences of being wrong. Rather, the cost in being wrong sets who has the burden of proof, but this burden can be met by a proponent of P if she discharges challenges to P. Furthermore, in assessing the epistemic effects of high-stakes, my view *requires* analyzing the strength of one's justification for P since doing so is required to assess whether the burden of proof is met. Far from setting aside one's justification, my view requires a fine-grained analysis of it.

On a related view, I should distance my position from what Elizabeth Harman refers to as Uncertaintism. Uncertaintism is the view that one's moral credences, the confidence with which one holds her moral beliefs, are relevant for determining how an agent should act (Harman, 2015, 53–54). On Harman's understanding, Uncertaintism is making merely a subjective moral claim that an agent is morally responsible only for what the agent believes; "Uncertaintism implies that being caught in the grip of a false moral view is exculpatory" (Harman, 2015, 57). I agree with Harman that a false moral view is not exculpatory; but I disagree that anything I say herein entails such a view. (I don't think Uncertaintism entails such a view either since being "relevant" to how we should act does not entail being sufficient for determining how one should act.) A false moral view is not exculpatory once one takes into account the frailty of our moral faculties (Chapter 2), the disagreements we encounter with conscientious interlocutors, and the high cost in being wrong about some of our beliefs. If, in adjudicating the epistemic status of one's own beliefs, one ignores any of these three features, one is being epistemically unjust.

Pragmatic encroachment is the view that knowledge claims are sensitive to non-epistemic factors such as an agent's practical interest in not being wrong (thus, *pragmatic* factors *encroach* upon knowledge attributions). Whether an agent knows P depends in part on the agent's interest in avoiding the costs in being wrong about P. The standard cases used to illustrate pragmatic encroachment are the bank cases (DeRose, 1992, 913).[23] In case A, Kermit and Piggy are driving home on a busy Friday evening. Kermit has just been paid and he is considering depositing the check in the bank that night. But as they drive past the bank they notice that the lines are exceptionally long. Kermit proposes waiting until Saturday morning to deposit the check, having remembered that the bank was open on Saturday several weeks ago. Piggy mentions that many banks are closed on Saturdays. Kermit continues to believe (suppose rightly) that the bank will be open on Saturday, relying on his memory of the moderately distant past. Case B is just like case A except that Kermit and Piggy have a very important mortgage payment that will be withdrawn automatically over the weekend and their account is insufficient without the deposit. If they do not deposit the paycheck, they will be evicted from their home. Kermit recalls that the bank was open on Saturday several weeks ago, and Piggy mentions her potential defeater to that belief. Does Kermit know that the bank will be open on Saturday in case B? Many authors have the intuition that Kermit does not know in case B, but he does in case A. The explanation is that the cost in being wrong that the bank will be open on Saturday in case B is too much to rely simply on memory of the moderately distant past. Banks could change their hours, it could have been opened on a Saturday just once a month, etc.

Cases involving practical costs can be interpreted in at least three different ways. First, one could say that Kermit does not know that the bank is open in case B, but he does know in case A. Second, he does not know in either case. Third, he does know in both cases but, for case B, he needs to be certain that the bank is open on Saturday to be justified in *acting* on that belief. On this third interpretation, knowledge does not require certainty, but he needs to be certain that the bank is open on Saturday because of the costs in being wrong in case B. All three interpretations grant that, in case B, Kermit's justification is below a threshold sufficient to justify the act of waiting until Saturday to deposit the check (see Reed, 2012).[24] The strength of justification sufficient for *knowledge* comes in degrees; and one can meet that threshold before meeting the threshold of justification required to justify *acting*. In cases involving high costs in being wrong, there is not enough epistemic justification to justify acting on p, but there may be enough to justify knowing that p. Reed's assessment of high-cost/low-cost dyads is that both "subjects have the knowledge in question, but only the subject with low stakes is rational to act on it" (Reed, 2012, 471). Reed and his critics agree that, in high stakes cases, an agent is not justified in acting on his beliefs with the strength and kind of justification ascribed to him. That agreement is the content of role 3, the justification role. I do not need to take a position on whether knowledge attributions are sensitive to pragmatic factors.

Discussion of pragmatic encroachment invites the question whether moral risk should be understood as subjective or objective given the problem of indifference. Return to Leibniz's example of the Caribs. Suppose a member of this society had a coherent set of beliefs which justified their heinous actions. It seems wholly implausible to suppose that there is no longer any cost to being wrong about their judgments that pediatric cannibalism is permissible. Of course there is a cost to being wrong; and a huge one at that. The most one can say is that members of the society do not themselves think that there is a cost to being wrong, or they think that their justification has met the higher epistemic bar that such costs set. But the idea that there's not a moral risk at all simply because they are certain that their judgment is permissible doesn't seem right. Everyone *should* agree to the following conditional "if your [a member of the Caribs] moral judgment is false, you would be engaged in serious wrongdoing." Hence, the presence of a moral risk does not require subjective epistemic agreement.

Conclusion

At the very incipient stages of one's inquiry, one may believe P with some justification.

Regarding this initial entry point for one's beliefs on a subject matter, Chapter 2 outlined certain non-alethic sources which can obfuscate our moral perception. Reasons for thinking that such sources are operant in the formation of one's belief gives one reason for thinking that the belief is a result of a questioned source. Suppose, however, I continue my inquiry to defend P, much like the subjects in the Lord, Ross, & Lepper (1979) death penalty study conducted their inquiry.[25] Here, I think I am acquiring supportive justification, but only by instantiating certain non-alethic motives which inform my inquiry.

I was clear in Chapter 2, however, that ubiquitous skeptical conclusions do not follow simply from the observation that some of our beliefs might be the result of non-alethic sources.[26] Rather, in this chapter, I specify the properties of the beliefs we should hold with diffidence. What kinds of beliefs may result from a questioned source?

The points in this chapter answer this question as follows. The risk in being wrong in P sets a higher burden of proof or bar of justification on P, or belief in P becomes more sensitive to defeaters (i.e., the bank *might* be closed, you saw only *one* brownie get misplaced). If a burden of proof is incurred, it requires a detailed assessment of one's justification for P. Importantly, such justification will be undercut by whatever justification there is that P is a function of a questioned source. The reason is that, if S judges that S has met the burden of proof, S is using the very faculty she may have reason for questioning. And, S has reasons for questioning its reliability in certain settings of peer disagreement. Peer disagreement on issues that exercise the upper limit of human capacity gives one reason for thinking she has made a performance error. The intellectually virtuous person would tailor her doxastic commitments according to an honest assessment of this possibility for her and others. This assessment would involve epistemic humility regarding one's own capacities vis-à-vis the domain/issue in question, and epistemic justice in regard to others' inquiry on the domain/issue in question.

Many of the issues discussed in this book involve intentionally killing human beings. If one thinks that doing so is permissible, there is a high cost in being wrong about such a judgment. But that itself is not a theory-neutral assessment of the dialectical situation in contemporary bioethics. The next two chapters argue that killing human beings at any stage in their development is a morally risky activity. The next chapter considers arguments to the effect that you and I come into existence early enough to be killed by abortion or embryo-destructive research, and in cases of covert or suppressed consciousness. And the chapter that follows argues that such killing is morally problematic. The two chapters taken together set the burden of proof on those who think that such killings are permissible.

Notes

1 Suppose that a lung biopsy is not indicated given how small the abnormality is and that a transbronchial scope will not go deep enough into the alveolae where the abnormality resides.
2 To avoid confusion below, I should be clear about my view since it is not co-extensive with current positions. I do not think peer or even superior disagreement should lead to suspending my belief or lessening my credence in it in all cases. So, I do not endorse Conciliationism as it has typically been understood. Following Jennifer Lackey (2010, 302), Conciliationism (and its corollary Steadfastness) have typically been understood as conjoined with a Unity thesis according to which the epistemic effects of peer disagreement are the same in all circumstances. I reject the Unity thesis largely on the grounds Lackey canvasses. Though, for reasons I address below, I do not hold to her justificationist view full stop. Thomas Kelly (2008 and 2013) recommends understanding peer disagreement as one piece of one's total evidence. For Kelly, encountering peer disagreement may involve no belief revision at all, since one's total evidence may still rationally support one's original belief. It could also justify reducing one's credence in the disputed belief, suspending the disputed belief, or changing the disputed belief. For my purposes in this book, my virtue account is compatible with Kelly's in that beliefs with a high cost in being wrong are more sensitive to defeaters. Peer disagreement in the setting of high costs in being wrong injects *enough* reason for caution, even on the total evidence view.
3 The fact that we are agents with a distinct will means that we can only take responsibility over our own epistemic house; my beliefs are mine, not someone else's. The implication of this rather banal observation, however, is that some privileging of my own beliefs must occur and it would be quite virtuous for me to do so. What is bad about dogmatism is that the privileging is done *simply* because my beliefs are mine.

4 This is true on matters that involve interpreting a complicated set of data or on matters that involve perspicuous perception as in the Radiology Case. Also, my point here is compatible with whatever position one takes on what evidence is, propositions vs data. Whether one holds that evidence is the proposition 'red spots on the stomach' or the data of there being red spots, one still needs medical knowledge to infer that measles is present.

5 Nathan King (2012) argues that, though disagreement might exert epistemic effects, we would never know it because one would need to compare, side by side, the character of one's own inquiry with the putative peer. But we do not have access to how another person processes his information. I only add to this that if biases do not announce their presence, as argued in Chapter 2, we might not have exhaustive access to the quality of our own inquiry either.

6 Of course, one may also double down by arguing for one belief and providing an error theory for the other. My point in the text is consistent with this response since one would not feel the need to inquire further and provide such reasons if both beliefs were not initially recognized as plausible.

7 The conditions under which I think disagreements exert epistemic effects are cases involving inquiry that exercise the upper limit of human cognitive capacity. So, extended inquiry on complex information is one species, but looking at X-rays and interpreting ever so subtle deviations from the norm are also cases even though the latter is not properly an *extended* inquiry.

8 A symmetry breaker (or a justification for asymmetry) is a term Christensen uses to refer to one's own justification that one's interlocutor is not a peer. It is a justification for thinking that one's own belief has superior epistemic credentials compared with one's disputant. For Conciliationism, the symmetry breaker must be independent of the specific beliefs in dispute so as to avoid circularity.

9 Michael Depaul notes that "having rational beliefs . . . is a matter of one's beliefs conforming to one's own standards, that is, of believing what one would take to be true upon reflection. Rationality is, therefore, subjective and correctly explicated along internalist lines" (Depaul, 1993, 74).

10 Lackey is explicit that she is externalist with respect to justification. I am setting this aside since the question regarding peer disagreement is how one may *rationally* respond, and epistemic rationality has typically been understood as internalist; the subject is held responsible for how things look from her own epistemic point of view.

11 Lackey's comments suggest that there might be a third notion of personal information according to which the agent is simply *confident* and has *justification* for her beliefs. But I do not see how this can be a symmetry breaker since one's interlocutor can realize those features just as well. This might not be a plausible understanding of the modified bill calculation case, since basic math problems are calculable by those of modest intelligence. Persistent disagreement about the shared amount starts to look like an idealized case of disagreement and one we would likely not encounter. But it does seem a plausible understanding of ordinary disagreements on complex issues requiring extended inquiry, such as discussed in this volume and in the Radiology Case which exploits our intuitions on needing refined faculties in order to discern the domain correctly.

12 Monitoring would not likely add to my evidence for the following reasons. First, monitoring cannot yield the conclusion that my faculties are reliable since that would be circular. The monitoring would have to take my evidence as its principal object. There are two options in this regard: I could (a) recheck whether evidence e in fact supports p, and/or (b) recheck whether I have considered all relevant evidence. Option (a) is not going to add to the

stock of evidence I already have, but it might take it away. That leaves (b). But what counts as relevant evidence is a function of my background theoretical commitments (again, see Longino, 1979). So, the threat of circularity looms, which would not add to my overall evidence.

13 See Bryan Frances's (2014) work, which is a survey of cases which push and pull our intuitions in different directions. No principle manages to capture our intuitions on all cases.

14 See Chapter 10 (n. 5) for a brief discussion on the relationship between intuitions on cases and principles.

15 Kelly (2013) gives a case of a Holocaust denier who is *ignorant* of the justifications most of us have for the Holocaust having occurred. But this is not a counterexample directed against all epistemologists who think that *peer* disagreement exerts a defeater for one's own belief (e.g., Thune, 2010). While there are problems in identifying whether my interlocutor is a peer, exposure to relevant facts is often mentioned as a necessary condition and it is verifiable (see King, 2012). In any case, Kelly's example illustrates the fundamental difference between our positions on disagreement. When confronted with an astonishing belief or report, Kelly's approach is to add up the evidence he has. That evidence will wash out whatever epistemic effect peer disagreement may have, especially in cases where one's interlocutor subscribes to an unconventional belief. My position is that when confronted with astonishing beliefs, a focus on the evidence I may have is myopic. One needs to consider whether further inquiry is just in the circumstances. Holocaust deniers and smoking-causes-cancer deniers are easy cases to reject without further inquiry and are not counterexamples to my view. Clearly, however, not all astonishing reports or unconventional beliefs should be rejected with exclusive reference to one's own evidence and inquiry. Coady (1992, 190 ff.) gives an example of a mariner's astonishing report that turned out true, but when the mariner sent his findings to the journals in his field, they rejected them without comment. Given the context and information provided by Coady, the editors were clearly closeminded and handled the new report unjustly. And yet, they did exactly what Kelly's total evidence view recommends. So, in focusing on the virtues, my account considers our reliability, motives – alethic or otherwise – etc., in assessing our own and others' inquiries. I do not focus merely on the evidence for p.

16 In understanding peer disagreement via the virtues I avoid the self-defeat objection to Conciliationism. Conciliationism recommends lowering my credence in a belief about which I know to exist peer disagreement. This includes my belief in Conciliationism itself for which there are those who disagree. My virtue approach recommends taking an attitude towards others' belief-forming mechanism that satisfies intellectual justice. Compatible with my view is also Elga's (2010) response to the self-defeat objection.

17 Unless the disagreement is with an epistemic superior, but even here there are counterexamples (see Frances, 2014).

18 It is true that Irving carries with him a background burden of proof for anything that he ingests, namely, he must be sure it does not have peanuts in it. But because presumptions are a type of cognitive attitude towards propositions, Irving cannot presume Mislabeled (whose propositional content is contextual) until he walks into the Starbucks and sees the arrangement.

19 Henceforth, the locution 'cost in being wrong about P' and semantically similar phrases should be understood to include an agent acting on P, or acting as if P were true.

20 Suppose Irving does not witness any misplacement but considers Mislabeled because of a general but flimsy suspicion of quality control measures. I am

inclined to think that Irving may still take a brownie. Suppose instead that Star Confectionery (a subsidiary of Starbucks) made the news that morning because it mislabeled its brownies with a customer experiencing anaphylactic shock. With this little evidence of which Irving is aware, he should have a muffin. These permutations illustrate the defeater role of risk.

21 For example, I do not discuss what is called vital conflicts (Rhonheimer, 2009) in OB/GYN practice in which one has an exclusive choice between saving the mother by ending a wanted pregnancy prior to viability or letting both die. I harbor doubts, however, that we have obligations in tragic dilemma cases. We do not have an obligation to act against significant goods. Since tragic dilemmas practically require acting against a significant good, we do not have an obligation to act one way or another in such cases – though acting one way or another may be permissible.

22 On this point I think that Moller should be understood as avoiding Boonin's critique given his first vector. But Moller does not tell us how one should go about assessing the quality of those reasons – in fairness, that was not his stated task anyway.

23 Much has been written on pragmatic encroachment. For book-length treatments, consult Fantl and McGrath (2009) and Stanley (2005). Important article-length work not discussed here is Guerrero (2007). Guerrero and I share numerous intuitions; my disagreement pertains almost exclusively to his discussion of abortion.

24 Reed's position avoids the problem of indifference according to which I can get knowledge simply by caring less. Though there are plausible rebuttals to this problem (Coss, 2018), avoiding this dispute with no other intuitive costs is philosophically economical.

25 Kelly (2008) thinks that what is epistemically suspect about what the subjects did is that they privileged the *initial* evidence they were exposed to in support of their beliefs. Kelly rightly observes that the order in which one accrues her evidence should not matter epistemically; what matters is apportioning one's belief to the total evidence.

26 On this point I am opposed to Sinnott-Armstrong (2008, 2006) because my skeptical conclusions are more parsimonious and local. But even if Sinnott-Armstrong is correct, so much the better for the sub-conclusion in this book, namely, that many of our practical judgments are subject to epistemic diffidence.

4   Persons and Human Beings

The previous two chapters attempted to limn an answer to the question 'how should we conduct our moral inquiry?' The rough answer is that we need to be epistemically virtuous to counteract the motivational dispositions that can distort our moral perception and to prevent reasoning like a lawyer instead of a judge (Haidt, 2001). Global skepticism does not necessarily follow, but local skepticism does when I am confronted with a putative peer who disagrees with me on an issue where there is a high stake in being wrong and the issue exercises the upper limit of human cognitive capacity. Again, I need to be epistemically virtuous to avoid dogmatism and flaccidity. Moral risk indexes the burden of proof (among other roles). This chapter and the next descend into the periphery of bioethical discourse and together argue that the burden of proof is set on those who think that killing human beings is permissible. I address in this chapter what is a human being and when does one come into existence. The next chapter addresses whether human beings have intrinsic dignity.

This chapter covers the topics of substance and personal identity. Any review of a standard encyclopedic entry on either topic will reveal that they are both complex issues with enormous bibliographies. Therefore, choices are made throughout in terms of what points/arguments I address in more detail and not everyone will agree with such choices. Views I choose for consideration, however, are standard. The level of justification reached in this chapter aims only to show that, given the current articulation of standard views, the burden is set on those who think that it is permissible to kill human beings – even those 'at the margins.'

In the next section I make explicit some common-sense intuitions about human substances, and from such observations build a plausible case that you and I are essentially human animals. If this view is correct, I explain in the second section why you and I come into existence likely before we develop exercisable psychological capacities. In the third section I explain arguments in favor of a psychological view of the person. In the fourth section I assess these arguments.

Human Beings and Substances

You exist now, you did in the past, and hopefully you will exist in the future. Through time *you* have undergone and will undergo numerous changes. The features and qualities that would accurately describe you when your mother held you in her arms are quite different than the ones that accurately describe you now. But you exist throughout all these changes. What are you then? You cannot be *identical* to those features that accurately describe you (whenever), since many of them may not accurately describe you at different times. This rather commonsensical thought is where we begin.

A plausible answer to the 'what are you?' question is that you and I are human animals/substances. What does this view mean? To say that you and I are substances connotes the idea that each of us is an individual *entity*. Traditionally, the language used was 'primary' substance, examples of which include individual entities such as Fido, Felix, Oscar, you and I.[1] A primary substance is an individual entity. Furthermore, primary substances have a nature, or, more accurately, a *way of being* (which includes its characteristic powers, developmental pattern, and morphological features). Traditionally, the nature or way-of-being is referred to as a secondary substance since its existence as a concrete thing is parasitic on the existence of a primary substance. Examples of secondary substances include, canine, feline, *hominoidea*, and *Homo sapiens*. Henceforth, what I mean by substance is a human primary substance, unless otherwise noted. And the term substance is interchangeable with 'an entity' or 'a thing.'

The language of primary substance may be foreign but it captures some common-sense intuitions about individual entities, especially human beings. Each substance has features, such as being bi-pedal, having blond hair, black skin, being smart, quick witted, etc. A substance and its features differ in an essential respect. Substances can *take on contraries* of various features; the features themselves cannot without loss of identity. You can have blond hair at one time, and black hair at another. But black hair cannot be white hair without ceasing to be black. Relatedly, a substance can exist *through* changes in its properties and relational features.

The idea that I can take on the contraries of features and survive changes in properties (broadly construed) might suggest an understanding of substance as a metaphysical pin cushion into which pins (i.e., properties and relations) are inserted and exchanged. That is not how to understand the substance view. There is no characterless bearer of characteristics. If substances are characterless and you and I are not characterless, then you and I cannot be substances.

The idea to abandon is that a substance is a characterless bearer of characteristics. One may think that we are required to endorse this idea in so far as substances have properties but are not identical to those specific properties, and the instantiation of those properties depends upon the existence of the substance (this latter conjunct is explained below). It would seem to follow that a substance is wholly different from its properties – a characterless bearer of characteristics. To clarify, a substance can never be without properties or relations. To say that a substance can survive changes in properties and its relations does not entail that a substance is something *entirely* without *any* properties or relations. It just means that I am not identical to any *specific* cluster of properties or relational features. Justin Broackes comments,

> When one squashes a ball of clay, something that *was round* now *is flat*; the clay has 'lost its roundness', not in the sense that one item (the roundness) has been detached from another (the clay); but only in that the clay was a certain way, is now another way . . . [I]t 'lost' one property only as it 'gained' another—the clay was always of one shape or another, and, in general, things are always one way or another.
>
> (Broackes, 2006, 149)

It is true that a substance is not identical to any one of its properties or even to the complete set of properties it has at a given time. In fact, it is not of the same ontological type as any of its properties since a substance is not a property at all. But this claim hardly entails that substances exist without having any characteristics or properties; for any concrete-spatio-temporal continuant is a certain *thing*.

However, some changes are substantial in the sense that they change the *nature* of the thing. A shorthand way of describing this fact is to say that substances can have both *accidental* and *essential* features. If a table were not extended it could not be a table – being extended is an essential property of table. Notice, however, that a table is not identical to the property *being extended*. An even more trivial example is being alive. If you were not alive, you could not exist. Being alive is an essential property of you.[2] An essential property is a property a thing must have in order for it to exist. But this does not entail that an essential property is unique. Crawford Elder (Elder, 2005, 4 ff.) tells us that chromium has an atomic number of 24. But suppose it also had the unique distinction of being mined in parts of Africa. The property of coming-from-Africa would still be an accidental feature of chromium. Chromium *could* have been mined elsewhere and still be the metal that it is. If a piece of metal had an atomic number of 79, we know it cannot be chromium; it must be gold. You and I have essential and accidental properties.

Care should be exercised in understanding the phrase 'you and I *have* essential properties.' Given the definition of essential property, the following count as essential properties (Plantinga, 1974, 60):

a   Being self-identical.
b   Being either a prime number or something else.
c   Being alive if one is an organism.

These are all properties that any existent thing has. Any existent thing is either a prime number or something else. Every existent thing has the property of being identical with itself. Essential properties, then, do not necessarily tell us anything about *the thing* that has those properties. More generally, since I cannot be a property (properties are existentially dependent upon things), I cannot be an essential property. Essential *properties* do not necessarily tell us what I am. To be sure, I can have an essence, so long as the term 'essence' is understood not to refer to a property, feature, or part of me, but to what makes me be the thing I am (Oderberg, 2008a).

I have been speaking of properties and features. The next intuition is that we are not a mere collection or aggregate of properties and features. When Felix the cat gets up and walks out of the room, the property of *walking*, of being *black*, of being *quadrupedal*, of having a tail 13 in. long, and of weighing 5 lb. etc., do not all get up and walk out of the room.[3] Rather, *Felix*, a black quadrupedal cat of such and such size, weight, and morphology, walks out of the room. We are individual beings, but we have multiple parts. You have the capacity to think, to be aware of your environment, to eat, to move, etc. Likewise, most of us have arms, legs, brains, a functional nervous system, organs, etc. We have both physiological components (organs and limbs) and metaphysical components (psychological powers or capacities, and a specific nature – we are not dogs, cats, or horses – we are *human* beings). You possess a multiplicity of both physical and metaphysical components. How then should we understand ourselves as being one thing?

Consider a methane molecule. Hydrogen and carbon are its component parts. But methane is not hydrogen plus carbon plus some metaphysical glue that bonds them together. Rather, methane is a unified whole whose parts we can abstract away mentally and identify individually as hydrogen and carbon. Likewise, a lemon is not made up of yellowness plus fruit plus sour plus some metaphysical glue. Rather, a lemon is a fruit that is colored yellow, is sour upon taste, etc. In general, a substance is "not color plus shape plus weight. It is a colored, shaped, heavy thing" (Scaltsas, 1994a, 151). The chief problem with understanding substances as being aggregates of parts is that the unity of the whole is left unexplained. Theodore Scaltsas explains the problem as follows:

> Consider any complex whole, such that the parts constitute a single whole, not as a heap but like a syllable is a single whole. Then the whole cannot be identical to the aggregate of its parts. The reason why is that if we disperse the parts, we still have the aggregate of the parts but we do not have the whole any more. This shows that the whole is over and above the aggregate of the parts. But it cannot be over and above the aggregate of the parts by an element that is like the parts, because then the same argument would apply again.

The new aggregate (of the parts plus the extra part that is supposed to turn the original aggregate into a substance) is preserved when its parts are dispersed. But the substance is not preserved when the parts are dispersed.

(Scaltsas, 1994a, 64)

If we disperse hydrogen and carbon, we no longer have methane, but we do have a hydrogen molecule and a carbon molecule. Co-present parts do not equal a unified whole.

The questions that needs answering, then, are twofold, 'what makes this thing be the kind of thing it is?' and, antecedently, 'what makes this thing be one thing?' To know the nature of a *this* (a particular substance), we need to have already identified the *this*. For Aristotle, the notion of a substantial form answers both questions:[4]

And this is the substance of each thing (for this is the primary cause of its being); and since, while some things are not substances, as many as are substances are formed in accordance with the nature of their own and by a process of nature, their substance would seem to be this kind of nature, *which is not an element but a principle.*

(Aristotle, 1941, 24–31, emphasis mine)

A substantial form is that which makes a thing be the thing it is, for example, a horse, a cat, a human being. It explains why the powers of a thing are in fact *characteristic* or *prototypical* powers, i.e., why a human being cannot see like a bat, and vice versa. Patrick Toner observes that an entity's substantial form explains why it has the capacities it has, why it develops those capacities and not others, when it is supposed to develop those capacities, "and it accounts for why we think it tragic for a baby to be born without an upper brain, and why we do not think it tragic when a tulip lacks an upper brain" (Toner, 2011, 69).

The key role that substantial form plays in making one thing a unity is not so much to explain how many things can *make up* a single thing, but rather how the many things *cease* being many (Scaltsas, 1994b, 109). It is important in this regard to understand that substantial form, for Aristotle, is not a distinct constituent along with the other physiological or metaphysical parts of the human being. Rather, the identity of those parts and powers as being parts and powers of one thing is dependent upon the substantial form. A finger separated from the human being is no longer a finger, insofar as it no longer functions as one. Similarly, the hydrogen molecule and the carbon molecules do not retain their independent identity when they are parts of methane. Their doing so would invite the idea that methane is simply a hydrogen molecule meta-physically glued to a carbon molecule. But that is clearly false. Rather, the parts of an organic whole are *re-identified* in accordance with their function in the whole. The substantial form, then, is not one among many relata. In fact, there is *no relation* between substantial form on one hand and whatever else on the other. The substantial form does not relate parts to one another; it re-identifies those parts as contributing to the functionality of the whole. 'Re-identification' means that we can abstract by a mental act the different components of the unified whole, but we cannot mistake the object of our abstraction as having independent identity in the thing of which it is a part. We can abstract away mentally and identify individually the parts of carbon and hydrogen, but this separation has no corresponding reality in methane. Those parts are re-identified as methane in the concrete particular.

These reflections apply equally well to metaphysical parts. So, if one thinks that human beings are composites of soul and body, one may be right if this is understood as a mere abstraction. There is no corresponding relation of soul (or a psychological power such as consciousness) and body (or functional brain) *in res*. When one thinks about the soul of Leibniz, one is no longer thinking about some independently identifiable thing *in Leibniz*; just as thinking about the properties of hydrogen does not involve thinking about some independently identifiable thing *in methane*.

To summarize, you and I are one thing. What makes us one thing, though with many parts and powers, is a substantial form. The substantial form makes us be the kind of thing we are, including our developmental trajectory (discussed below), specifying powers (e.g., rationality), and characteristic properties (e.g., morphological features such as bipedal). Explaining this view further, P. M. S. Hacker illuminates saying, "if it is a living being, its morphological features, characteristic organs, pattern of development, and characteristic modes of behavior are non-derivative properties of the creature, *and are determined by the nature of the organism which it is*" (2010, 43, emphasis added). Michael Loux makes a similar observation:

> Kinds . . . cannot be reduced to properties. It is, of course, true that in virtue of belonging to a kind [such as human being], a concrete particular will possess many properties. . . . Aristotelians will concede all these facts; what they will deny is that a plant's belonging to the kind *geranium* can be reduced to or analyzed in terms of its possessing these properties. As they see things, it is because it belongs to the kind that it possesses these properties and not vice versa. The kinds to which concrete particulars belong represent unified ways of being that cannot be reduced to anything more basic.
>
> (Loux, 1998, 119–120)

We may appeal to such properties and attributes to discover or know what kind of thing it is, but the properties do not make the thing be what it is, its nature does. The explanatory arrow moves from the nature to the entity's specifying powers.

Our powers, features, and qualities are all *ontologically dependent* upon the existence of the substance – on the entity that *has* or *possesses* these powers, features, and qualities. Having blond hair cannot exist without an *entity* that has blond hair. But that same entity can exist without blond hair. The substance Felix was born and weighs 5 pounds, but none of Felix's *properties* were born or weigh 5 pounds. Another way to think about this notion of dependence is to consider the distinction between subject and predicate. Both Fido and Rover are dogs. As such, 'is a dog' is predicated truly of Fido and Rover. But neither Fido nor Rover can be predicated of anything else. Fido is not a *feature* or *quality* of something else.

Substances are concrete, individual things as opposed to abstract universals. A mathematical number is abstract; you cannot bump into a prime number; but you can touch, bump, see, and point to in space and time a concrete object. In this respect, substances are continuants, they occupy space, and endure through time. Because substances endure through time, they should be distinguished from events or instances. And because they are particular, they are not universals. (Universals are abstract things that are multiply realizable such as redness, risibility, or powers such as rationality.) Powers and properties do not exist, at least not concretely, except with a substance that bears such powers and properties. *The power* of rationality does not think; but a *human being* with that developed power thinks. Typically, only concrete entities can do concrete activities. The power of rationality is not a concrete thing, but an abstraction from the thing that has rationality. The power of thinking cannot exist without a thinker. Likewise, actions do not exist without agents. In general, one cannot build a concrete particular by metaphysically gluing together abstract universals. A set of abstract properties is itself abstract. This is not to say that abstract things do not exist. All that is said here is that abstract things do not exist *as* concreta. A psychological capacity considered in itself is an abstract thing. A psychological capacity *of* me is concrete. But its status as concrete is wholly dependent upon me existing. The implications of these points are enormous and are noted below and in later chapters.

This intuition, namely, that we are concrete spatiotemporal continuants, seems quite strong, so much so that it is stronger than the intuition that we are identical to a certain set of psychological properties (for example, having certain thoughts, beliefs, and intentions). Suppose that one's thoughts, beliefs, and intentions were reducible to neurological correlates. And suppose that we were able to develop synthetic neurons and populate them with specific propositional content – per impossible on my view.[5] We could then create a cyborg with your exact thoughts, beliefs, and intentions. If this is too far-fetched, consider brain fission cases. Stroke patients, when they have a stroke to one hemisphere, retain most of their thoughts, beliefs, and intentions. And we know from seizure patients that severing the corpus callosum is not life-threatening. It is conceivable, then, to take one half of your brain and place it in a decerebrate but functional body. There is now another human being that has your exact thoughts, beliefs, and intentions. And yet, you are not identical to (i.e., the same human being as) this other human being.[6] And one very natural way of explaining this intuition is that you still occupy *this* concrete spatiotemporal line of existing and that other human being over there is occupying a different concrete spatiotemporal line of existing.

A substance does not admit of degrees. Either Fido exists or he does not. Of course, Fido can become smarter, more obedient, more mature, i.e., develop from puppy to adult. The qualities or features of Fido admit of degrees, but not Fido himself. After all, we can always ask, what is it whose features are possessed more or less?

Lastly, it is intuitively plausible that infant, toddler, child, juvenile, and adult can refer to one and the same human being. As such these are called 'phase' concepts; whereas human being is a substance concept. The important point to observe about phase concepts is that you survive the transitions from one phase to the next. *You* were an infant and *you* were a toddler, etc. Conversely, you are not now the toddler you once were because you are not now a toddler.

In summary, there are four desiderata that an account of human substances must meet. These include accounting for: (1) our individuality, though we share properties with other persons, (2) a person's substantial unity, we are not heaps or aggregates, even though we each have many parts (Scaltsas, 1994a, 59–96); (3) our identity through change; and (4) our characteristic way of being—we are not eagles or horses. With these desiderata in mind, human persons are (i) particular (ii) entities (iii) that have developmentally indexed causal powers, specifically rational ones, and (iv) they have a certain nature. Characteristic (ii) is meant to highlight that persons are things, not states, properties, or even powers. Characteristic (iii) is meant to indicate that when an entity develops a species-specific power, no new entity comes into existence. To do so would identify the new entity with a power, and this would be a categorical error. Characteristic (iv) is meant to highlight the fact that there is no bare thingness, but that things have characteristic states, properties, and powers. We *have* certain powers, qualities, and features but we are not identical to them. The expression of rationality (however one may define this power) can be evidence for being a person, but you and I cannot be identical to either the power of rationality or its exercise. We are spatio-temporal continuants that endure through changes in our powers, qualities, and features. The argument for these claims depend on two intuitions, one phenomenological and the other conceptual. When I think a thought and then communicate that thought to others, it is one and the same thing that does thinking and the communicating. When I think about running and then run, it is the same thing that thinks and runs. Conceptually, you and I are concrete entities; powers, capacities, and properties are themselves abstract. You and I cannot be identical to a power, but we can *have* a power.

When Do You and I Come into Existence?

Devin Henry (2005) asks us to imagine a paper cup lying on the side of the road. After a few months that cup will have broken down into its constituent parts. It will be, after a while, merely pieces of paper and no longer a cup. But then imagine that these pieces of paper suddenly organize themselves into another paper cup, or even a lampshade. Suppose further that this amazing feat happens with surprising regularity. Paper particles organize themselves into paper cups. Henry's thought experiment is meant to direct our attention to how amazing self-organization is. It is precisely this property of self-organization that is evinced by embryogenesis. Not only are early-stage organisms self-organizing, but they also hit their mark – the embryo seems to "know exactly what it wants to be" (Henry, 2005, 8). So, the embryo organizes itself, not in any direction whatsoever, but in a very controlled and precise endpoint, namely, the mature form of its nature. In explaining how this can be, one must avoid two errors. The first error explains these features with reference to a self-conscious homunculus inside the embryo who directs development. A second error might explain self-organization and developmental success at the expense of maintaining the unity of the entity that develops. The importance of obeying this unity constraint can be seen by considering the development of an embryo's organs including her digestive tract and reproductive organs. By definition, the organism is now a fetus; but it is still the same human being that persists through this change. Developing all my organs did not give rise to another entity. So, any explanation of self-organization and developmental success must explain why it is *one and the same thing* that is doing the developing. If not, one wonders whether an explanation for development has really been offered.

Mechanistic views will account for the development in terms of the biochemical matter causing ever more higher levels of organization, complexity, and powers.[7] But for Aristotle, order at any lower level of material order cannot cause ever higher levels of organization. Jonathan Lear remarks that, "What is needed in addition is form as a basic irreducible force – a developmental power" (Lear, 1988, 39). The substantial form is not merely the mature adult form of an organism, it is certainly not another part such as a homunculus, and it is not reducible to genes as on genetic determinism; but it is that which accounts for why the organism is what it is and develops as it does. Again, Lear is on point,

[I]t is a force in the organism for attaining ever higher levels of organization until the organism achieves its mature form . . . the idea that the order which exists at the level of flesh would be sufficient to generate the order required for human life was as absurd for Aristotle as the idea that the order that exists in a pile of wood would be sufficient for the pile to turn itself into a bed.

(Lear, 1988, 39–40)

In explaining this view, Aristotle often exploits analogies with artifacts and craftsmen. The analogies are apt insofar as they tell us what it is to come into being and in virtue of what. The difference between artifacts and natural objects is that natural objects have their cause internalized. Nature is an inner principle of change and rest, making the thing be what it is. A thing's form is what this nature is. It follows that a natural object has its form from its beginning (Lear, 1988, 17).

If you and I are individual entities with a nature/form, you and I exist when that entity does. Development does not introduce new entities; when you develop arms, legs, fingerprints, and psychological powers, other things do not come into existence. Reaching a developmental milestone does not change the nature of that which reaches it. Mathew Lu recently states the point as follows,

The relevant issue here is that any (putative) potential must belong to a substance with a particular nature. To say that a particular substance has a potential to develop in some way is not to make a prediction about the *future*, but to make a claim about that thing's nature *right now*.

(Lu, 2018)

As a human being develops through the embryonic, fetal, neonatal, etc., phases, *it* develops rational abilities. To say otherwise is arbitrary. One can distinguish among *exercising a capacity well or poorly, actually exercising a capacity, possessing an immediately exercisable capacity* (that awaits a decision to exercise it), *possessing a readily exercisable capacity* (such as once impediments are removed—one wakes up, the fog of alcohol wears off, and so forth), and *possessing a remote capacity* (such as the ability to learn Icelandic after a lot of effort), and *possessing a very remote capacity* (such as the zygote's ability to grow a brain and body that can learn Icelandic). To insist that any of these capacities except the last divides a human substance from a non-human substance is arbitrary.

The plausible intuition is that development does not change the identity of the thing that develops. Why not? The change is internal in the sense that the human being causes its own changes with a view towards survival, growth, and maturation of its prototypical powers. A tree does not develop into a bookshelf; but a sprouted *platanus orientalis* seedling develops into a voluminous mature tree. A Polaroid picture of a jaguar develops from a brown amorphous smudge into a visibly clear representation of the jaguar (Stith, 2014). Blank film does not develop into anything. The second idea is that development into ever more mature stages is indicative of a nature/form actually being present. This is not to suggest backward causation in which a mature human causes the immature human to develop. Rather it is to suppose that purposefulness exists in things, and the truthmaker for why this thing is the way it is and develops the way it does is its formal nature (Pruss, 2013). A mature organism of its kind manifests more species-typical powers than its immature counter-part; but those powers/capacities *express* what kind of organism the thing is, but do not *cause or make* that organism be what it is. Those powers are ontologically dependent upon the substance, not vice versa. Consider the maturity from infant to adult. Significant cognitive and bodily changes take place of one and the same thing. The end towards which x develops, tells us what x is all along. The human being at the embryonic stage is not a potential person but a person who is developing potencies.[8]

Persons are not Human Beings

In this section I consider an alternative view to the substance view. There are numerous alternatives, but the one I pick is a function of its popularity, philosophical persuasiveness, and relevance to healthcare ethics issues. For lack of a better term I will refer to the alternative view as the 'functional brain view.' This view focuses on the fact that you and I have *exercisable* psychological capacities. The idea that I exist, or could exist, without any exercisable capacity for consciousness or rational thought strikes proponents of this view as counterintuitive. One proponent of this view is Jeff McMahan. McMahan focuses on consciousness stating that,

> The corresponding criterion of personal identity is the continued existence and functioning . . . of the same brain to be capable of generating consciousness or mental activity. This criterion stresses the survival of one's basic psychological *capacities*, in particular the *capacity for consciousness*.
>
> (McMahan, 2002, 68)

And elsewhere he says,

> We begin to exist when the fetal brain develops the *capacity for consciousness*, which happens sometime between twenty-two and twenty-eight weeks after conception, when synapses develop among the neurons in the cerebral cortex. Only after the development of the capacity for consciousness is there anyone who can be harmed, or wronged, by being killed.
>
> (McMahan, 2007, 186)

The view entails that persons (functional brains with exercisable psychological capacities) and human beings (living human organisms) are distinct things.

More recently, Campbell and McMahan have clarified their view to avoid the too-many-thinkers problem – discussed below. They emphasize having an exercisable capacity for consciousness as a necessary condition for being a person but capture this condition in terms of a *functional* brain. Functional brains and mere brains are different substances that never overlap or share matter:

> [F]unctional brains and mere brains are never temporally or spatially coincident, but . . . the matter that composes a functional brain comes to compose a mere brain when the functional brain loses the capacity to generate consciousness. On this view, the functional brain is not a mere brain in a functional state. *It is one substance with a certain set of identity conditions that include the retention of the capacity for consciousness*, and the mere brain is a different substance with a different set of identity conditions that do not include the capacity for consciousness.
>
> (Campbell & McMahan, 2010, 290, emphasis added)

The intuitive argument for this view is straightforward. You and I are essentially persons. Persons are those beings who can exercise psychological capacities (which may include self-consciousness or cognition). Human beings do not necessarily exercise psychological capacities, such as human beings at the embryonic or fetal stage or those in a persistent vegetative state. It follows that persons and human beings are different kinds of things since they have different persistence conditions. Therefore, you and I, if we are essentially persons, are not human beings. We may be constituted by human beings (Baker, 2000) or be parts of human beings (McMahan, 2002, 92ff.), but we are not the *same thing* as a human being.

Of course, the key premise is the second claim, i.e., persons must be able to exercise psychological capacities. The chief support for the functional brain view comes from various thought experiments, namely, the brain transplant (BT) examples and the dicephalic twin example.[9]

These examples aim to highlight the intuition that we are not identical to our bodies, but rather to our psychological capacities rooted in a functional brain. The strategy in each example is to envision someone without corporeal properties while leaving one's psychological capacities intact and ask if one still exists. If the answer is 'yes' then our existence is dependent upon having exercisable psychological capacities. Having just those capacities would seem to be essential to who we are. Here is McMahan's rendition of a BT example:

One's entire brain is extracted and transplanted into the body of one's identical twin, who has just suffered brain death and whose brain has been removed. One's brain is appropriately connected to the nerves in one's twin's body, so that after the operation a person is revived in one's twin's body who is fully psychologically continuous with oneself as one was before the operation. Most people believe that one would survive this operation and would continue to exist in what was formerly the body of one's identical twin.

(2002, 20)

Suppose that Jack's brain is transplanted into John's former body. The intuition is that Jack continues to exist because where Jack's thoughts, beliefs, memories, desires, and feelings go, there he goes also. Certainly, if we were to ask the person post-transplant what his name is, his interests are, his beliefs are, etc., he will answer each question exactly as Jack would have before the transplant (Shoemaker, 1963, 23–24). At the very least, McMahan has established that a condition for one person being identical to another person at a later time must include psychological criteria.

Once a largely psychological account of the person is motivated, McMahan moves on to motivate specifically an "embodied mind" account.[10] For McMahan, the specific contents of one's psychology – her beliefs, memories, etc. – are sufficient but not necessary for being a person. Considering cases of deprogramming, whereby a person loses her specific memories and beliefs such as with progressive dementia, suggests that the person is not thereby destroyed. Demented patients are often still aware of their surroundings. In this regard, the embodied mind account

stresses the survival of one's basic psychological *capacities*, in particular the capacity for consciousness. It does not require continuity of any particular *contents* of one's mental life. This allows that one may survive the deprogramming of one's brain and that one continues to exist throughout the progress of Alzheimer's disease, until the disease destroys one's capacity for consciousness.

(McMahan, 2002, 68)

Summarizing the account, McMahan notes that,

There need be only enough physical and functional continuity [of the brain] to preserve certain basic psychological capacities, particularly the capacity for consciousness. This, I believe, is a sufficient basis for egoistic concern; it should, therefore, be a sufficient basis for identity, other things being equal.

(McMahan, 2002, 69)

Functional continuity is defined as "the retention of the brain's basic psychological *capacities*" (2002, 68); and physical continuity requires "either the continued existence of the same constituent matter or the gradual, incremental replacement of the constituent matter over time" (2002, 68).

I find this a very elegant presentation, and it receives some support from our intuitive judgments in response to the BT and deprogramming examples. I do not, however, think we should accept it as an account of what we are.

There is an interpretive issue when assessing McMahan (2002) and Campbell and McMahan (2010). Following the lead of (2010) one might say that, if the functional brain thinks my thoughts and I think my thoughts, it follows that I am a functional brain. Eric Olson (2007) notes that, so long as there are no other candidates for something thinking my thoughts, it would follow from Campbell and McMahan (2010) that I am a functional brain. Olson observes,

> [b]ut isn't it obvious that I think in the strictest sense? Surely it couldn't turn out that it is something other than me that thinks my thoughts . . . It follows that I could not be anything other than my brain. If the true thinkers of our thoughts . . . are brains, then we must conclude . . . that we are brains.
>
> (Olson, 2007, 79)

Whereas in McMahan (2002) it appears that he is more concerned not with the 'what are we?' question but with the persistence question of personal identity. Let me explain.

As observed by Olson (2017), there are different questions when one discusses the metaphysics of persons. There is the 'what are we?' question which asks what is necessary and sufficient for being a person. More specifically, the 'what are we?' question may turn to ask what is *it* (e.g., a property, feature, or fundamental ontological status) that distinguishes persons from non-persons? The answers to the 'what are we?' question may be wholly different from the persistence question. The persistence question asks 'what is it for one person at time t1 to persist through to time t10?' The persistence question presupposes that the relata are already identifiable persons – it asks what it is for one thing to persist *as a person*. Olson further specifies a third question pertaining to what kinds of evidence are relevant for answering one of the questions already noted. For the persistence question, one might ask, "What evidence bears on the question of whether the person here now is the one who was here yesterday?" (Olson, 2017). The evidence question has to be distinguished from the other two. Again Olson explains:

> What it takes for you to persist through time is one thing; how we might find out whether you have is another. If the criminal had

fingerprints just like yours, the courts may conclude that he is you. But even if that is conclusive evidence, having your fingerprints is not *what it is* for a past or future being to be you.

(Olson, 2017)

For example, proponents of the substance view might say that the evidence for identifying whether S is a person will refer to S's DNA and what we know empirically about things that have such and such DNA. Or they will say that having human parents is evidence for being a human being since like produces like. But no proponent of the substance view will say that you and I are DNA codes or, worse, that you and I just are our parents! Having a certain DNA is an empirically informed marker for being a substance with a rational nature as is human patrimony. (Relatedly, critics of the substance view conflate that view's answers to the evidence question and the 'what are we?' question. Thus they often misunderstand the view to involve the claim that you and I just are things with a specific DNA or members of the kind *Homo sapiens*.[11])

The present interpretive issue is that, in using BT examples to motivate McMahan's position, one is led to believe that the key concern is to answer the persistence question. As Olson notes, the "usual question [in personal identity] is when a *person* picked out at one time is identical with a *person* picked out at another time" (1997, 77). And the chief concern for the substance theorist is to answer the 'what are we?' question. As such, there may be *no* disagreement between McMahan and me once we index our reflections to their respective questions. I explain below why I think one should accept as correct McMahan's commentary on the BT examples as illustrating what criteria are sufficient for persisting. I argue that they do not motivate a plausible answer to the 'what are we?' question. (McMahan's claim quoted above (2007) about *when* you and I come into existence presupposes that you and I are essentially minded beings. Whether this can be argued for is addressed below also.) The task for now, then, is circumspection in identifying how that view differs from the substance view on the question of 'what are we?'.

The substance view holds that each of us is identical to a human animal, there is no *other* thing that is a person and to which you and I are identical. If one wants to use the term 'person' to refer to one's psychological properties or powers, and 'human being' to refer to one's corporeal properties or features that is innocuous enough. But just as identifying hydrogen or carbon are abstractions from methane, so too with person and human being. The human substance is one concrete continuant that has both psychological and corporeal aspects.[12] Understood as an answer to the 'what are we?' question, the functional brain view denies this. Human beings and persons are different *things* that may not even share the same biological matter (e.g., your body, brain, cells, tissues).[13]

It is not McMahan's view that you and I are phase sortals. You and I, on his view, are substances whose existence essentially depends on having exercisable psychological capacities. The key claims, then, that separate the functional brain and substance views are the following propositions about persons:

> (Cap): You and I are persons at t *iff* you and I *can* exercise psychological capacities at t.

Proponents of the functional brain view accept (Cap) – for capacity. Proponents of the substance view deny that exercisable psychological capacities are necessary for you and I to exist. What is necessary is that you and I are rational animals, and being a rational animal requires having a nature that disposes one to *have* or *develop* rational capacities. Relevant to this point, Ronald Tacelli and Stephen Schwarz observe a distinction between being a person and functioning as one. One can be a person before one is able to manifest the developed psychological functions of persons. For them, it is the nature that makes you be the thing you are, not the functioning of a developed power. They say that "there is development and the gradual unfolding of a nature – *your nature* – bit by bit in time. But the nature is always actually there, controlling its own development" (Schwarz & Tacelli, 1989, 93). I concur, and we can stipulate this view as follows.

> (Concreta): S is a person at t *iff* S is an individual with a rational nature at t.

Given my comments above on nature (or substantial form), what makes us be the kind of entity we essentially are is that the matter composing our respective bodies is informed by the same kind of substantial form which, among other things, endows us with the potency for rational thought.[14] So the distinction between the two views is whether it is enough for you and I to exist that we are individuals with a rational *nature*, or must we be able to *exercise* rational *capacities*.

Critique of the Functional Brain View

Following Snowdon (2014), there are three arguments against the view that you and I exist only when an exercisable capacity for consciousness exists. I discuss here the first two as they form a coherent unit. Snowdon gives us two *reductio ad absurdum* arguments, the target assumption is that a person P is not identical to a human being H. On the functional brain view, you and I are persons, but 'human being' refers to one's body. The first step in Snowdon's argument is to suppose that P has both psychological (P is conscious) and physical features (P has a body). It also seems plausible enough to suppose that H has physical features. But does H also have psychological features? Snowdon answers as follows,

[I]t seems that H can see its environment, can reason, remember, talk, and think of itself. This all seems true because it is, quite simply, *obvious*, and also a necessary part of our explanation of the successful interaction of the animal H and its environment.

(Snowdon, 2014, 93)

Continuing with this line of thought, it also seems obvious that human beings talk, communicate, walk, and run. Human beings can see, feel pain, hear, and smell. A human being has the same brain and neurological system as the person appears to have. A human being's successful and adaptive behavior in her environment is explained best by her being able to perceive, think, desire, and intend. These are all psychological abilities. Olson states the point as follows.

The psychological-continuity view implies that that animal is not identical with you. Yet the animal would appear to be rational and intelligent. At any rate it has a normally functioning adult nervous system. It is physically indistinguishable from you. It has the same surroundings and history. What more does it take for a thing to be able to think? What could prevent the animal from thinking?

(Olson, 2002, 190)

The punchline is this: the psychological abilities and states of H seem to be the exact same abilities and states of P. "It appears to follow that if ~(P = H) then there are two [different] things which are leading the same psychological lives located at a certain place, and *that* seems absurd" (Snowdon, 2014, 93). Likewise, Olson concludes that "there would appear to be *two* rational, thinking beings within your skin: a person with psychological identity conditions, and an animal with non-psychological identity conditions" (Olson, 2002, 190). The functional brain view, therefore, entails an absurdity. If two things share the same physical and psychological features, we would expect them to be the same thing not two different things.

Snowdon's second *reductio* argument grants for the moment that on this view persons are identified with certain psychological capacities or states. If what makes the difference between S coming into being and not being is having a capacity for consciousness (McMahan, 2007, 186), S is a brain with an exercisable capacity for consciousness. But human beings have certain psychological capacities and states too since they have the same functional brain as the person does. So, human beings with psychological capacities are candidates for being persons as well. But if the person is not identified with a human being, then there must be two persons where we thought there should only be one. And this is absurd for several reasons mentioned by Snowdon. I'll mention one he does not address. The consequence that there are two persons suggests that 'person' is multiply realizable. Recall, however, that there cannot be two Fidos or two Rovers. You and I are concrete individuals. An *individual* entity cannot be *two* at the same time and in the same respect. The substance view does not face the too-many-thinkers problem because it does not reify one's exercisable psychological capacities into a separate thing.

Snowdon's *reductio* arguments serve as defenses of a key premise (premise 3 below) in a broader argument for the identity of you and me to human beings *at every stage in which we exist*. The emphasis here is meant to argue that you and I come into existence before the onset of exercisable psychological capacities. I call this the Unity Argument, and it follows closely Olson's argument (1997 and 2002).

If the functional brain view is correct, human being and person are two different things, specifically, if you and I are essentially persons, you and I come into existence sometime after conception when our brains become functional enough to generate conscious states. We can ask what happens to the organism at the fetal stage when it experiences the onset of consciousness? There are only two options: either it dies or it lives. It does not die for three reasons. There is no corpse,[15] organisms do not die because they *gain* abilities as a result of their natural developmental processes,[16] and our intuitions on pre-conscious harms.[17] It must, therefore, live. But if 'human being' and 'person' are distinct entities, the person at the onset of consciousness exists, *and* the human being continues to exist. There are now two things in the same space at the same time. It is precisely here that Snowdon's *reductio* arguments rebut the plausibility of this suggestion. The brain view must suppose that the person is a different part, such as the functional brain, and the human being is the rest of the body. But Snowdon's arguments show that this is absurd since the human being has every right to say that it has a functional brain, and the person has every right to say that it has a body. Here is the argument in detailed outline:

1   If the human being at the fetal stage (hereafter fetus)[18] ≠ me, then I came into existence sometime after conception.
2   If I came into existence after conception then either the fetus dies or continues to live.
3   Neither is it the case that the fetus dies nor does it continue to live. (The defense of this premise is made explicit below.)
4   Therefore, it is not the case that I came into existence after conception. (From 2 and 3, MT.)
5   Therefore, it is not the case that the human being at the fetal stage is not identical to me. (From 1 and 4, MT.)
6   Therefore, I am identical to the human being that existed at the fetal stage. (Negation rule applied to 5.)

Defense of premise 3:

(3a) If the human being at the fetal stage **died,** then it died because 'it' *gained* an ability to think, and this ability is the working out of the fetus's *self-directed development,* and there is *no corpse.*

(3b) It is not the case that things die when they gain an ability and this ability is the working out of its developmental program, and there is no corpse.

(3c) Therefore, the fetus did not die. (From 3a and 3b.)

(3d) If the human being at the fetal stage continues to **live** (and he/ she is **not** the same thing as me), then there are two different things with the same physical (*this* body) and psychological features (*this* thought/intention).

(3e) It is absurd to think that two *different* things can have the same psychological and physical features. (Snowdon's arguments canvassed above.)

(3f) It is not the case that the fetus continues to live. (From 3d and 3e, MT.)

(3g) Therefore, it is not the case that the human being continues to live and it is not the case that it dies. (From 3c and 3f, Conj.)

Premise 3: Neither the fetus lives nor does it die. (From 3g, DM.)[19]

Premise 1 is an assumption given the functional brain view. Premise 2 is an exclusive disjunction given premise 1. Premise 3 is the key premise and is defended in the arguments running from 3a–3g. Premises (3d) and (3e) are the only premises open to dispute – important objections to premise 3b are addressed in previous footnotes. Premise (3e) is defended above via Snowdon's *reductio* arguments. Premise (3d) is committed to the idea that if the existence and persistence conditions of two things A and B differ, A and B must be different things.[20] On the view that I come into existence after my human being does, human being and person have different persistence conditions and are, therefore, two different things on such a view. An important assumption supporting (3d), however, is the idea that the human being shares the same psychological properties because the human being also has a functional brain. This entitles it to have psychological properties on the assumption that material organic things with a certain type of neurological configuration can think.

McMahan thinks that his account does not entail that there are two thinkers when there should only be one. We should understand the relation between ourselves and our organisms as a relation of part to whole, not a constitution relation. McMahan gives several examples to illustrate.

When a limb on a tree grows, the whole tree is said to grow. The limb (the part) grows, and (the whole) tree gets bigger in virtue of the limbs growing. It is not absurd to say that there are two things that are growing, the limb and the tree. The tree is not constituted by the branch (cut the branch and the tree still exists), but the branch is certainly *part* of the tree. Likewise, the horn in my car makes a noise, but the car makes a noise in virtue of the horn making a noise. "In the same sense in which the tree grows because its limb does, and in which the car honks because its horn does, my organism may be said to think, feel, and perceive because I do" (McMahan, 2002, 92). And he states that these "analogies help elucidate the sense in which there are two conscious entities present where I am. My organism is conscious . . . only by virtue of having a conscious part" (McMahan, 2002, 93).

It is important to understand the desiderata McMahan needs to meet in responding to the Unity Argument. He needs to tell a plausible story in which all the following commitments make sense: I and my organism are not the same kind of thing; there are not two thinkers where there should only be one; and radical dualism is untenable. (Radical dualism would hold that the organism has *no* psychological properties and he rejects this position.) McMahan wants to hold that my organism has psychological properties but only in virtue of having me as a part of it.

The following dilemma will show that McMahan fails to avoid the absurdities that the Unity Argument highlights. The cornerstone of McMahan's response is that there exists a relation between me and my organism and that the psychological properties of my organism are had *in virtue of* me.

The 'in virtue of' relation can be understood in two different ways. Consider the following two propositions:

(Causal):   the airplane moves *in virtue of* the engines.
(Mereological):   the engines fly *in virtue of* being a part of the airplane.

On the causal understanding, the airplane moves in virtue of the engines; i.e., the engines cause the airplane to move. On the mereological understanding, the engines fly only because they are attached to the airplane. Without the empennage and wings, the engines cannot go airborne. Applied to persons and their organisms we can say the following. On a causal understanding of the 'in virtue of' relation, my organism is caused to think by me every time I think. This suggests that my organism has psychological states and properties every time I think – thus avoiding radical dualism. It is agreed, however, that my organism is not the same thing as me on the embodied mind account. Since I have psychological states and properties, it follows that there are two different things that have the same psychological states and properties. When I cause my organism to think, it thinks. But what does it think? Presumably, it thinks the very same things I do. But if my organism and I are two different things, McMahan must still grant 3d.

Suppose that the 'in virtue of' relation is understood as mereological. My organism thinks only because I (the thinker) am a part of the organism. Does my organism have any psychological properties if we imagine it without the thinking part? Either it does or it does not. If it does, then what psychological properties does it have and why be so sure that it cannot be a person? If it does have psychological properties, where are the corresponding psychological powers? Armstrong observes that all properties bestow a power (active or passive). He says "it is only in so far as properties bestow powers that they can be detected by the sensory apparatus or other mental faculty" (1980, 45). Now we can ask whether the organism has the property of being a thinker. If it does then it would have the power to think. On the supposition that organism O and person P are different things, there would be two thinkers. Hence, the too-many-thinkers problem remains.

If it does not have psychological properties, i.e., being a thinker, then it would not have the power to think. On this latter supposition the organism would not have any psychological states, properties, or powers, and this is to court radical dualism of which McMahan rightly rejects. What generates the problem for the mereological interpretation is that being a thinker or being conscious is something a thing either possesses or it does not.

So, if the 'in virtue of' relation is understood as causal, McMahan is still committed to a key premise in the Unity Argument. If the 'in virtue of' relation is understood as mereological, he is implicitly committed to radical dualism, which he explicitly rejects. Either way McMahan in (2002) fails to meet the required desiderata.

As noted above, Campbell and McMahan (2010) have clarified their view to address directly the too-many-thinkers problem. They deny that you and I are *at all* spatially coincident with our respective organisms. You and I are identical to *functional* brains according to which "when the brain irreversibly loses the capacity to generate consciousness, we cease to exist" (2010, 289). The functional brain, on their view, is "one substance with a certain set of identity conditions that include the retention of the capacity for consciousness, and the mere brain is a different substance with a different set of identity conditions" (2010, 290). So, if our functional brains lose the capacity for consciousness, we go out of existence. This offers a response to the too-many-thinkers problem because that problem is generated only on the supposition that there *can* be thinking animals. Campbell and McMahan's revised view denies this.

What might be the initial problem with this view? A functional brain is a mature brain that has developed the requisite synapses, the proper functioning of which can generate consciousness. It should be pointed out here that although we know what neurological architecture is sufficient for generating consciousness, we cannot say what is necessary except that some level of neurological organization is required (Howsepian, 2011). Let's suppose, then, that an immature brain is one that is not able to generate consciousness because it has not developed the requisite organization – whenever that might be. On the functional brain view, the mature brain (Bm) is not identical to the immature brain (Bim).

For the functional brain view, Bm ≠ Bim because Bm is capable of consciousness and that functionality defines it as a different substance with distinct identity conditions from the mere brain. Campbell and McMahan must suppose that Bm and Bim are necessarily different because they are different things – just as chromium can never become gold. So, we should understand this claim symbolized as follows, P: □ (Bm ≠ Bim). To falsify P all one needs to show is that it is possible that Bm is identical to Bim: ◊ Bm = Bim. It appears easy enough to do so. If it is possible that the development of an entity does not change the identity of that entity, then P is falsified. Since it is possible that development of an entity does not change its identity, namely, development does not change the *what* that it is (Stith, 2014), then P is falsified. I should note that the BT experiments described above do not justify holding that it is *necessarily* the case that Bm is not identical to Bim. The intuition is that *once Jack's brain matures*, his capacities, thoughts, beliefs, etc., serve as reliable evidence for tracking Jack through time and change. Nothing follows about whether or not Jack could have preexisted the actualization of consciousness.

The Unity Argument aims to show that there are good reasons against dissociating human beings and persons. In what follows I argue that there are no persuasive reasons *for* the dissociation. In this regard I return to the BT experiments and address the lessons learned from them. My aim is modest in what follows, which is to show that the balance of plausibility is on the side of the substance view, enough to set the presumptions noted later on abortion and embryo-destructive research.

Critique of the BT Experiments

The intuition that Jack survives is wholly dependent upon there being a continuity of Jack's thoughts, beliefs, and intentions. McMahan rightly notes that we should resist thinking that Jack is *identical* to a set of thoughts, beliefs, and intentions for we can easily imagine that Jack exists, believes, or thinks something different from what he does. We might appeal to Jack's beliefs as evidence that the person he is persisted through the brain transplant operation. So far, we learn that BT examples motivate what counts as sufficient conditions for one person at t1 being identical to another person at t2. McMahan is sensitive to this train of thought, which is why he exploits the deprogramming example. What is necessary for being the same person is the persistence of one's functional brain which must include an exercisable capacity for consciousness.

But which one of the thought experiments motivates the intuition that the persistence of exercisable psychological capacities is *necessary* for being a person? Neither the brain transplant example nor the deprogramming example invite us to have the intuition that having *exercisable* psychological capacities is an essential feature of being a person. If Jack were to suffer deprogramming of the specific contents of his mental life but retain a capacity for consciousness, we would say that Jack still exists. But this too seems only to support a sufficiency condition – if Jack retains his exercisable capacity for consciousness he still exists. We might have the intuition that Jack ceases to exist if he permanently loses this capacity – for example, if Jack suffers whole-brain death. But there is no disagreement between psychological accounts and the substance theorist on *that* claim.

Maybe the thought experiments are not meant to motivate necessary conditions at all; rather, reflection on the meaning of terms does that. Mary Anne Warren (1973) suggests this when she says that "I consider this claim [that persons must have consciousness and a developed capacity to reason] to be so obvious that I think anyone who denied it . . . *would thereby demonstrate that he had no notion at all of what a person is*" (Warren, 1973, 56, emphasis added). The intended use of BT examples may not be to motivate necessary conditions for being a person. The real reason why psychological criteria are necessary for being a person is because of one's own intuitions on what 'person' means. For the purposes of my overall argument in this book, it is enough to observe that such basic intuitions on what counts as a person are rebutted by the intuitions highlighted in the too-many-thinkers problem. There is no privileged status that one's semantic intuitions should hold *after* exploring the conceptual consequences of those intuitions.

The chief lesson I wish to convey, however, is that the intuitions the BT examples generate are innocuous. We already know prior to the BT examples that the developed human brain supports consciousness. That Jack survives due to a continuity of his psychological powers is an interesting observation but fails to motivate a specific view of personal identity. Most views on personal identity will grant that continuity of one's psychological powers is a sufficient condition for personal identity. When Sydney Shoemaker first proposed the BT example, he observed that the intuitions it generates are consistent with materialist conceptions of persons. The behaviorist could accept the transplant intuition and yet maintain "that all the properties of persons can be regarded as physical properties (behavioral dispositions and so forth) and that there is therefore an important sense in which persons are material objects" (Shoemaker, 1963, 26). And we may suppose that the intuitions we learn from the BT examples are consistent with a Cartesian dualism. The only conclusion that follows is that psychological continuity is a sufficient condition for remaining the same person. Nothing in the BT examples, however, entail that human beings *just are* functional human brains.

BT Examples as Arguments against the Substance View

I have argued that the BT examples do not motivate the functional brain view on personal identity. But maybe the BT examples are not arguments for this view but rather arguments against other views, like the substance view. If the intuitions the BT examples invite us to have cannot be accommodated by the substance view, then the functional brain view wins by default. So, can the substance view accommodate the intuitions that the BT examples invite us to have?[21]

For the substance view, an entity has a nature, i.e., a substantial form that makes that entity be the kind of thing it is with the proto-typical powers of that kind. When we transplant Jack's brain into John's (former) body, we only know it is Jack that wakes up after the transplant because he can tell us what Jack thought, believed, and intended prior to the transplant. The intuition that Jack still exists is readily explained by the persistence of his psychological powers. Such persistence is sufficient for personal identity on the substance view. The brainless body left behind differs from the human embryo in that the former cannot develop psychological capacities, but the latter regularly does.

A proponent of the substance view can concur with all these observations in so far as there is a continuity of Jack's psychological powers and these are sufficient for personhood. The only twist is that on the substance view, powers do not exist without a concrete substance that realizes these powers. What is important for the substance view is that those powers themselves, in this entity, need explaining. The reason this entity has such capacities in the first place is that it has a rational nature. The nature of a substance *S* explains why *S* is the way it is, develops the way it does, and has the capacities it does. As Lear remarks, "'The why' is an objective feature of the world; it is that about which we *ought* to be curious if we wish to understand a thing" (Lear, 1988, 26). In the BT experiments, the concrete substance is Jack, not a psychological power. And we know it to be Jack because he shares his thoughts – i.e., the evidence question. The conclusion that Jack's existence requires an exercisable capacity for consciousness rooted in a functional brain simply does not follow. Jack is not a functional brain, he is an entity with a functional brain.

At the very least, the intuitions we have in response to the BT examples are not *exclusive* motivations for the functional brain view. The substance view would agree that it is in fact Jack who wakes up post-transplant, *and it would explain that intuition simply by noting that there is a continuity of Jack's powers characteristic of a developed human being.*[22]

The difference between substance and functional brain accounts of the person should not be understood as the former emphasizing bodily continuity and the latter emphasizing psychological continuity. Both accounts recognize that to be a human person, rationality is essential. The difference is that for the substance view, why S is the way S is, and develops the way she develops, is metaphysically fundamental. S's formal nature is the principle of change and development, and makes S be the kind of thing S is, i.e., a rational entity. The explanatory arrow moves from the thing's nature to the capacities it develops and has. The functional brain view privileges the actual exercise of psychological powers; the substance view privileges the entity that has those powers.

What is the ontological status of the decerebrate body once the brain has been removed? On the substance view, it no longer exists as a human being. It undergoes a substantial change in virtue of permanently losing those powers prototypical of human beings. Does this concession entail that the substance view is a functional brain view after all? The answer is no. Whereas you and I are not capacities, you and I may go out of existence if we permanently lose certain capacities.[23] What you and I are on the one hand, and what functional potencies the loss of which serve as evidence for death on the other, are two different ontological categories for the substance view. If I permanently lack a heart rate, one may infer that I am dead; but I am not identical to a heart rate.

The differences between the substance and the functional brain views become more apparent when we consider issues at the beginning of life. The substance view is compatible with the functional brain view that Jack is John, and that the reason for thinking so is because there is a continuity of his psychological capacities. But sharing these convictions does not entail that persons do not come into existence *until* they can exercise rational activity. For the substance theorist, development does not introduce other distinct entities as its species-specific powers become exercisable, nor does it destroy the immediately preceding entity. It is even plausible to suppose that for any thought experiment which exploits our intuitions on *adult* persons, the substance theorist can agree with the functional brain view and psychological accounts more generally on almost every detail and with the explanations for our intuitions (i.e., where the rational capacities go, there the person goes also). But the substance theorist can admit all of this while rejecting the idea that the development of an entity involves the coming-to-be of another distinct entity.

Regarding the overall argument in this book, the principal problem with the BT and dicephalic twin thought experiments is that they underdetermine the positions on practical matters (e.g., abortion) that many proponents of the functional brain view think are permissible. A popular argument for the permissibility of abortion is to argue that unborn human beings are not persons. The notion of 'person' is a psychological one according to which a person is identified with having a set of psychological capacities: i.e., self-consciousness. As we have seen, this position is motivated by these thought experiments. Neither experiment, however, provides *exclusive* motivation for a psychological account; the functional brain and substance views are on epistemic par vis-à-vis these experiments. The lessons learned from such experiments are compatible with alternative accounts of the person: accounts which do not entail that unborn human beings are not persons. Consequently, the functional brain view is underdetermined vis-à-vis its use as a justification for permissible killing (Napier, 2015). (By underdetermined I mean that there is a view that is on par with its motivations that does not provide a justification for killing.) This argument assumes that all human beings, however nascent, should not be intentionally killed. To this premise we turn.

Notes

1 There may be non-living primary substances, e.g., Zeus. The emphasis throughout is on living ones since my concern is *bio*-ethical.
2 Two clarifications. First, the example of being alive stretches the notion of property beyond what I think is plausible, but my skepticism does not affect the main point in this chapter. Second, if post-mortem survival is possible, this claim might need more parsing such as understanding '*you* being alive' post-mortem as requiring a bodily resurrection (see Eberl, 2009).
3 This example and several others mentioned here come from Scaltsas, 1994a.
4 The notion of form is synonymous with a thing's nature. A thing's nature makes an entity be the kind of thing it is with its characteristic powers (for humans, rationality), developmental pattern (embryo–fetus–infant–, etc.), and morphological features (heart, lungs, bipedal, etc.). So, by form I do not mean merely shape or figure.
5 See Plantinga (2007 and 2006). I am inclined to think that something like belief transfer is either irrelevant or impossible. It is true that you and I can have the same belief in terms of its propositional content. Both of us can believe that 'it is raining outside.' But it is unintelligible how *you* can have *my* belief that it is raining outside. If what gets duplicated is simply the content, we did not need a thought experiment to tell us that. If what gets duplicated is *my* belief, we are asked to imagine the incoherent.
6 Throughout this chapter, I understand X is identical to Y as X is the *same thing* as Y. I should also note that I am assuming Wiggins's defense of absolute identity (2001, chs 1 and 6).
7 For why Aristotle's teleological views are compatible with modern biology, see Austriaco (2004).
8 See Napier (2015, 670 ff.) for a reply to McMahan's dilemma (2002, 11 ff.) for substance accounts of the person. See Henry (2008) and Bertalanffy (1952) for why the account I describe here is neither preformationist nor epiphenomenalist. See Tollefsen (2011) for further commentary. See Burke (1996) for why the potential for development as understood here is not subject to counterexample from parthenogenesis.
9 For my analysis of the dicephalic twin example see Napier (2015, 666ff.) and my website for supplementary materials on this book.
10 "Embodied mind" is McMahan's term, but his view is a species of psychological accounts in so far as McMahan makes having an exercisable psychological capacity an essential feature of being a person.

11 Examples include Warren (1973, 53) and Boonin (2002, 23ff); though, to Boonin's credit, he surveys other more faithful understandings.

12 It may be the case that the notion of person has greater extension than the notion of human being. That is, it may be the case that there are alien life forms or rational parrots that manifest rational capacities (which is sufficient evidence for believing that they are persons) but they do not have the same morphological features or developmental trajectory as human beings (and therefore are not human substances). Likewise, McMahan's Superchimp (2002, 147) receives a genetic enhancement after birth which enables it to develop rational capacities parallel to the trajectory of normal human infants. His handling of this case invites further clarifications made below about distinguishing the 'what is it?' question from the evidence question.

13 I say "may not" to respect the diversity within psychological accounts of the person (i.e., Baker, 2000).

14 For further defense of these claims see Garcia (2008) and Oderberg (2008a).

15 The relevance of there not being any corpse is that we are concrete embodied entities. Because the dilemma involves whether the *organism* at the fetal stage dies or lives, the relata are both organisms. When organisms die, they typically leave behind corpses or at least we can discern an absence of functionality. Neither is the case for the organism post consciousness. It is irrelevant to point out potential counterexamples of the following sort: if persons are identified with psychological capacities, and the brain loses its capacity to support psychological capacities the person would die without leaving behind a corpse. What is the error? The issue is not whether a person understood psychologically would leave behind a corpse – of course it would not. The relata of the dilemma are organisms, so changing the kind of relata changes whether there being any corpse is relevant. Closer in relevance is nuclear annihilation of an organism. But this is not a counterexample either because annihilation is something *more than* mere death.

16 Tooley's kitten (1972, 60ff.), which receives a serum that causes it to develop rational capacities, seems to cease being a cat when it gains those rational capacities. This is not a counterexample since injecting a serum is not a natural developmental process. Another potential counterexample might be the extraction of a totipotent cell from the 4-cell embryo. Suppose the cell begins development qua human organism. Here it appears that the cell dies because 'it' acquires an ability to function as a multicellular organism. I think that it is correct to say that the totipotent cell ceases to exist when an organism begins to exist. But the counterexample is not available to the embodied mind account of persons which grants that persons are parts of bodies – i.e., the organism continues to exist. To other theorists (possibly Lowe, 1991), I would say this: the gaining of an ability is not evidence that that thing which gained the ability has *died*. Granting that the person can come into being when an ability becomes actualized does not entail that the body the person now inhabits dies. Put another way, there is no reason to suppose that the evidence set for persons coming into being is identical to the evidence set for thinking that the pre-conscious organism dies.

17 Suppose a pregnant woman abuses drugs and as a result the child that is born suffers serious cognitive defects. If the organism dies, then how can the harms caused by the illicit drug use persist? Presumably, the deleterious effects of the drug use affected the organism prior to consciousness. So if it died, there are no grounds we have for saying that the child was harmed by the mother's drug use. But clearly he was.

18 Locutions such as 'the fetus' can be confusing. Properly speaking, the fetus refers to *the human being* at the fetal *stage* of development. It is a phase

concept much like infant, toddler, juvenile, etc. So, every occurrence of 'fetus' should be understood as '*human being* at the fetal stage.' It would be too cumbersome and with no gain in clarity to state the latter for every occurrence of the former. On this same point, the symbol = should be interpreted per Wiggins (2001) as 'the same substance as' and ≠ as 'not the same.'

19 DeGrazia (2005) and Boonin (2002) would agree with me to this point. They hold that you and I come into existence either at conception or shortly thereafter, but we do not have a right to life at every point in our existence. Our moral views differ as will become apparent in Chapters 6 and 7.

20 I do not discuss Baker's constitution views (2000 and 2005). This is a decision based strictly on space. See my website for supplementary material.

21 In what follows, I am indebted to Hershenov (2011, 469ff and 2008a, 491ff.).

22 In anticipation of our discussion on abortion, I should also observe that the BT examples do not motivate a view that you and I come into existence only *when* we develop exercisable psychological capacities. That Jack survives the transplant *after* he has developed psychological powers (in virtue of a continuity of such powers) does not entail that he does not exist *prior* to the development of those powers. If, for example, the nature of an entity is not identical to the exercisable capacities it has but to the thing that develops and has those capacities, BT examples tell us nothing about when you and I *begin* to exist. I suppose that in order to motivate 'beginning' intuitions, one might consider brain transplants at the fetal stage of existence. I doubt the plausibility of such a project. Consider abortion survivors who were severely injured by the attempted abortion. They survive, but with lifelong disabilities and injuries. The intuition is that such abortion survivors were harmed by the abortion. But if they were harmed *by* the abortion, they must have existed when the abortion was attempted. Genetic manipulation of a gamete is not a counterexample to this if we keep straight the kinds of harms suffered. I can be harmed by congenital malformations to my father's sperm prior to my existence. But I cannot suffer battery prior to existing.

23 PVS patients are not dead on my account for several reasons, one of which is the possibility of covert consciousness (see Owen, 2013, and Monti et al., 2010). So, even on psychological accounts, one cannot be sure that they do not exist as persons.

5 Human Dignity

The reflections so far support the view that you and I are essentially human beings. We develop certain capacities in accordance with the developmental plan prototypical of our species – but *we* are doing the developing. One might say correctly that we have the potency for consciousness as soon as we come into existence, since we are at that point the kind of thing that self-develops to the point at which that power is exercisable. Though we are not identical to our capacities, it is correct to say that we *have* such capacities. You and I no more come into existence when we developed the capacity for consciousness than an eagle comes into existence when it flies away from its nest for the first time. The key question confronting us now is whether you and I have dignity or inherent worth whenever you and I exist? Can you and I gain or lose *inherent* worth?

There are at least two difficulties facing any commentator on the notion of human dignity. The first is that it is questionable whether human dignity picks out a *single property* or feature that *makes* humans worthy. Pre-theoretical intuitions indicate that there are any number of things, properties, or features that are valuable about the human person. This suggests that human dignity might be a covering concept that functions like the notion of justification in epistemology. In epistemology, what counts as a justified belief varies widely. Some say that a justified belief requires having been produced by reliable cognitive faculties, by properly functioning faculties, or by acts of intellectual virtue, or that it must have adequate grounds, etc. Each of these properties of a belief (e.g., adequate grounds, produced by a reliable faculty, etc.) picks out a valuable property or feature of what we want in our beliefs. They are as Alston (2005) notes, epistemic desiderata. But rather than thinking that justification is reducible to any *one* property or feature, justification should be viewed as an umbrella concept which includes any number of epistemic desiderata the realization of which helps us attain truth. It is implausible to suppose, for example, that a justified belief must have adequate grounds and any other property (such as being reliably formed) is completely irrelevant.

A similar line of thought applies to dignity. Those commenting on dignity – broadly construed – have widely divergent views on what marks or 'grounds' human worth (Sulmasy, 2008; Dworkin, 2013; Lee & George, 2008; McMahan, 2002) and a similar diversity regarding what moral injunctions follow from such worth (Rosen, 2018, 100ff.). What each proposal identifies is one aspect of human worth, like looking at a majestic mountain from different sides and altitudes. Human worth is spherical, if you will, and any inquiry into its nature and scope requires orbiting it and appreciating the different aspects of it. It is not false that human beings are rendered worthy in virtue of having interests, but that is not the only aspect of our worth. Instead of thinking that our worth is grounded in any one property or feature, we should see it as an umbrella concept that covers several aspects of our value. In what follows I wish to take the reader around the mountain and orbit the human person to piece together a more comprehensive view of our worth. In so doing, my treatment emerges as much more ecumenical than accounts that focus on any one property or feature because my treatment does not deny that those features are valuable. The present account pays attention to our irreplaceable value and preciousness – explained below. So, whereas human *worth* functions as an umbrella concept; for my purposes here *dignity* refers to our irreplaceable value and preciousness. My focus distinguishes my project from related discourses on well-being, welfare, and happiness (see pages 101–103 below).

A second difficulty in thinking about dignity specifically is how to frame the inquiry from the start. Typically the metaphor of 'grounding' is used to frame the discussion. What *grounds* human dignity?[1] What *makes* a person have human dignity? In virtue of what does a person have dignity? The terms 'grounds,' 'makes,' and 'in virtue of what?' invite the idea that the worth of a person is based on something *else* that makes the person worthy. As such, the metaphor of grounding, etc., invites answers that attempt to pick out a property or feature of the human person. If one assumes such a starting point, a human person may not have the 'right' property or feature. As such the very way in which the question is asked presupposes that it is possible for a person to lose or gain dignity specifically and moral worth generally. The metaphors of grounding or making, then, assume controversial answers to important questions right from the start; and they necessarily constrain the answers we can offer to the question.

Change the metaphor and one changes the trajectory of inquiry. This can be seen more clearly on the issue of organ donation. Consider the following way in which we can understand the ethics of organ donation: how can we increase the supply of organs without violating a stakeholder's *rights*? By focusing on rights, answers to the question are already constrained and the inquiry focuses on what rights there are. We can increase the supply by any means that do not violate a stakeholder's rights.

This may include any number of options from selling one's organs to routine salvaging post-mortem (Delaney & Hershenov, 2009). Notice how differently one thinks about the issue if we ask the question the following way: how can we *love* our *community* better? When the notions of love, the common good, and gift are central features of the ethical frame, a different set of answers are brought into relief.

In what follows, I avoid asking the question about what grounds human dignity since that invites answers in the form of properties or features, which the person may gain or lose.[2] The question already presupposes that dignity is an accidental feature of you and me, and not inherent in the fact that we are. By asking the question that way one presupposes that a human being could exist without having dignity, an incredible assumption to make at the start of one's inquiry.[3] Furthermore, the end result of such an inquiry cannot but place dignity in the wrong place, namely in the properties or functions of the person but not in the person. Following Brewer (2009) and Gaita (2004) I avoid phrasing a starting question at all and instead focus on narratives and certain emotive states as a way to shine a light onto the preciousness and irreplaceability of the human person. In this way, the metaphor of orbiting the person is more apt to describe my procedure.

Two Tasks and a Note on Method

Suppose I believe that it is wrong to do x on a human being in circumstance C. Suppose I explain my moral intuition by grounding it in the notion of intrinsic dignity. For example, the reason why it might be wrong to rape a patient in a persistent vegetative state (PVS) is because human beings have inherent worth that does not go away simply because she or he is unconscious. My interlocutor has a choice on whether to agree with my intuition and explanation, or to disagree with either one or both. For the latter disjunct, she could reject the notion of intrinsic dignity and hold that it is permissible to rape PVS patients if they are in fact *permanently* unconscious. She could agree that it seems impermissible, but our intuitions on such a case are subject to an error theory.[4] As such, our intuition that the action is immoral does not support the idea that the patient really has intrinsic dignity. Third, she could explain our intuition that it is wrong with reference to the rape being a violation of the patient's ideal interests. Finally,[5] she could say that it is a case of harmless wrongdoing much like it would be wrong to disrespect a dead person's body – no *one* is harmed, but it is a wrong action nonetheless. All explanations except the first are consistent with the intuition that it is wrong to rape a PVS patient but explaining why does not necessarily involve invoking intrinsic dignity.[6] If this were our dialectical situation, adjudicating our disagreement would be onerous indeed, but this hardly entails that dignity is not in truth the best explanation (see Diamond, 1982).

One subtext of my argument in this chapter is to suggest that the dialectical situation is not as intractable as I have just described. The primary tasks in this chapter are to motivate through narratives and certain emotive states (e.g., grief, remorse, etc.) the presence of dignity in every human being. The second task is to argue that those accounts of human worth that focus on having certain exercisable abilities or interests do not rebut or challenge the account of dignity that I offer in this chapter. They only function as rebuttals or challenges if they claim that human worth is *only* a function of having certain exercisable abilities or interests. The arguments for this 'only' clause are, however, insufficient and recapitulate the problems of a monistic account of justification. As such the presence of intrinsic dignity in every human being is a much more ecumenical position than has previously been recognized.

The method used to get to this conclusion is through narrative and reflection on certain emotive states. A satisfactory defense of why such a method will deliver the promised epistemic goods I leave to Stump (2010, chs 2 and 3), Nussbaum (1990, chs 2 and 5), and the discussion on acquaintance knowledge in Roberts and Wood (2008, 50ff.) and Baldwin (2003). Presently, I follow Gaita's work (2004) because it incorporates these methods in his account of human dignity (i.e., preciousness and irreplaceability). Gaita illustrates this method nicely quoting from Simone Weil, "if I light an electric torch at night out-of-doors I don't judge its power by looking at the bulb, but by seeing how many objects it lights up" (2004, xxx). His point is that saintly love, his term, performs this function of lighting up the inherent worth of those around us. This is clearly not a method by which one picks out properties or features, but it is meant to attune one's own moral perception to the person. Another way to understand the difference in methods is that the typical approach focuses on propositions about value, but the focus revolves around propositions, not persons. What narratives and emotive states offer is to shine a light on the human person in order to see our preciousness and irreplaceability *in vivo*, so to speak.

But there is another advantage to providing narratives as a means of contact with the values to which those narratives point. As pointed out in Chapter 2, we are not detached observers who reflect without any potential brumous influences on our ability to see value. We judge something as good or bad because we resonate with it or we have lived our lives in light of such values. But the faculty by which we assess value may need sharpening. Narratives and reflecting on emotive states can function as acuminating our perception of moral value (see Little, 1995).

Dignity: Three Aspects

Whatever has dignity has at least three aspects to its worth. First, things with dignity have *inherent* worth, which means that a thing has this worth whether the thing believes it or not. Assuming human beings have dignity, human beings have a worth that does not go away when we become sick, disabled, or even unconscious. It does not go away in the grips of suicidality. Remy Debes observes that "Human dignity, if it exists, and whatever else it may be, isn't something that must be earned or bequeathed" (Debes, 2009, 47). Similarly, Gómez-Lobo and Keown (2015) entertain an analogy between eyesight, intelligence, and one's life. Eyesight is inherently good even if I come to see horrible things, intelligence is inherently good even if I come to believe falsehoods, and I am inherently good even if I come to experience bad things. Thus, a person's inherent worth is not affected by the quality of the person's life experiences, it is unearned and not bequeathed by other human persons. The love lost teenager, though depressed and possibly suicidal, retains inherent worth. Inherent worth grounds why a suicidal patient's assessment of his own worth can be false.

Having inherent worth is not a gradable worth; it only captures the intuition that our worth is an objective feature.[7]

Second, human dignity entails having *equal* worth, which means that your worth is the same as any person's worth no matter what their or your social position is. This is not to say that relative to some measures, certain people in society are more important. Triage protocols in the setting of a pandemic give preference to health care workers, police officers, and fire fighters. On my view the notion of dignity should capture the idea of equal worth across all things that have dignity. The claim about equal dignity is simply that it would be equally wrong to insult a police officer as much as it would be to insult a homeless person; or to murder a health care worker as much as to murder a patient. The virtue of commutative justice for Thomas Aquinas or the emphasis on impartiality in modern moral theory assumes this very feature of dignity. Focusing on properties and features of the person do not figure in our thinking on justice and fairness. In fact, we avoid indexing a person's worth with respect to them; racism and sexism are examples.

If all human persons did not have equal worth, treating them impartially or in light of commutative justice would not make sense. Dignity plays no favorites. Leon Kass has an instructive observation about the equal worth of human life applied to medicine.

> In clinical medicine, a primary ethical focus is on the need to respect the equal worth and dignity of each patient at every stage of his or her life—regardless of race, class or gender, condition of body and mind, severity of illness, nearness to death, or ability to pay for services rendered. Defenders of human dignity rightly insist that every patient deserves . . . equal respect in speech and deed and equal consideration regarding the selection of appropriate treatment. Moreover, they also rightly insist that no life is to be deemed worthier than another and that under no circumstances should we look upon a fellow human being as if he or she . . . deserves to be made dead.
>
> (Kass, 2008, 300)

Pairing these two features of human dignity together supports the intuition that human dignity explains a number of our moral intuitions including why discrimination, of any sort, is wrong; why murder and rape, of any one, are wrong; and even why arrogance or hubris towards anyone is wrong.

The latter two are interesting in that other accounts of human worth cannot explain why these *attitudes* are wrong. For example, the value of autonomy cannot account for why arrogance is wrong since it is not obvious that being arrogant would necessarily involve a deprivation of one's own autonomy or that of others. Suppose I simply harbor an arrogant attitude towards others but never act on it in ways that limit their autonomy. If our worth were wholly exhausted by having autonomy, it would seem permissible to act on my arrogance towards those who really are compromised in their autonomy, e.g., the mentally disabled, the socially disenfranchised, etc. Similar things can be said about interests. It would not violate someone's interests to *think* of them as inferior to you. In fact, if we focus on interest-satisfaction as being solely valuable, not acting on one's arrogance or hubris would violate the other's interests if the other had interests to be treated in inferior ways, e.g., a dwarf consenting to being thrown for amusement or a prostitute. Such a result is deeply counterintuitive. Dwarf-throwing and prostitution are cases of someone consenting to be treated as inferior but a violation of interests cannot account for why the arrogance of *the throwers* and the exploitation by *the 'Johns'* is immoral.

There is a third aspect of dignity according to which you and I are precious and our worth is irreplaceable. This aspect will take longer to explain but represents the distinctive features of Brewer's (2009) and Gaita's (2004) projects. In what follows I consider, in order, remorse, grief, and love as vectors by which we can apprehend someone's irreplaceable value and preciousness.

Remorse, Gaita argues, shines a light onto the irreplaceable worth of the one who has been wronged. We can see this in a backhanded way by first considering whether the typical explanations for wrongdoing in modern moral philosophy capture precisely what the remorseful person responds to. We cannot imagine the remorseful person responding, without parody, as

> What have I done? I have violated the social compact, agreed behind a veil of ignorance. What have I done? I ruined my best chances of flourishing. What have I done? I have violated the rational nature in another? What have I done? I have violated the ideal interests of an autonomous agent.[8]

Such responses border on parody if they are meant to account for the content of a person's remorse. Rather, the remorseful person comes to have a lucid grasp of having wronged *a person*. And what a remorseful person understands as wrong need not be reducible to harm, but could involve, as with a repentant arrogant person, a lucid realization that others are fundamentally equal to oneself.

The nature and etiology of this lucid realization can be seen clearly regarding a woman who regrets her abortion. I deliberately choose a controversial example to illustrate the point that the lucid realization is in some sense basic – one cannot argue to it, but rather from it – and it bypasses mockery. As recounted in Abby Johnson and Kristin Detrow's (2016) book *The Walls are Talking: Former Abortion Clinic Workers Tell Their Stories*, one worker recounts her experience with a patient whom she names Angie. Angie was in her mid-30s and had shown up for her ninth abortion procedure. As recounted, the clinic workers were disturbed not only that this was her ninth abortion, but also with Angie's levity and rather picayune manner with which she conducted herself. Angie was such a seasoned veteran that she refused any sedation for her procedure and conversed with the doctor throughout it, at one point saying "be careful down there Doc. I might want to have children one day" (Johnson & Detrow, 2016, 72). Angie seemed proud of her indifference and jovial manner, which made even the veteran abortion workers uncomfortable. After the procedure, Angie asked to see the remains saying "I've had it done so many times, I might as well know what it looks like" (Johnson & Detrow, 2016, 74). Apparently, Angie had not asked for this before. The worker proceeded to the "products of conception" lab, located the thirteen-week-old baby, arranged the pieces, and placed the remains on a table next to Angie's recliner for her to see. As recounted by the worker,

> When her eyes traveled to the container, she gasped sharply, and for the first time since she had arrived, Angie was utterly silent. A few moments later her entire body shuddered and gooseflesh was raised on her smooth brown arms. When she reached out her hand to touch the baby, I tried to pull the dish away. She grabbed my wrist and stopped me. We were both silent for a few moments as she continued to stare at the contents of the dish. I stepped back, Angie fell forward to her knees, her fingers still wrapped around my wrist. The other girls in the recovery room began to take notice, and my discomfort level rose exponentially . . . She remained frozen on the clinic floor. "That's a baby," she said, barely audible at first. "That was *my* baby," she said. Her volume steadily increased as a torrent of words poured from her mouth.
> (Johnson & Detrow, 2016, 75)[9]

The feeling of remorse for Angie, who had no prior pro-life sympathies, corresponded to a lucid grasp that the remains in the dish was *her* child.

'What have I done? I have killed something with weak psychological unity relations' hardly captures the content of Angie's remorse. What Angie's remorse lit up for her was the preciousness of her child. Whether Angie's remorse is apposite will have to be settled below (Chapter 6). What is uncontestable is that Angie saw her baby, and this from someone who, seconds before, considered abortion rather perfunctory and beyond moral critique. One should not be too quick to discount or invalidate Angie's perceptions.[10]

Gaita's point in analyzing remorse is to bring into relief the fact that various accounts of wrongdoing on offer in contemporary moral theory border on parody. The principal reason why is because "the individual who has been wronged and who haunts the wrongdoer in his remorse has disappeared from sight" (2004, xxii). The preciousness of the individual is lit up by the remorse of having wronged him or her. The argument here is that remorse is a common emotion that is apposite in many cases. If the object of remorse turns out to be the preciousness of the person, remorse functions as a periscope by which one glimpses human worth.[11] We might be submerged in a theory of rights, or in a time-relative interest account, but remorse lights up the worth of this human being in ways untouched by these theories. Talbot Brewer observes that if we were to express our remorse by saying "what have I done? I have killed a sentient being capable of forming and pursuing long-term projects and commitments" (2009, 172) we have given a response that borders on parody.

A potential contender to Gaita's reflections might be interest accounts of harm. As Beauchamp and Childress (2001, 148) observe, "These arguments [for what counts as wrongdoing] suggest that causing a person's death is morally wrong, when it is wrong, because an unauthorized intervention thwarted or set back a person's interests." At issue is not whether we feel remorse. The challenge is to argue that the remorse or regret is a function not of some nebulous preciousness of the person, but simply a function of having violated the person's interests.

In reply, the interest accounts of harm and wrongdoing fail to avoid parody or are simply counterintuitive. Consider friendship or parenting in which the growth of the friendship or parent–child relationship requires, at times, confronting and even thwarting the interests of the friend/child. When we do not try to dissuade a loved one from a wrong-headed decision and the friend/child is injured or significantly harmed from it, we feel apposite remorse precisely because we did acquiesce to their interests.[12] In such a case remorse cannot be understood as lighting up the value of someone's interests – quite the opposite. The only way to avoid such a result is to argue that the friend and parent in such cases ought not to feel remorse. That would be a counterintuitive position. Again, consider a penitent murderer who appreciates the wrongness of her actions. If the object of her remorse is expressible as having countervailed the interests of another, she has missed the moral reality of her action. Whereas, if she understands her actions as having killed *him*, "I have eliminated *his* existence," we should be content with her response as being accordant to the gravity of her offense. So, in many cases, remorse lights up the individual preciousness of the one wronged.

Consider next, grief. Brewer (2009, 174) observes that "mature grief at the death of a loved one involves an awareness . . . that nothing could represent a compensation for what has been lost. Consolation might be possible, but compensation is not." We do not mourn the loss of a person's capacities, properties, or features. A person might be risible, gregarious, and affable, but we do not mourn the loss of risibility, gregariousness, and affability. Nor is it necessarily the case that we love the person because of those features. "But grief is not just a generic pro attitude towards an irretrievable entity with a certain set of *natural properties*; grief lights up its lost object as having had a very particular sort of value" (2009, 176, emphasis mine). Brewer's point is that the object of grief cannot be a property or feature of the person, but must be the person herself. Grief presupposes that something of value has been lost, not just the absence of good experiences. It follows that grief lights up the individual preciousness of the person.

Finally, consider love. When someone loves me, he does not love a feature or a property of me, but he loves *me*.[13] Gaita recounts a story from Primo Levi who relates the story of his last days in Auschwitz when Russian artillery rounds could be heard in the distance. After years of suffering, liberation was a few weeks away. One of the prisoners below his bunk was named Ladmaker. Ladmaker was a 17-year-old Dutch Jew who suffered from typhus and scarlet fever in succession, and a cardiac anomaly was developing. Additionally, because of his sickness and malnutrition he was bedbound and formed bedsores such that he could only lie on his stomach. He was always hungry, in spite of his fevers, and no one in his compound could understand Dutch which made caring for him difficult. One night, Ladmaker crawled out of his bed in an attempt to make it to the latrine. He was so weak, he fell to the ground sobbing in despair and pain. Levi then tells us how a bunkmate named Charles responded.

> Charles lit the lamp . . . and we were able to ascertain the gravity of the incident. The boy's bed and the floor were filthy. The smell in the small area was rapidly becoming unsupportable. We had but a minimum supply of water and neither blankets nor straw mattresses to spare. And the poor wretch, suffering from typhus, formed a terrible source of infection, while he certainly could not be left all night to groan and shiver in the cold in the middle of the filth.
>
> Charles climbed down from his bed and dressed in silence. While I held the lamp, he cut all the dirty patches from the straw mattress and the blankets with a knife. He lifted Ladmaker from the ground with the tenderness of a mother, cleaned him as best as possible with

straw taken from the mattress and lifted him into the remade bed in the only position in which the unfortunate fellow could lie. He scraped the floor with a scrap of tin plate, diluted a little chloramine and finally spread disinfectant over everything, including himself.

(Gaita, 2004, xvi)

Gaita observes that Charles's actions could be classified as supererogatory, which they were. But the goodness of the action is not exhausted by the concept of duty, or supererogation. It is not exhausted either by the consequences of the action, namely, Ladmaker's comfort to the extent that he could possibly be comforted. An SS officer could have provided such comfort but still think all along that Ladmaker should die in the gas chambers. What Charles did was act *tenderly* towards another human being in the midst of extreme hardship and suffering. "Goodness, wonder, purity, love" (Gaita, 2004, xvii) are concepts that better capture the moral landscape than concepts that describe Charles's actions as beyond duty, or results in good outcomes, or satisfies Ladmaker's interests. "The wonder of what Charles did is that he responded fully to Ladmaker's degradation . . . *while affirming Ladmaker's undiminished humanity*" (Gaita, 2004, xix, emphasis mine). Narratives like the one Levi hands down to us invite us to *see* through affliction and disability to the irreplaceable worth of the sufferer. What did Charles see? To what did he respond? A plausible explanation is that he saw clearly that the suffering of Ladmaker was bad; but with greater acuity he saw that Ladmaker retained inherent worth. Speaking specifically about affliction, Simone Weil makes a similar observation; seeing the other's value – to love the afflicted *without condescension* – is a "miracle greater than walking on water" (Weil, 1968, 172). Weil and Gaita are urging us to look more closely at the *irreplaceable* person as being animated with inherent value while at the same time immersed in affliction or disability.

What is it to condescend? Loving the afflicted without condescension involves apprehending the inherent worth of the person despite the brumous effects of the person's sufferings or 'low quality of life' as we say. Conversely, to condescend involves the following.

To look on a life as one in which it is unintelligible that there should be meaning is to see it as empty of what is distinctively human. It is worse than merely to see it as empty of goods and opportunities . . . If we find it unintelligible that anything could matter to someone living such a life, then we cannot think that any evil done to him, or by him, can go deeper with him.

(Gaita, 2004, 194)

This is not to say that condescension is not understandable. In response to patients experiencing terminal delirium, for example, it is tempting to see *nothing but* their affliction. However, like Ladmaker, and many others, there exists some*one* with undiminished humanity.

The reason this insight is a "miracle" for Weil is because it requires such perspicuous moral acuity. Loving the afflicted and disabled without condescension involves not having the thought that the afflicted would be better off dead or not having been born at all. Reflecting on Saint Theresa of Calcutta's work, Gaita notes that her compassion "expressed the denial that affliction could . . . make a person's life worthless" (Gaita, 2004, 202). Such a love without condescension invokes wonder for Gaita and is miraculous for Weil not merely because the *actions* are meritorious, supererogatory, admirable, or that they issue from good motives or intentions. "The wonder which is in response to her [Saint Theresa] is not a wonder at her, but a wonder *that human life could be as her love revealed it to be*" (Gaita, 2004, 205). What Charles's actions and Saint Theresa's life advert us to is just how valuable those persons are about whom their loving activities were oriented. There is an adaequation between Saint Theresa's love for the afflicted and the beloved's preciousness. Her love reveals to us what might have been obfuscated otherwise, namely, the depth and comprehensive value 'still remaining,' if you will, in the afflicted and disabled. Saint Theresa's love reveals that her patients were "fully our equals" (Gaita, 2004, xiii). Saintly love performs a revelatory role. Certainly, saintly love provides fodder for philosophical reflection on moral heroism and supererogatory action. But it would be cutting the inquiry short if we stopped there. Saintly love is meant to sharpen our own moral acuity. "Sometimes we see that something is precious only in the light of someone's love for it" (Gaita, 2004, xxiv). Recounting stories of love is primarily meant to have us see more lucidly what the lover sees.

What is it, then, that has dignity? Quite simply, you and I do. Endorsing a similar view but defending it by other means, Patrick Lee and Robert George remark that, "all human beings have real dignity simply because they are persons" (2008, 411). So long as we exist, we are precious, irreplaceable, inherently valuable, and equally worthwhile. What then is the relationship between dignity and our existence? Following Gloria Zuniga, I hold that dignity and the person are a two-item *Sachverhalte*. Zuniga, following Wittgenstein, "describes *Sachverhalte* as thinkable configurations of objects that stand in a determinate relation to each other . . . A speck must have some color, a tone some pitch, and an object of the sense of touch some hardness" (Zuniga, 2004, 122). Dignity is in the person as pitch is in a tone or hardness in an object of touch. Our inherent worth may be absent only if we do not exist. Though the object and its hardness are not identical, so too having worth is not identical to existing – the two are co-extensive but not co-intensive. One cannot be found without the other. Certain valuable functions, such as reasoning, and taking an interest in certain projects and plans, are valuable. And those who are able to engage in such functioning are certainly valuable. But the dignity of the person cannot be localized to actualizing a function or property. Dignity is, rather, a *dimension* of the individual person.

We should be careful in saying, however, that you and I have inherent dignity *because* we are individuals with a rational nature. There are at least three ways to understand the 'because' in such a claim. First, 'because' can be understood as referencing a cause, as in 'Joe hit a homerun because he hit the ball hard.' 'Because' may also reference an explanation as in 'Neo took the red pill because he wanted to get out of the Matrix.' Finally, 'because' may delineate a more comprehensive understanding of a thing as when we say that this child will develop functional rational capacities because it is a human being; this piece of metal is gold because it has atomic number 79; and x boils at 212 degrees at sea level because it is H_2O. The relationship between, for example, having atomic number 79 and being gold is entirely unlike the relationship between hitting a ball and scoring a home run. One might say that discourse on moral status uses 'because' in the first or second senses as in 'this person has moral status because she takes an interest in continued living.' Having an interest causes or explains why she has moral status. On my view, dignity is something that we have because of what we are, not because of what we can do.

Arguing for this claim cannot be done by asking what is it that 'makes' us have dignity since doing so already assumes that you and I could exist without it; such a question assumes a bifurcation between properties or functions that are valuable on the one hand and persons on the other. The argument for my claim proceeds by tuning our moral antenna to the moral frequencies, if you will, that dignity sends out. Such tuning requires recapitulating narratives and reflecting on certain emotive states – on the assumption that certain emotions are ways of apprehending value (Pizarro, 2000; Little, 1995; Zagzebski, 2004). Properties, functions, and the capacity to take an interest in x are all abstract and impersonal, Ladmaker is not. Narratives and reflection on emotive states bequeath a knowledge of persons as worthy.

Discharging Misunderstandings

There are several misunderstandings of this view of dignity that I should address before relating it to alternatives. The first misunderstanding is that human dignity as I understand it here is specieist which, to some, is just as bad as being racist or sexist. Properly understood, an account of human dignity according to which all human beings have inherent and equal worth can be perfectly compatible with a view that all nonhuman animals have inherent and equal worth as well. One can say where dignity is without saying where it isn't. Thus, in giving an account of human dignity, one is not necessarily tied to a project of *comparing* the worth of human beings in relation to other nonhuman beings.

Consider another misunderstanding. Jukka Varelius says,

> Possessing the same moral status assumedly entails possessing the same basic moral rights . . . as the doctrine of human dignity entails that all humans have the same moral status, denying that all humans have the same basic moral rights would seem to be incompatible with endorsing the doctrine of human dignity.
>
> (2013, 91)

The idea is that if human beings have inherent worth at every developmental point in our existence, we must have the same rights at all points in which we exist. But we can easily think of counterexamples to such a claim; for example, infants do not have a right to vote, but they would on this (mis)understanding of human dignity.

Why is this a misunderstanding? (It would not be a misunderstanding if we focus on the notion of *basic* moral rights. But the typical counterexamples offered by proponents of this claim do not suggest this interpretation, e.g., voting.) Inherent dignity can ground or explain why we have certain moral rights; and even why we all have the same moral rights – the infant has the same right not to be intentionally killed as you and me. But it does not follow that it would be immoral not to *fulfill* certain rights (the same cannot be said for *violating* someone's rights). For example, two conscious healthy patients may have an equal right to health care, but it may not be immoral to withhold health care from one of them in a triage situation involving scarce resources.

The misunderstanding results from a failure to distinguish between *having* the same rights and *being such* that one's rights can be violated. The latter pertain to the conditions under which my rights can be violated. For example, both a PVS patient and a conscious patient *have* a moral right not to be raped; and both satisfy *the conditions for violating* that right, namely, insofar as you exist, you should not be raped. The same goes for slander, battery, and any number of violations. However, both a temporarily comatose patient and a healthy patient *have* a right not to be lied to, but only the healthy patient satisfies *the conditions for violating* that right, since being lied to requires an active ability to form (false) beliefs. So, some rights require certain abilities to be 'online' in order to ground claims in which one's rights are violated. With this distinction in hand (and it is not ad hoc as indicated by the lying example) we can obviate most putative counterexamples. A person can have inherent and equal dignity as anyone else, and this dignity can ground one's moral rights; but certain violations of those rights depend upon the development of one's species-typical powers. Of course, the right not to be intentionally killed is violated precisely when one is killed. The violation does not depend on whether you can experience your own dying or whether you can form an interest against it (as illustrated by the Meiwes case, see Chapter 11).

Varelius also asserts (2013, 91) that having equal and inherent human dignity would entail that patients in a minimally conscious state (MCS) or even PVS patients would have an equal claim to receiving healthcare as less seriously injured patients, but they clearly do not. I agree, but nothing pernicious to my account of dignity follows. We do not list MCS patients on transplant waiting lists, and we do not in virtue of the fact that they will not benefit from a replaced organ as much as someone who is more functional. We do not list certain conscious adult patients either, whom Varelius considers to have full moral status. For example, we do not list patients in heart failure over a certain age (suppose 65) on heart transplant lists, but this hardly entails that heart failure patients over 65 do not have inherent dignity, much less does it permit intentionally killing them. We do not list such patients for similar reasons for why we do not list MCS patients: they would likely not benefit as much from the replaced organ or there are contra-indicating comorbidities.[14]

A related misunderstanding holds that, on my view, patients need to be kept on life support at all costs. Suppose Joe is in a permanently unconscious state. According to some, such an existence is "no better than death" (Goldman, 2010, 77). If Joe's *life* retains dignity, as proponents of this view understand dignity, we should have to say that we keep him alive at all costs.

In response, it is important to make a distinction between two different moral claims in such examples. One could say that *continuing to live* in an unconscious state is not valuable, or one could say that Joe has no *dignity*. The first claim does not entail the second. I can have the moral intuition that Joe should not receive any further aggressive life-support measures as he is in a permanently unconscious state. But this concession hardly entails that Joe no longer has dignity. There are many conscious patients for whom we judge that further aggressive measures would not be morally warranted but they have dignity on anyone's view.

To be sure, we think it sad and grieve the fact that Joe is in an unconscious state partly because he ought not to be in such a state. We do not mourn the fact that a tulip is not conscious, but that is because of the kinds of things tulips are. We do mourn the fact that Joe is in a permanent unconscious state because of who Joe is, namely a human being. The fact that we mourn that Joe is in a permanently unconscious state indicates that he has suffered an *injury* or an *assault* on who he is by nature.[15] We should resist inferring from our mourning that Joe has no worth at all; my view holds that our mourning is a sign that we are countenancing Joe's dignity. We do not grieve the absence of consciousness per se, but that *Joe* has lost consciousness. Again, the various states, abilities, and capacities of a person are parasitic on the person. We do not mourn *their* absence but mourn because *the person* is deprived of them.

A further misunderstanding of the position that all humans have dignity is to understand it as saying that there is something morally special about being a "member of the species *homo sapiens*" (Douglas and Savulescu, 2009, 310), or that having a certain genetic code is worth conferring (Warren, 1973, 53; Brown, 2007), or that having a natural capacity to reason is the worth-conferring feature (Stretton, 2008, 795). I consider these misunderstandings together since they make a species of the same error. To see this consider Stretton's understanding of what *he* thinks is Patrick Lee's position (which is similar to my own). Stretton grants that, "all human beings are equally human beings, just as all dogs are equally dogs. But it does not follow that the natural capacities of all humans, or all dogs, are precisely equal" (Stretton, 2004, 272). From this general observation Stretton offers the following riposte. "Since natural capacities for higher mental functions exist in substantially varying degrees, and since the right to life, on [Lee's] view, arises from such capacities, therefore . . . the right to life must also exist in substantially varying degrees" (Stretton, 2004, 273). What is the error?

On the position I am advocating, natural capacities and having a certain DNA are markers or indicators of what kind of thing something is. The subject of value is not a genetic code, nor is it even having a capacity to reason. The subject of value is a person, you and me. Consider a species of the same error though directed against my interlocutor's position. My interlocutor might say that having the capacity for consciousness is what 'confers' worth. Suppose I offer the riposte that there is nothing morally significant about P 300 event-related potentials (which is the putative neural marker for visual consciousness (Rutiku, Aru, & Bachmann, 2016)), local gamma band responses (another marker for consciousness (Aru & Bachmann, 2015)), or the presence of synapses (McMahan, 2007). Clearly, such responses would not understand the position so much as mock a strawman. So too would understanding my position as locating our inherent worth in the markers or evidences for knowing what kind of thing you and I are.

Nevertheless, there is something morally relevant about membership in a class. I treat my daughter radically different than I treat my dog. I love my daughter best by *not* treating her as a dog – suppose my dog, in spite of training, attacks children in the neighborhood. It would not be obviously immoral to put him down, but it would be obviously immoral to kill human beings for battery. I have no spat about eating sustainably caught fish, but I would never eat a human, sustainably caught or otherwise. More generally, I love something best by loving it *as* the thing it is. We all have this intuition I might add. If I set as my *summum bonum* money making, I have loved something (an instrumental good) in radical disproportion to how my will should be oriented to money making – what *kind of thing* it is does not warrant such intense love. Christopher Kaczor offers several examples on this point.

> [O]nly those in the class of living beings can have a right to life, only those in the class of sentient beings can have a right not to be tortured, and only those in the class of intelligent beings can have a right to education.
>
> (Kaczor, 2013, 19)

Membership in a kind is morally relevant.

In any case, the riposte that there is little moral relevance to being a 'member of a kind' works both ways. There isn't anything particularly morally significant about an interest being satisfied: we would need to know what the interest is about, and an interest qua interest (abstract universal) is not especially important either (Lemos, 1995, ch. 2). Moreover, there is little especially important about a capacity for consciousness (qua universal) in the absence of a subject who realizes that capacity. There is, however, something enormously morally important about you, me, Ladmaker, and any other individual person. If my interlocutor asks '*in virtue of what* are you and I morally important?' she has already assumed that you and I can exist without having dignity.[16]

One final misunderstanding of my view is rooted in James Rachels's famous and influential distinction between being alive and having a life (similar to the distinction in contemporary clinical ethics between life itself and quality of life). He states that "to be alive is to be a functioning biological organism . . . Human beings not only are alive; they *have lives* as well" (Rachels, 1986, 24–25). He then proceeds to understand that human dignity – what he refers to as sanctity of life – places the worth of the human being in merely being alive.

> The sanctity of life can be understood as placing value on things that are alive. But it can also be understood as placing value on *lives* and on the interests that some creatures . . . have in virtue of the fact that they are the subjects of lives.
>
> (1986, 25)

Rachels criticizes the view that being alive is a basis of inherent value as follows.

> From the point of view of the living individual, there is nothing important about being alive except that it *enables* one to have a life. In the absence of a conscious life, it is of no consequence to the subject himself whether he lives or dies.
>
> (1986, 26)

Rachels thinks that it follows from these claims that we should be concerned primarily about lives, and only secondarily about things with life.

Though Rachels's views are addressed in Chapter 8, I note here why his view is not a competitor to mine. The distinction between being alive and having a life is not exhaustive. If having a life means some sort of narrative, then I could have *many* lives. I could have made numerous different choices in my life and would have lived a radically different narrative, but I would still be me. This point is rather simple: I am not identical to a particular set of experiences or narratives. Likewise, if being alive means simply a functional biological organism, then Ladmaker was not *merely* alive. But he also suffered much and so, on Rachels's view, his narrative life was horrible. But on my analysis above, there is more than just Ladmaker's functional body, and Ladmaker is not identical to a specific set of experiences or narrative. There is also *Ladmaker* who is precious and *that* life is irreplaceable (Zagzebski, 2001; Meilaender, 1998). Narratives and interests are not irreplaceable. We can conceive of different subjects having the exact same experiences as Ladmaker, and Ladmaker having a wholly different set of experiences had he not been seized by the Nazis.

With her usual insight, Linda Zagzebski sets out to answer why we might think that persons are inherently valuable. Along the way she motivates why Rachels's dichotomy is false. She takes as a starting assumption Kant's notion of dignity which,

> implies two different things. One is that anything that has dignity is more valuable than any number of other things that have a price. . . . The other is that things with dignity cannot be compared in value to anything else. . . . That means that we can never make up for the loss of a thing with dignity by *replacing it* with another or even many others.
>
> (Zagzebski, 2001, 402, emphasis mine)

On the assumption that persons have dignity, she goes on to find in virtue of what persons have these two features of worth. Zagzebski is right when she notes that any account of irreplaceable worth *cannot* refer to any shareable property such as having a capacity or having a certain nature. "Surely we love and value other persons primarily because they are who they are, not because they have the *capacity* to love us or other persons" (Zagzebski, 2001, 411). Further on she notes,

> If someone is irreplaceable in value, I assume that means that if we lose her, no one else, no matter how similar to her, can replace her. That must mean that part of her value comes from something about her that nobody else has.
>
> (Zagzebski, 2001, 413)

And that something is, on Zagzebski's account, simply the subject herself as an incommunicable being. What has irreplaceable value is the incommunicable subject herself, you and me. When a person dies, something of irreplaceable worth is lost, and the loss of this worth is not dependent upon or reducible to the loss of 'joys, achievements,' etc. The value of a person's plans and projects borrow their value from the person who realizes them. The plans and projects do not matter in a way that is not dependent upon the fact that the person matters. "To take substance as primary for ethics is to take the person—the person as she really is—as the main end, or one of the most important ends, of moral activity" (Chappell, 2004, 72).

Kenneth Henley, too, motivates these intuitions by noting that we love and care for someone not strictly in virtue of their qualities or characteristics, but we love the person. We would "in at least some cases deny that caring for that individual consisted just in valuing those characteristics. Sometimes we value the individual as an individual, and we would not accept as a replacement even an exact duplicate" (Henley, 1977, 345). Our worth as persons must include, as a desideratum, our irreplaceable worth.

Does the view of life as merely an enabling good capture the worth we have *as individuals*? The answer is clearly no. If Jones's life is merely an enabling good, the only things of intrinsic worth are the joys, achievements, and pleasures that one experiences while being alive. But this position has counterintuitive results. Here again, Henley is on point,

> The ending of a human life [on the enabling view] could rationally be considered a loss only in so far as it carries with it the deprivation of joys, accomplishments, and pleasing or useful characteristics – all of which are in principle replaceable.
>
> (Henley, 1977, 346)

But this would make it irrational to mourn *the person's* death since there would be "no reason to mention in the description of the losses the individual who would have had the valued items" (Henley, 1977, 346). If life is merely an enabling good, the badness of death reduces to the absence of the joys, experiences, and functions that the individual no longer can have. Reference to *the person* being dead drops out. But that is the principal reason for our lugubrious reactions to death. We do not mourn the absence of Joe's experiences, we mourn the absence of Joe. The result here is counterintuitive because we clearly do value individuals as individuals and, if someone were to die, the description of the loss would refer essentially *to that person* and not specifically to the cessation of pleasures or accomplishments. Thus, the irreplaceable person is neither identical to a mere body, nor to a biography in Rachels's senses.

Alternatives: Interests and Autonomy

In this final section I address putative competitors to the claim that all of us have intrinsic dignity in virtue of being human beings. The view I offer locates the inherent dignity of the human person in the person. Putative competitors to my view either locate the source of value in the person's abilities, or, more accurately, in the exercise of those abilities, or the view is not a competitor upon analysis since it is simply referring to a different dimension of human worth – a different angle on the mountain if you will. The chief problem with the former option is that it locates our fundamental value in a specific functional ability, and not the thing that has the ability.

A rather clear statement to the effect that autonomy is the only value to consider comes from Taylor (2016).[17] For Taylor acting autonomously is a sufficient condition for achieving a person's well-being.

> The link between the value creating approach to analyzing autonomy and the protection or promotion of her well-being should be clear: insofar as a person is autonomous if she is acting to satisfy those pro-attitudes that are truly her own and thus whose satisfaction would create value for her, then she will be acting to protect or promote her well-being. A person with BIID [body-identity integrity disorder], for example, would, *if the strong desire to amputate his left leg that existed in his motivational set was truly his own, promote his well-being by having it amputated.*
>
> (Taylor, 2016, 99, emphasis added)

It seems that on Taylor's view, S choosing x entails that x promotes or protects S's well-being.

It is hard to see how this view can be true, or it is not a view about whether human beings have inherent worth. In charity, I interpret Taylor according to the latter disjunct, discussed below. To defend why the former disjunct should be discarded consider the following argument. Either I cannot be mistaken about what constitutes my well-being or I can be. If I can be, then me willing x is not sufficient for promoting my well-being. If I cannot be mistaken, anything I choose for myself is congruent with my well-being. This includes suicide and cutting off one's healthy limbs or other choices that might stem from delusions, psychosis, or a personality disorder. These are examples of people who can be mistaken about what is good for them.

It will not do to retort that such patients are not rational or are not competent since the only argument for why they are not is that they are willing something that is not good for them. And the criteria used for judging what is 'good for . . .' are objective criteria. We know, for example, that a patient suffers from anorexia nervosa when that patient refuses to maintain enough nutritional intake due to a distorted body-image. And a sufficient amount of nutritional intake is not a function of what the patient chooses to consume, it is an objective feature for that patient's body type, metabolism, and size. So, if they are not competent, and yet they are making a choice that is "truly one's own," it must be because of objective features about their choice, namely, that choice does not redound to the person's well-being.[18] If they are competent, then why *treat* them? Why even try to dissuade them for on one interpretation of Taylor's view, that would be encouraging them to act contrary to their well-being? Clearly, however, it is permissible to dissuade and treat such patients, and help them will what is truly good for them.

Importantly, this 'desire-satisfaction theory' also seems to fall prey to the following peculiarity: if S desires for his well-being to *diminish*, i.e., desires to be unhappy, then, if he succeeds in bringing about the object of his desire, his well-being will *increase*. But it increases by being unhappy.[19] It is rather simple to avoid this peculiarity: either admit that 'getting what we want' doesn't always fulfill us or accept the Aristotelian dictum that a person wills what *appears* to produce happiness – viz., it is impossible to desire what is understood as contrary to one's happiness. Both options depart from the desire satisfaction theory. The first for obvious reasons. The second because many desire what is *objectively* contrary to their well-being apart from how things may appear. Consequently, satisfying one's desires does not entail well-being.

According to the second disjunct, Taylor or those who may follow him are not addressing the same question as I am in this chapter. In defense of this, note the change in language from dignity to well-being.[20] Answers to the question whether S has well-being will refer to things like a happiness quotient, health, fortune, etc. (see Haybron, 2008). Referencing these items indicates that well-being refers to the *ways* in which one might flourish (Koch, 2016, 8ff.). But dignity focuses our axiological reflections on *the one who* is (or is not) flourishing. Furthermore, a thing's well-being may be understood unidimensionally, e.g., a person's physical or spiritual well-being; but the same unidimensionality makes little sense when discussing dignity (e.g., physical *dignity*?). Conversely, my plants may be said to fare well, but they do not have dignity. So, dignity is not unidimensional when referred to a specific person, but it is likely that not everything that exists has it. We might say that dignity is not unidimensional but is indexed to the agent herself; but also it may not be predicated of all species types. Disaggregating happiness and dignity can be done along similar lines. Roughly, happiness refers to an achieved state, whether a specific state of mind or as applied to one's narrative life. Again, dignity on my view refers to the value of the one who is (or is not) happy. A PVS patient and Ladmaker may not be able to be happy (the former due to loss of function, the latter due to circumstance), but both have dignity on my view. Though more can be said, these distinctions and the edges on which they are made is enough to illustrate that Taylor and possibly others (Steinbock, 2009) are not competitors to my view on dignity since they are focused on the question of *how* one may flourish, or on what are the constituents of a flourishing life. But they do not appear focused on whether the entity that is flourishing (or not) is precious or has irreplaceable worth.

Conclusion: The Ecumenical Nature of Dignity

Implicit in what has preceded are the reasons why I think my understanding of human worth is much more ecumenical than other discussions. At most stages in the above dialectic, I have granted that various features such as interests, autonomy, a quality life, are all valuable things – suitably qualified and in context, e.g., interest satisfaction qua interest appears neutral at best. I have not encountered an argument, however, for why interests, or autonomy, or a quality life are necessary conditions for having preciousness or irreplaceable worth. Ladmaker lacked a quality of life, but at no point did he lose his preciousness. When we orbit the human person and catch a glimpse of the person's worth through the periscopes of remorse, grief, and love, a more pluralistic view emerges. Human dignity is not incompatible with the values of fulfilling one's interests, or acting autonomously, but our worth is hardly exhausted by these as well. Given the parasitic nature of having interests and possessing the capacity for autonomous action on being a person, it is the incommunicable and irreplaceable individual that is the most fundamental subject of value. Dignity is the value that *the concrete individual* has.

More specifically, I suggest that after having entertained various narratives and in reflecting on emotive states, intentionally killing Ladmaker, you, me, or any other innocent human being is prima facie wrong.[21] Such killing would end our existence. The moral principle that it is wrong to intentionally kill an innocent human being[22] is provisionally exceptionless (putative counterexamples are addressed as we proceed, particularly in Chapter 8).

James Rachels thinks that in accepting this principle one is begging the question. If we have not already decided that abortion or euthanasia are impermissible, "then we would have no reason to affirm" (Rachels, 1986, 69–70) the principle that it is impermissible to kill innocent human beings.

On this point Rachels misunderstands the dialectic. The moral principle is accepted on two more fundamental ideas: (a) a moral principle is only as strong as the goods it aims to protect or promote. The principle I am accepting as provisionally exceptionless aims to protect the good of our lives. Our interests and desires are not unqualifiedly good, our choices might be downright bad, but you and I can never *be* bad (Fagerberg, 2010; Meilaender, 1998). (b) The exceptionless quality of one's strongest moral principles is justified by one's commitment to nondiscrimination. Limiting the scope of the moral principle requires argument. We do not reason from 'it is impermissible to kill me, and there is no apparent morally relevant difference between me and my colleagues, my neighbors, and my fellow citizens, etc.' to 'it is impermissible to kill all human beings.' Rather we start with an open scope on principles that aim to protect such important goods. The one who wants to limit such protections needs to argue for such limitations. Neither of these commitments requires already deciding on euthanasia or abortion.

Notes

1 The emphasis could just as easily be placed on 'human' as 'What grounds *human* dignity?' The emphasis is no longer on 'something *else*,' but rather on 'what it is to be' human.

2 For this reason, I do not consider the voluminous literature on 'moral status' to overlap with my concerns here since the former typically asks what 'confers' moral status. The text adumbrates why this starting point is unwarranted.

3 Brown (2007, 593ff.) is one instance where this assumption is made without apparent defense. He saddles his interlocutors with the problem of an explanatory gap according to which one must argue that "biological properties" or "species identity" explains why something has moral status. To even think there is a gap must make the assumption I note in the text.

4 Error theories aim to explain why our moral intuitions can be so strong yet with no corresponding moral fact.

5 I do not mean for these examples to exhaust the number of rejoinders. The point in the text is not what to think about dignity, but how to think about it.

6 I happen to think that all such explanations are execrable and resemble Beauchamp and Childress's commentary on the Pirates Creed of ethics. This creed they say, "is a coherent, carefully delineated set of rules" meant to govern the Pirates' relationships to one another and to their spoils. "This body of substantive rules and principles, although coherent, is a moral outrage. Its appeal to 'spoils,' its awarding of slaves as compensation for injury, and the like involve immoral activities" (2001, 400). Likewise, thinking that it is permissible to rape PVS patients or thinking that it is not permissible but explain that judgment with reference to abstractions like ideal interests avoids the moral reality confronting one. For discussion see Diamond (1995, 23ff., chs 13 and 14).

7 It is consistent with this claim that two different *kinds* of things can have inherent worth but differ in terms of *how* worthy each item is, e.g., a human being versus a tree or non-human animal. But it is not gradable within the human family.

8 Adapted from Gaita (2004, p. xxi).

9 We are led to believe from this story and other accounts of abortion workers that abortion clients are not told the facts of prenatal development. For an extended analysis of remorse and the possible psychic mechanisms preventing one from experiencing it, see Mitscherlich and Mitscherlich (1975).

10 To the riposte that many others do not react like Angie, it is apparent from the workers' stories that showing the women the remains was a violation of a protocol which is typical across abortion clinics.

11 In exploiting the metaphor of a periscope, I am suggesting two ways of considering the epistemic effects of remorse. It might be that one is submerged, so to speak, in a theory and the remorse allows one to glimpse the moral reality which the theory had occluded. Or, if moral perception is theory laden we might say that the remorse introduced a new datum or intuition that does not sit well with one's current theories or beliefs (on analogy with anomalies as

understood by Kuhn (1996, ch. 6)). Therefore, one must bring about a new and different 'reflective equilibrium' that takes account of the new datum. Whatever we may assume to be the background epistemic position, remorse has the same epistemic effect. Thanks to Ben Richards for pointing out these different interpretations.

12 Ideal interests do not help since the one who is wronged has then 'disappeared from sight' since ideal interests might not be held by anyone; they are not necessarily occurent interests.

13 See Vlastos (1973, 30ff.) who critiques Plato's view of love along the lines I address in the text.

14 Varelius also constructs a rescue case to illustrate the limited value of MCS patients. Rescue cases are dealt with in Chapter 7.

15 The *subject* of dignity is Joe, the *explanation* for why he has dignity is because of what he is, how we *know* what he is, is by way of various markers such as exercised rational capacities, DNA, or human patrimony.

16 For further related clarifications see Lee (2004) and Chappell (2004).

17 For the brief discussion that follows, I'm setting aside treatment of why autonomy is a value. I am doing so because I think it is obvious why it is *a* value; I argue simply that it is not the only value, and that it is not a necessary condition for having dignity.

18 Adding conditions such as full-knowledge or ideal agent conditions to handle such counterexamples does not help the monist view of autonomy either. What prompts the addition of such conditions is our intuition that such choices are bad and yet are chosen. The features that make them bad are independent from the feature that they are chosen. See Murphy (1999).

19 I thank Ben Richards for drawing my attention to this peculiarity.

20 This paragraph relies heavily on Peter Koch (2016, 4ff.).

21 Denying this intuition might not be a sign that my method is defective, but that my interlocutor's conscience is not yet attuned to the values at stake. Certainly one can provide an objectively good argument that fails to convince, or a poor argument that does convince. Moral knowledge is a function of one's basic moral sensitivities (see Chapter 2). On these points I follow Diamond (1995), Anscombe (1958, 17), McDowell (1997, 157ff.), Blum (1994), Little (1995), and Depaul (1993, 137–186).

22 For further defense and commentary, see Gómez-Lobo (2002). My own view is that moral principles are only as good as the goods they aim to protect or promote. Apprehending the gravity and plausibility of a principle, then, is parasitic on a clear apprehension of the goods at stake. Of course, a principle may *be* exceptionless because the goods at stake should never be destroyed. I believe this for certain goods, but it is not necessary to defend this view. My concern in this chapter is primarily epistemic. Therefore, my procedure moving forward is to entertain whether there are good reasons for killing or harming persons in light of its *prima facie* impermissibility.

Part II

Dignity at the Beginning and End of Life

6   Abortion

The penultimate chapter argued that you and I are essentially human substances. I argued that this position avoids the too-many-thinkers problem and that it accommodates our intuitions on brain transplant thought experiments. Such intuitions are not, then, exclusive motivations for psychological accounts of persons. As such, the view that you and I are human substances is plausible and there are few theoretical costs to holding this view. The previous chapter highlighted the view that human worth is multidimensional, which includes having inherent worth. Views that are more unidimensional (focused exclusively on autonomy or interests) identify sufficient conditions for why it may be wrong to kill one of us; but these are not necessary conditions. So, thinking that autonomy and interests are important values is consistent with thinking that inherent human dignity is also a sufficient reason for not killing someone.

This chapter represents our first practical issue that the previous ideas may illuminate. The aims of the chapter are to answer the following questions. What is abortion? Why might one think that it is impermissible? Why might one think that abortion is permissible? After giving plausible answers to these questions I conclude with the argument for epistemic diffidence applied to the act of abortion.

What is the Act of Abortion?

Assessing the moral quality of a human action requires knowing what the action is, and why it is done. Concerning a definition of abortion, a plausible starting point is that it is the intentional killing of an unborn human being. To avoid any aura of begging questions, some time is given explaining it.

There are at least two key terms in the definition of abortion: intention and human being. Discussed in this chapter are those actions in which the agent intends, i.e., sets out as one's goal, to end the life of an unborn human being. The idea that abortion is an intentional killing can be seen from the perspective of the person performing one. If one were to ask a doctor who is performing an abortion what she or he is doing,[1] the answer must refer to the goal of ending the life of this human being. If the child survives, as some do,[2] the abortion is typically documented as a failed or unsuccessful abortion indicating that the goal of the abortion is to end the life of the human being. Of course, a doctor performing an abortion may not understand his action as one of intentional killing of a pre-born child, or unborn human being. For this and other reasons, if abortion were immoral, it may be that many abortion-performing doctors are non-culpably ignorant of that putative fact (Fagerberg, 2010, 144–145).[3] As discussed in this chapter, abortions are cases of intentionally ending the life of a human being. Actions taken in which the child's death is not the aim (e.g., salpingectomy in cases of ectopic pregnancy, or other species of vital conflicts (Rhonheimer, 2009)) are not considered in this chapter.

The second key term is that an abortion kills a *human being*. On this point there appears to be some confusion. Eugene Mills, for example, thinks that conception involves the *oocyte* changing from unfertilized to fertilized. He states,

> Review some sex education materials; watch, via microscope, the fertilization of an egg. You see an unfertilized oocyte—the one-celled human egg. A sperm approaches and, after traversing the corona radiata and zona pellucida, contacts the egg's cell wall. The sperm breaches that wall, enters, and dissolves, discharging its contents. The breach in the cell wall is immediately sealed. *The most natural description of these events is that you've watched one egg become fertilized, not the annihilation of one organism and the creation of another.*
>
> (2008, 328, emphasis added)

Mills's observations invite the question whether the sperm or the oocyte each are different *cell types* from the zygote.

To avoid arbitrary decisions on distinguishing cell types, two criteria are used: composition and behavior.[4] Cells with different composition will have different genetic composition and gene expression, and different proteins will be produced, etc. Behavior refers to the developmental pathway that an organism manifests, which is largely a function of having a different composition. Maureen Condic states,

> When cells are classified into specific types, differences in either composition or behavior are the bases for all *scientific*, as opposed to *arbitrary*, distinctions. If, for example, scientists were to propose that during embryonic development a novel cell type exists between a neural crest and a sensory neural progenitor cell, they would have to *prove* this assertion by pointing to specific material or behavioral characteristics.
>
> (Condic, 2008, 3)

Different organisms will develop along different developmental pathways and will be composed of different molecular components. Such is the case between zygote and unfertilized oocyte.

Furthermore, we need to distinguish between a human *cell* and a human *organism*. On this distinction Nicanor Austriaco notes that a cell cannot survive on its own and requires a human organism for its existence.

> Even when severed from the organism and isolated in a tissue culture dish, the human cell relies upon a human organism, either the scientist or the lab technician, to maintain the appropriate laboratory conditions it needs to live. In contrast, the human organism is self-sustaining and able to survive as an independent entity throughout its lifespan.
>
> (2002, 664)

The importance of this second step (distinguishing cell from organism) is that at issue is whether the behavior and composition of the zygote distinguishes it from the unfertilized oocyte *and* whether the zygote is an organism. If you and I are human organisms, and the zygote is not, you and I cannot be identical to a zygote. Austriaco's observations however, indicate that the zygote is an organism. In addition to having independent existence and the ability for self-repair, two other important properties that organisms possess but cells do not are growth and development (Richardson, 2000). Growth refers to the size and maturation of the organs in the organism itself. Development refers to the organism's ability to have its distinct parts ordered to the end of species-specific maturation. This includes not just survival, but also development of species-typical abilities. This is exactly what we see with the human being at the zygotic stage; we see growth and development, not the behavior of a stand-alone cell.

Understood as such we can see why Mills's description of the events of fertilization is accurate but insufficient. He is right to point out that the sperm and oocyte "contact the egg's cell wall" (Mills, 2008, 328). More technically, the membranes of these two cells fuse forming the zygote[5] which now has molecular material from *both* sperm and egg. The 'egg'[6] now has a different biochemical composition than what it had prior to the sperm dispensing its DNA into the egg. Condic notes that "because the zygote arises from the fusion of two different cells, it contains all the components of both sperm and egg, and therefore the zygote has a unique molecular composition that is distinct from either gamete" (2008, 3). This new molecular composition initiates a series of changes in the newly formed zygote, namely, chemical modifications are made to the zona pellucida which prevent fertilization by more than one sperm (except in the case of triploids). The significance of this is that the new zygote loses a key property that the unfertilized oocyte[7] had, namely, the ability *to be* fertilized. Since the zygote cannot have that ability, we can say that there is a different organism in virtue of its not having a defining potency of the oocyte. Second, the zygote manifests potencies associated with coordinated growth and development, self-repair, and sustained metabolic activity. Some might say that the organism does not come into being until syngamy, but that would ignore the coordination necessary to even make syngamy possible (Condic, 2008, 7 ff). Each of these behaviors is not indicative of the gametes alone – the unfertilized oocyte dies within 24 hours, and the sperm dies within 1–5 days; but the new living system may live on for 70 to 80 years. "Clearly, then, the prior trajectories of sperm and egg have been abandoned, and a new developmental trajectory—that of the zygote—has taken their place" (Condic, 2008, 3).

The Moral Analysis

Arguments for the Impermissibility of Abortion

Arguments for the impermissibility of abortion are a combination of scientific facts about the development of human beings, the fact that abortions are intentional killings from the perspective of the agent, and an ethical claim about the inherent worth of each individual human being. What remains to explain is what this ethical claim is and whether its scope includes unborn human beings.

The relevant ethical claim pertaining to abortion is the idea that it would be wrong to intentionally kill *you* (Gómez-Lobo, 2007). The moral prohibition against being killed is one of the most basic moral commitments we have about our fellow human beings. Whereas it is not wrong to drive on the right-hand side of the road in America as opposed to England, it is wrong everywhere to be intentionally killed. Children do not have a right to vote, but they have a right not to be killed even if they cannot understand the propositional content of a moral right or a future of value. The idea here is sensible: we should be protected against acts that eliminate our existence. Any weakening of the moral protection against being killed requires justification. The onus of proof is on those who would either reject this as an ethical claim altogether or limit the scope of its applicability.

So let's understand the ethical claim as the claim that it is impermissible to kill (henceforth intentionally is understood) any human being and you are a human being. Gómez-Lobo summarizes the point this way.

> To claim inviolability now is a shorthand way of saying that it would
> be morally wrong to deprive *me* of my life, and to deny inviolability
> at earlier stages would be a short-hand way of saying that it would

not be morally wrong to deprive *me* of my life. However, my life is the same life, indeed, it is *I*, at both points in time. A claim of inviolability now and lack thereof in the past would indeed behave like P—"it would be wrong to kill *me*"—and not P—"it would not be wrong to kill *me*."

(Gómez-Lobo, 2007, 314)

Limiting the scope of the moral claim involves a practical contradiction. To avoid it, one must show that there is some feature about a sub-set of human beings which makes it permissible to kill them. Such features are discussed in the next section. It is enough to observe that the argument depends on arguments already presented. The penultimate chapter argued that you and I exist throughout development and maturity – and that includes our development prior to birth. The previous chapter argued that you and I have inherent worth. Since the ethical claim is that it would be wrong to kill me (or you) it would not matter when that killing takes place in our life span for that act to be impermissible. In this sense, the pro-life position is non-discriminatory.

The pro-life argument can be summarized as follows:

1   Abortion is the intentional killing of an unborn human being.
2   Intentionally killing a human being is impermissible.
3   Therefore, abortion is impermissible.[8]

Premise (1) is plausibly true. Premise (2) is plausible given the arguments already presented and a non-discriminating application of the ethical claim to all human beings. The dangers of boundary drawing as pointed out in Chapter 2, among other considerations discussed in this chapter on pages 121–129 below, set the onus of proof on the argument for limiting the scope of the ethical claim.

Arguments for the Permissibility of Abortion

Any chapter-length treatment of the abortion issue must make decisions on which ideas or arguments receive attention. A comprehensive discussion is not possible. Readers familiar with the abortion issue will likely disagree with the arguments I choose to address or ignore but that is expected. To be clear about which arguments I am selecting for attention, a brief conceptual map is necessary.

Arguments for the permissibility of abortion are split into two broad categories: (I) the no-person strategy and (II) the person-but-lacks x strategy. The former class of arguments argue that unborn human beings are not persons and non-persons may be killed. Different arguments are presented for what counts as a human person but, for all of them, unborn human beings – especially at the embryonic or zygotic stage – are not persons (Warren, 1973 and 1992). The latter class of arguments typically grant that unborn human beings are persons in an ontological sense (Degrazia, 2005) – they may grant the truth of the claim 'my mother first felt *me* kicking when I was 18 weeks old.' But proponents of (II) argue that unborn human beings lack some morally important feature the lack of which makes it permissible to kill us even if we are already born (Singer, 1979) or only prior to birth (Degrazia, 2005, 290). Two types of features have been proposed: interests and bodily rights (Boonin, 2003; Thomson, 1971). So, under category II, there are two different claims. (IIa) Unborn human beings typically do not have the capacity to take an interest in continued living. Therefore, they do not have a right not to be killed. Such interest-based arguments typically entail the permissibility of infanticide (McMahan, 2002) since infants lack the ability to conceptualize themselves as existing into the future; however, Degrazia (2005, 290ff.) demurs. (IIb) Bodily rights advocates argue that *during pregnancy* the unborn human being does not have a right to further use of the mother's body.[9] On this strategy, the permissibility of infanticide does not follow since the emphasis is on the *bodily* right of the mother. Once born, the child is no longer in the body of the mother.

With this map in mind, I address IIb. The first strategy was addressed in Chapter 4. I pretermit treatment of IIa for at least two reasons. Such criteria (e.g., interests) were addressed in the previous chapter. The basic riposte is that having an interest in continued living is a sufficient reason not to kill the person, but there is no good argument for why having such an interest is a *necessary* condition for impermissible killing. Second, the claim that interests are necessary falls prey to plausible counterexamples – the implications of this point are discussed in the concluding section.

Unborn Children are Persons but Lack Bodily Rights

Judith Jarvis Thomson was likely the first philosopher to put forth a plausible and compelling argument for the conclusion that even if unborn human beings are persons in the full moral and ontological sense, it is still permissible to end a pregnancy by means of a direct abortion. The reason is that having a right to life does not entail a right to the use of another's body. The key premise in support of this conclusion is the idea that pregnancy is viewed as the mother's body providing life support to the baby. If one thinks that it is permissible to withhold life support from patients, an intuition most people should grant, then it is permissible to withhold life support (i.e., one's body) from the baby.

Thomson's argument centers on her "famous violinist" example. The purpose of the example is to construct a case in which it is intuitively plausible that a person with a full right to life may be allowed to die. Here is how she describes the case:

You wake up in the morning and find yourself back to back in bed with an unconscious violinist. A famous unconscious violinist. He has been found to have a fatal kidney ailment, and the Society of Music Lovers has canvassed all the available medical records and found that you alone have the right blood type to help. They have . . . kidnapped you, and last night the violinist's circulatory system was plugged into yours, so that your kidneys can be used to extract poisons from his blood as well as your own. The director of the hospital now tells you, ". . . To unplug you would be to kill him. But never mind, it's only for nine months . . . ." Is it morally incumbent on you to accede to this situation? No doubt it would be very nice of you if you did, a great kindness. But do you have to accede to it?

(Thomson, 1971, 56)

Most will agree that there is no moral obligation to remain plugged into the violinist (but also that it would not be impermissible to continue being plugged in). If the violinist has a right to life, how is it permissible to unplug yourself from him? On Thomson's view, having a right to life does *not* entail having a right to another's body. Thomson states, "I am arguing only that having a right to life does not guarantee having either a right to be given the use of or a right to be allowed continued use of another person's body" (Thomson, 1971, 56).

From the example and the intended conclusion, we can piece together Thomson's argument as follows.

4   If a person F is *dependent* upon another person's body M to *live* and M does not consent to or want F to be dependent upon her, M has no obligation to support F.

Premise (4) is supported by the violinist example. The generalization from the violinist case to 'for any M and F' is mediated by paying attention to the feature of being a world-famous violinist. If it is permissible for me to unplug myself from this valuable person, certainly it is for any other instantiation. Furthermore, consider an analogy with organ or blood donation. It may be laudable for me to donate my blood or a paired organ, e.g., kidney, to save the life of another. But no one *else* has a right to take my blood or kidney from me without my consent. The next premise simply pinpoints the relevant feature of an unwanted pregnancy using F for fetus and M for mother.

5   An unwanted, unborn person F is dependent upon M's body to live.
     From (4) and (5) it follows that,
6   Therefore, unless M consents to or wants F to be dependent upon her, M has no moral obligation to support F.

If we want the conclusion that an *abortion* is permissible from what has been stated so far, we need to make precise at least one more claim.

7   If M has no obligation to support F, then it is morally permissible for M to have an abortion.

8   Therefore, if F is unwanted by M, it is morally permissible for M to have an abortion.

This argument has been subjected to extensive criticism (Hershenov, 2001; Kaczor, 2011; Finnis, 1973). Despite an attempted reboot (Boonin, 2003, ch. 4; and Manninen, 2010), it remains a dubious argument (Eberl, 2010; Trotter, 2010; Beckwith, 2007, ch. 7). Notably, as B. Jessie Hill (2010) points out, courts routinely permit doctors to perform cesarean sections on women to save the child and, in some cases, to save both. So, the law does allow disruptions in one's bodily integrity to preserve significant goods, i.e., the life of the child. And in the cases it does, that justification *can* be duplicated to justify seriously limiting elective abortions. Even so, briefly recapitulating the dialectical development of this argument and its defeaters will motivate the argument from epistemic diffidence.

Reply to the Bodily Rights Argument

There are at least two points to consider in response to Thomson's argument. First, the violinist example is not analogous to abortion and pregnancy. And, second, if the mother has bodily rights, so does the baby. I explore these points in turn. There are at least two important disanalogies: one pertaining to abortion itself, and the other pertaining to pregnancy and parenthood. David Boonin (2003, 3) appears to agree that finding analogies with abortion and/or pregnancy is a delicate task. He states that "the moral problem of abortion is difficult because it is unusual" and its unusualness is a function partly of the unique relationship between mother and child, and the incipient development of the child.

To make the violinist example analogous to abortion, not only must I unplug myself, but I must dismember and kill the violinist. When we change the violinist example to comport with actual abortion procedures, our intuitions are that it is not permissible to dismember and kill the violinist. David DeGrazia appears to concur, noting that current "methods of abortion involve killing the fetus" and that "it is . . . dubious that you may kill your child in order to avoid the burden . . . of providing assistance that you have caused her to need" (2005, 285). So, the example, when made analogous to abortion, no longer supports the conclusion Thomson wants.

The same idea applies to the organ donation example. I may refuse to donate my blood or kidney to a person in need, but it is a radically different act if I were to proceed to dismember and kill that person. In most abortions, the goal in view is to end the life of the unborn human being. The target or aim of an abortion is the death of the unborn child.

The problem here might be illuminated if we keep in mind that neither Thomson nor Boonin are framing their arguments from the perspective of the abortionist who is performing the abortion. From such a perspective the abortionist is intending to destroy the baby even if the mother is double-minded about her decision or is decidedly opposed to the abortion but feels pressured into it.

Some philosophers have granted these points and note that the violinist analogy works only for cases of hysterotomy, namely, cases in which the unborn child is not dismembered or directly attacked but is instead removed or prevented from implanting. Boonin explains, "in both of these cases [i.e., hysterotomies], abortion seems simply to be a means by which a woman who has been providing needed life-support to the fetus she is carrying can effectively discontinue her provision of such support" (Boonin, 2003, 193). The bodily rights argument can still function as a defense of abortion but only for those methods that remove the unborn child. DeGrazia concurs, noting that such an argument justifies "abortion in only a small range of cases" (2005, 285).

But even this pollarded position is mistaken. Consider an infant neglect case.[10] Suppose a woman gets pregnant prior to modern abortion methods. When the child is born, she neglects giving him or her any sustenance. The child dies. Here there are at least three analogies with Thomson's case: (a) The child is *unwanted*; (b) s/he is unwanted because of the *burdens* of caring for and keeping the child alive; and (c) the mother *withholds sustenance* leading to the child's death. Ancient methods of infant exposure and modern-day cases of intentional neglect are clearly immoral. Furthermore, there do not seem to be any morally relevant differences between being dependent upon someone's body versus their behavior (see note 9).

Boonin claims that unplugging yourself from the violinist is not morally different from a hysterotomy, and neither is morally different from the infant neglect case. He states, "surely a person who fails to feed a hungry infant allows it to die and does not kill it" (2003, 199). On his view, when you unplug yourself from the violinist you are allowing the violinist to die, likewise when you intentionally neglect to feed a hungry infant. If the former is permissible, so is the latter.[11] It is clear, however, that intentionally neglecting a hungry infant is impermissible.

Before continuing, the previous point is important in appreciating the argument from diffidence. If the defense of abortion rights depends upon granting the intuition that it is permissible to intentionally neglect infants, the argument from epistemic diffidence becomes that much stronger. For consider the dialectical exchange up to this point: we start by granting the intuition that it is permissible to unplug yourself from the violinist. We then observe that, even if this is permissible, the permissibility of intentionally killing an unborn child does not follow. The problem is simply to find analogies between two radically different contexts of relationship, namely, the pregnancy-mother-child-intentional killing context and the stranger-bedbound-letting-die context. Once we come remotely close to identifying an analogy, namely, hysterotomy, we lose the intuition that such an act is permissible. This was illustrated by the infant neglect case. As quoted above, Boonin seems to grant that Thomson's argument entails the permissibility of infant neglect. Now we can ask whether it is more plausible than not to suppose that it is permissible to neglect infants? The weight of plausibility is on the side of impermissibility – the burden of proof is hardly met. The epistemic situation here would be like Irving taking a brownie from the 'no-peanut' basket after he sees *several* people moving brownies from the 'peanut' basket to the 'no-peanut' basket, the only difference being that it is not Irving's life but his own child's life who has the same allergy.

To this point, I have been challenging premise (7) because the violinist analogy is not applicable to abortion procedures themselves. The second class of disanalogies I noted pertained to pregnancy and parenthood. Regarding these analogies we turn to assess premise (4).

Premise (4) states that our obligations to support the lives of others is discharged if the lives of others *depend on our bodily functioning* and we did not *consent* to this dependence. Consider consent first. Our obligations to others do not depend on consenting to them. If I come upon someone who is bleeding profusely and will die without a ride to the nearby hospital, I should drive her there, even if my new car seats get a little dirty (Unger, 1996). If my only sibling and his wife die in a freak car accident leaving behind my niece and nephew needing care, I am obligated to care for them. If a desperate new mother leaves her recently born child at the hospital, someone has an obligation to care for that child. It may not be you or me, but the *child* is owed care and love. What these examples show is that consent is not a necessary condition for having an obligation toward another. Rather, our moral obligations to others are a function of the *goods* we ought to protect and promote (Goodin, 1985). Because an individual's life is such a great good, her protection from violence or assault on the one hand and help in leading a flourishing life on the other are so important. This was precisely the argument in the previous chapter, namely, dignity is not reducible to promoting this or that particular good but it adjures or importunes a moral regard for the *person* herself.

What might strike us as attractive about the violinist analogy is that it captures our intuitions on autonomy. But there are any number of other values in the vicinity such as caring for the vulnerable, the defenseless, and the voiceless. Moral obligations can come upon us even if they are not chosen. Consider that, instead of being plugged into a world-famous violinist, you are plugged into your own child. To unplug oneself in this setting is being a bad parent (Pruss, 2017). Coming to be a parent generates obligations (Prusak, 2013). On this point Schwarz and Tacelli are right.

So imagine a child – a baby boy – who is being raised by his mother alone. The mother, we agree, has certain special obligations. But why is that? Why does she, and not some other woman, have these obligations to him? There can be only one answer: Because *she*, and not some other woman, conceived him; because *she* is the biological mother.

(1989, 83)

Schwarz and Tacelli are creating a contrast case, "why does she and not some other . . .?" to bring into relief our intuitions that the parents of a child inherit special moral obligations and enjoyments. The parent–child relationship cannot be compared without obfuscation to a stranger-type relationship. Don Marquis (2010) argues correctly that pregnant women are *mothers* to their unborn children. Since all mothers are parents and parents have special duties of care towards their children, pregnant women have special duties to care for their unborn children.

That parents have duties to their children is true even if the pre-born child may have no right to the mother's body. Hugh McLachlan supposes that even

if no one [else] had a right to our bodies or a right to a particular performance from them, we might still have duties regarding our bodies. We might have a duty to keep our bodies healthy even if no one [else] has a right that our bodies are healthy.

(McLachlan, 1977, 202)

If I am a vowed religious person, for example, I incur a duty not to do violence to anyone including an aggressor. So, I have a duty not to harm such a person even though the aggressor who would be harmed by my just defense has no claim on me *not* to defend myself. Duties to one's child might be one-sided in this respect: we may have a duty to the child, even if the child does not have a claim on us. For all of what Thomson and Boonin argue, it may still remain contrary to duty qua parent to kill an unborn child.

So it is true that bodily support is morally relevant; but it is morally relevant in that it generates a moral orientation aimed to ensure the good of the child. A pregnancy that is not wanted does not discharge our obligation not to kill human beings, just as caring for orphaned children may be unwanted and burdensome, but that does not justify harming them.

I turn to consider the second point, namely, that Thomson's argument grants that the unborn child is a person. As such he or she has bodily rights as well (Kaczor, 2011, 151ff.). Recall that Thomson's argument grants that the unborn child can have a right to life but not a right to the bodily support of the mother because the mother has bodily rights. But if the mother has bodily rights because she is a human being, and the unborn child is also a human being, it would follow that the unborn child has bodily rights as well. And now we have the necessary ingredients for the following argument:

9   All human beings have bodily rights.
10   If a being has bodily rights at all, they include a right not to be dismembered or directly killed. (Assumption.)
11   An unborn child is a human being (granted by Thomson).
12   Therefore, an unborn child has bodily rights (from 1 and 3).
13   Therefore, an unborn child has a right not to be dismembered or directly killed (from 9 and 10).
14   Abortion is the dismemberment and direct killing of an unborn human being (factual description of most abortion procedures).
15   Therefore, an unborn human being has a right not to suffer an abortion.

Premise (9) is plausible since being a human being is sufficient for having bodily rights and premise (11) is granted by Thomson. Premises (10) and (14) are very plausible. The other statements are conclusions that follow from the premises. The basic point of the argument is this: human beings have bodily rights because all human beings are *embodied*. Since even unborn human beings have bodies, it would come as a shock to find out that they did not have *bodily* rights. And it would come as a shock to find out that of the bodily rights we do *not* have is a right not to suffer bodily dismemberment.

There are two objections to this bodily rights argument. First, the argument only applies to those abortion procedures that dismember or directly attack the unborn (e.g., D&E). The argument does not seem to apply to procedures that remove the unborn from the mother's womb (e.g., hysterotomy). The reply is to recall what we learned with the infant neglect case, namely, that intentionally omitting to provide a person with sustenance in order that the child die is just as wrong. One need not directly attack the body of a child to treat him disrespectfully. Neglecting his needs is just as wrong. The same can be said for the unborn. *Location* inside the womb versus outside does not discharge or eliminate a parent's obligations to their child. And the *burdens* of childrearing do not justify intentionally omitting care in order that a child die. I am *not* suggesting that bearing a child in one's womb is not different from caring for a child already born; but those differences do not justify a moral difference between killing the unborn child on the one hand and the born child on the other.

A second objection is to deny premise (9) by arguing that you and I are essentially persons, understood according to the psychological view described and analyzed in Chapter 4. But this is not a plausible reply to premise (9) even if one holds such a view. If you think that you are essentially a person and you understand personhood in psychological terms, that still does not entail that your body does not have bodily rights. A bodily being can still have bodily rights even if it may not be a person at the time it has those rights. The proponent of the psychological view would have to argue that we have bodily rights *only when* we are persons. But the clause 'only when' is challenged by rather simple counterexamples such as raping PVS patients (Watt, 2000) or doing risky medical research on nonconsenting comatose patients. So again, the weight of plausibility is on the side of premise (9).

In the remaining sections of this chapter I explain and defend the argument from epistemic diffidence in more detail.

The Argument from Epistemic Diffidence

Indexing the Burden of Proof

The moral risk of being wrong sets who has the burden of proof. For Irving (introduced at the end of Chapter 3), the cost in being wrong that the brownie is not made with peanut flour is enormous. The presumption is in favor of Mislabeled and a corollary is that non-Mislabeled bears a burden of proof because of the greater cost in being wrong. Consider, then, the following proposition:

(p): Abortion is permissible.

Suppose that S is an OB/GYN and believes (p), acts as if (p), and is mistaken about (p). S would perform a gravely immoral action. If the pro-life argument is correct, the child is voiceless, powerless, and is killed where the child should be the safest, i.e., the mother's womb. (I am self-consciously using affective descriptions to capture the gravity of the moral costs, *if* the pro-life position is correct.) Abortion requires pretermitting the moral stance one should have towards human vulnerability. (One might be tempted to add the likelihood of fetal pain but killing is not wrong because it is painful or, conversely, permissible because it is painless). Now suppose that we quantify across all S's in which they mistakenly believe (p) and act on it. The consequences here are clearly enormous, namely, the unjust killing of millions of vulnerable and innocent human beings.[12]

This is enough to motivate the weight and kind of risks; but who bears those risks? For the issues of abortion and embryo-destructive research, it is the nascent human being.[13] Why is this relevant? Suppose I am out hiking with my daughter and we happen upon what looks like a deep creek. I want to dive in for a swim but I am uncertain of its depth. Whereas I might be justified in risking it myself, to ask my daughter to jump in first is risible. The point is that delegating risks to others looks *prima facie* haughty, arrogant, or cowardly. Being clear about who bears such risks further elevates the bar of justification needed to justify acting in spite of such risks.

Consider the negation of (p) and its moral risk.

~(p): Abortion is not permissible.

Suppose S believes ~(p), acts as if ~(p), and is mistaken. Does S *perform* a gravely immoral action? If S is an OB/GYN and acts on ~(p) by refusing to perform an abortion, S has not done anything wrong, and this is so for any S. Acts of omission are wrong only if we *ought* to have acted. But to say that an abortion ought to be performed would commit a deontic fallacy for no one has argued that an elective abortion is obligatory. Furthermore, some abortion rights advocates concede the legitimacy of conscience rights.[14] If S is the mother and mistakenly believes ~(p) she does not perform an immoral act either since there is nothing wrong with continuing a pregnancy. Ted Lockhart remarks that *not* having an abortion is considered morally permissible by most parties (2000, 53) and possibly heroic in some circumstances as depicted in the movie *Precious* (2009). Giving birth to a baby is not morally problematic; ending the life of the baby is.[15]

Suppose S is an OB/GYN except that we quantify across all OB/GYNs. And suppose again that, for all S, S believes ~(p), and acts on it, and is mistaken, thus, they refuse to perform any abortions. According to Boonin the burden that is symmetrical to widespread killing is the "unjust burdening of women with unwanted pregnancies" (2003, 322). In the following sections I consider three arguments for symmetry: the unjust burden of unwanted pregnancies, social consequences of mass refusal, and constraint on choice. I argue that none count as symmetrical burdens.

Pregnancy Itself as an Unjust Burden

The argument that bearing an unwanted pregnancy is a moral cost observes that incurring an unwanted burden is unjust. An unwanted pregnancy is burdensome. Therefore, an unwanted and burdensome pregnancy is unjust.[16] One might locate the 'burden' in the fact that it is unwanted or in the bodily effects of pregnancy or both. Where the burden is located does not matter for my critique; what matters is the claimed connection between being an unwanted burden and being unjust.

Not all unwanted burdens are unjust. Let's agree that a wanted pregnancy that is viewed as burdensome is not an unjust burden. An unwanted pregnancy that is viewed as burdensome is also not an unjust burden – at least not without assuming that all *unwanted* burdens are *unjust*. Certainly not all are. A mother may choose to continue an unwanted pregnancy for other reasons, e.g., to place for adoption, and few think that this is immoral, unjust, or that one is obligated *not* to place for adoption. I may not want to care for my brother and sister-in-law's children upon their deaths in a freak accident, but that unwanted burden is not an unjust one. Examples abound of unwanted burdens which are not unjust simply because they are not wanted.

Of course, some unwanted burdens are unjust, e.g., slavery. But even here, the reason for the injustice has more to do with the violation of human dignity than in the fact that a slave's labor is burdensome.[17] One would have to argue that *some* unwanted burdens are unjust and that unwanted pregnancies are in that class of unjust burdens. Doing so, however, would have to import a premise which specifies that unwanted pregnancies have a moral property that unjust burdens share and that such a property makes or justifies that burden as unjust. Since that moral property cannot be the property of being unwanted (per arguments above, that is insufficient), one must search elsewhere. A candidate property is not immediately obvious. To see why, consider one possible candidate such as the lack of moral status in the unborn child. The lack of moral status in the child doesn't make bearing a pregnancy unjust – for then all pregnancies would be unjust. Thus, for x to be unwanted and burdensome does not provide any reason for thinking that x is unjust.

One might argue instead that even if continuing a pregnancy is not unjust, preventing one from ending it is unjust, assuming neutrality on (p). In response, consider what would make the prevention unjust. To recapitulate motifs previously noted, the source or reason for being an injustice cannot be a function of the pregnant *state* being unjust, since it is permissible to continue with a pregnancy. Another possible source might be that it is preventing a person from *willing* to end the pregnancy. I concede that this is a cost, but it is not symmetrical in gravity with the costs in being wrong about (p). If *what* is being willed to end is not itself a bad thing (i.e., pregnancy), preventing someone from ending it does not appear to be a grave evil. Suppose it is permissible to eat Chilean sea bass (suppose they have made a slight comeback from being endangered) but that it is also permissible to continue a moratorium on harvesting this fish. Because I am a cautious restaurant owner, I prevent you from ordering any. It is permissible to serve and not to serve this fish. Preventing you from ordering any due to false caution may be a cost in being wrong, but it is hardly a grave matter. Consider the point more generally: when we do not know what x is, there is nothing morally significant about willing x. This is because we do not know what x is. When we add that what is being willed is ending something for which it is both permissible to end or continue, preventing one from ending it (analogous to not serving the sea bass) does not compromise significant goods. The point is that preventing someone from *willing* that which is permissible, even if erroneously, does not compromise significant goods, when the other option is also permissible.

If abortion is actually permissible and S is prevented from procuring an abortion then the cost in being wrong about abortion is this: one is being prevented from doing what is permissible. If, however, abortion is not permissible and S is allowed to procure an abortion, the cost in being wrong is this: one is allowed to do that which is obligatory not to do – namely, to intentionally kill you or me at a nascent stage in our existence. So, although Boonin may be right to say that there is a cost in being wrong, his argument does not justify a symmetrical cost.

Maybe the injustice is not a function of one's will and pregnancy, but a function of one's will and access to a medical procedure. One might say that, if all OB/GYNs refuse to perform abortions, this would be depriving many pregnant women of a medical procedure to which they are morally entitled. On the assumption that ~(p) is erroneous, the objective moral risk in performing an abortion would be nil and preventing one from getting an abortion would be an unjust restriction on one's bodily and autonomy rights.[18]

Two points attenuate the weight of autonomy risks. First, it is doubtful that one has an autonomy right for a particular medical procedure. Even if a person has a right to health care, it does not necessarily follow that a person has a right to a particular procedure. Even if I were to have cancer, I do not have a right to ipilimumab if it were contraindicated. I do not have a right to a procedure that will compromise my health. So, if I have a right to health care, I still do not have a right to a specific procedure. Of note, abortion is the only procedure in all of medicine declared a constitutional right (Forsythe, 2013, 10).[19] Without being viciously circular, the point stands that there is no right to *elective* procedures.

Second, even if one were to argue that a person has a right to a procedure, the justification for that right would have to be a function of the goods of health and welfare that are at stake. The procedures would have to be *clearly beneficial*. (The riskier the procedure, the more inclined we are to say that preventing access to it is not unjust.) But if continuing a pregnancy is not itself either immoral or an illness or a disease, then a procedure that *ended* pregnancy would not necessarily cause a state of health or welfare. Ending cancer brings about the good of health, because cancer is a disease; but if pregnancy is not a disease, ending it does not necessarily bring about the good of health (cases of vital conflicts aside). Of course, on the assumption that abortion is permissible, ending the pregnancy would be consistent with health. What we need to generate intuitions that the unavailability of a procedure is *immoral* is that the procedure bequeaths a benefit not otherwise accessible. Since pregnancy is not itself a disease, ending it cannot itself be considered a promotion of health or welfare.

A more fundamental problem with understanding the 'burden of pregnancy' as a symmetrical moral risk is that it is irrelevant when we consider the empirical evidence. Mothers who choose abortion experience a higher incidence and gravity of regret than mothers who choose to continue their pregnancy (Fergusson, Horwood, & Boden, 2009). The psychological cost of having an abortion versus continuing a crisis pregnancy is on the side of abortion. This evidence suggests that bearing an unwanted pregnancy does not have the devastating psychological sequelae that ending it does. Second, the typical burdens mentioned by mothers seeking abortions include interference with education or career, or not being able to afford the baby (Finer et al., 2005). Notably, these burdens occur *after* the child is born.[20] Pregnancy itself is rarely referred to as being a burden that initiates seeking an abortion.[21] This evidence suggests that 'the burden of pregnancy' is an empty moral risk in the sense that few seeking an abortion consider it a sufficient justification for having one. I will agree that restricting access to a medical procedure that is morally permissible has moral costs. My argument to this point is that these drawbacks are hardly symmetrical with the costs of being wrong about (p).

Social Consequences as Moral Risks

Continuing with the assumption that S is quantified across all OB/GYNs who refuse to perform abortions, other consequences might be social such as overpopulation. But this too does not justify a moral risk that is symmetrical with the risk of mistakenly believing (p) and acting on it quantified for all Ss. We do not solve overpopulation concerns by killing off enough people to the point of sustainability. The reason why is because that is a morally horrible solution. We would rather work to distribute resources as best we can (or should), even if the effects of overpopulation persist. This indicates that if forced to choose, we would rather avoid mass killing than avoid overpopulation.

Referring to broad social consequences to identify the burden of proof has other problems associated with it. To be clear, at issue is identifying who has the burden of proof in light of the objective moral risks at stake. In this regard, it is instructive to look at parallels with slavery (Willke, 1984). Pre-Garrison justifications for slavery noted the socio-economic consequences of abolishing it (Eltis, 1987). But the idea that the abolitionists bore the burden of proof is not justified simply by referencing the bad social consequences that might follow. Those consequences are not necessarily the moral risks at stake with continuing the institution of slavery, but are practical effects given contextual features. Thus, even if it were true that abolishing slavery would lead to serious socio-economic consequences, it would do so only by assuming as constant pre-Garrison practices, institutions, and economic systems. The abolitionist could easily observe that the burden of proof then shifts to proponents of those very practices and institutions that, when *paired with the abolition of slavery*, lead to the bad consequences. The point is this, when confronted with bad consequences of abolition given contextual features, we have a choice. We can use the bad consequences as reasons against keeping constant those features or as reasons against abolition. We can see in the slavery case how ridiculous the latter option is.

Formally, the same dialectical situation faces the abortion issue when indexing the burden of proof. Abolition of abortion might lead to what we all agree are bad social consequences, but only if we assume as constant certain institutional policies or common behaviors. The burden of proof then rests on why one would hold as constant those policies and behaviors that, when paired with the abolition of abortion, lead to bad social consequences. Suppose that the abolition of abortion when paired with current institutional policies leads to discrimination against pregnant women in the workplace. There is nothing about the absence of abortion that causally entails such discrimination, the institutional policies do so. But such discrimination is a reason to change the policies rather than to continue to permit abortion. At least, there is not a morally neutral argument to hold as normatively constant those policies.

An example of a behavior might be sexual promiscuity. If abortion were not available, this would be a reason for tailoring one's sexual decisions to avoid crisis pregnancies for oneself or one's partner. Persons who choose chaste lives do not report serious psychological dysfunction, thus there is little risk to avoiding the 'need' for abortion at all. Whereas disagreement exists as to whether a promiscuous lifestyle leads to disvaluable psychological sequelae, there is agreement that those who choose chaste lives do not suffer dysfunction (Nettleman, Ingersoll, & Ceperich, 2006; Armour & Haynie, 2007).

So, just as the abolitionists for slavery did not assume a burden of proof simply because its abolition would lead to bad consequences, so too all OB/GYNs who refuse to perform abortions need not assume a burden of proof.[22] Any bad consequences that might follow do so because of certain practices, behaviors, and institutions about which there is no normative reason for holding as constant. Therefore, we do not have a reason for thinking that serious moral risks would follow from all Ss refusing to perform abortions *specifically*. The burden of proof remains on the proponent of (p).

Constraint on Choice as a Moral Risk

Thomson (1995) appears to think that the risks in being wrong about (p) or ~(p) are asymmetrical with *more risk* in being wrong about ~(p). If successful, her argument shifts the burden of proof onto a pro-life argument. Her argument is succinctly stated as follows.

> First, restrictive regulation [of abortion] severely constrains women's liberty. Second, severe constraints on liberty may not be imposed in the name of considerations that the constrained are not unreasonable

in rejecting. And third, the many women who reject the claim that the fetus has a right to life from the moment of conception are not unreasonable in doing so.

(Thomson, 1995)

The value of liberty paired with some notion of 'not unreasonable' are taken by Thomson to set the dialogical burden on the pro-life argument. If Thomson is right, any pro-life argument for which it is reasonable to reject one of its premises is enough to permit someone to act as if the argument is incorrect. I hope to show that her argument is subject to reasonable rejection.

Because I refer to specific premises in what follows, enumerating her argument is necessary.

A   Restrictive regulation of abortion severely constrains women's liberty.
B   Severe constraints on liberty may not be imposed on the basis of arguments that *the constrained* might reasonably reject.[23]
C   Some of those who might be constrained reasonably reject arguments for the restriction of abortion.
D   Therefore, restrictive regulation of abortion should not be imposed.

Premise (B) as stated by Thomson refers to the women who might be constrained by restrictive abortion policies. And it says *of them* that they might be reasonable in rejecting pro-life arguments. It is not clear what counts as being reasonable for Thomson: is it coherence, justification with no known defeaters, reliably formed belief, etc? Aside from these details, one can *understand* why a woman faced with a crisis pregnancy would find abortion as an attractive option. If reasonability is defined as means-end reasoning, those facing crisis pregnancies would be reasonable in considering abortion. But this is not what Thomson needs for her argument. I might fail to appreciate the weight of the reasons for a coercive taxation policy – because I have an interest in keeping my own hard-earned dollars. But that would hardly justify the state in not imposing such a taxation policy. Premise (B) needs to say that pro-life arguments can be rejected based on reasons that are objectively plausible. To motivate why, imagine the following parody of Thomson's argument understood without this objective feature.

A1 Restrictive regulation of slavery severely constrains slaveowners' liberty.
B1 Severe constraints on liberty may not be imposed based on arguments that the constrained might reasonably reject.

C1 There are those who reasonably reject arguments for the restriction of slavery.
D1 Therefore, restrictive regulation of slavery should not be imposed.

Notice, all I have done is swap out abortion for slavery in this parody. (Notice also just how unpersuasive the argument would be if we included the original 'not unreasonable in rejecting' criterion.)

Maybe Thomson understands 'reasonable rejection' objectively in the sense that opponents to restrictive abortion policies have objectively good reasons for their position. So, her argument from risk must include the following conditional or one trivially different.

- (O1) If there are objective good reasons for *opposing* restrictive abortion measures, abortion should be allowed. ('Allowed' because in premise (B) reasonable rejection is said to justify non-imposition.)

  The chief problem is that this conditional does not consider whether there are objective reasons for *endorsing* restrictive abortion policies. Suppose those reasons are good ones. For example, if true, the idea that human beings maintain their ontological identity through development qua persons would be a good reason for restricting abortion access. Conversely, if true, the idea that unborn human beings are not persons would be a reason for opposing restrictive abortion measures. It is in *this* setting of good objective reasons on *both sides* that one mounts a moral risk argument. Again, to avoid Boonin's challenge (Chapter 3) one cannot set aside the justification one has for one's beliefs *or for others' beliefs*. So, we should understand the key conditional as follows.

- (O2) If there are good objective reasons for both opposing and endorsing restrictive abortion policies, abortion should be allowed.

Once we have captured the dialectic on abortion accurately, (O2) is hardly apparent. If the objective reasons are good ones on both sides, it simply does not follow that abortion should still be allowed. (Consider the counterintuitive ring of a hunting version of O2: if there are good objective reasons for opposing and endorsing restrictive hunting practices, unrestricted hunting practices should continue).

That pro-life arguments inherit the initial dialogical burden would follow only if the liberty involved in exercising *this* choice (the choice to have an abortion) is a value that outweighs all other value considerations (i.e., the values referred to by the arguments for restrictive policies). But that axiological claim is neither obvious nor true. Furthermore, how would one argue for such a claim? We do not endorse the killing of our children even if taking care of them severely restricts our individual liberties. The value of our liberty is circumscribed. Importantly, the value of that liberty does not itself justify a moral difference between born and unborn children, since that would be irrelevant. The value of an abortion choice is parasitic on the arguments for a moral difference, and therefore it is a value that is neither independent nor can it be presumed. So, the life of one's child functions as a value the elimination of which can be considered a significant error; and that value putatively trumps the value of one's choices.

Finally, there is an equivocation on the notion of liberty between premises (A) and (B). The value of liberty referred to in (A) is the putative value of making this choice for abortion – restrictive regulation would prohibit making *this* choice.[24] Conversely, premise (B) is plausible only when 'liberty' is taken to refer to one's *capacity* to make choices.

Now consider the counterintuitive ring of understanding premise (B) as: severe constraints on *one's specific choices* may not be imposed on the basis of arguments the constrained might reasonably reject. We do this all the time and justifiably so (see 45 CFR 46 Sub-part D). For example, environmental regulation constrains our choices, but those who are constrained (i.e., the energy industry and those who own Hummers) might have *coherent* reasons for rejecting these constraints. Rephrasing premise (A) is even less intuitively persuasive. Consider, "restrictive regulation of abortion severely constrains women's *capacity* to make choices." Whatever restrictive regulation of abortion does, it certainly does not impugn one's *ability* to make decisions. So, when Thomson claims that restrictive abortion policies "severely constrain women's *liberty*," an equivocation is being made between (A) and (B). Two different values are being conflated: the value of having free will at all, namely, the *capacity* to make choices and the value of *this* specific choice.

But more needs to be said about how the two values, the value of a specific choice and the value of the capacity to make choices, can come apart. Consider a pregnant woman and her liberties and freedoms. Presumably, simply being pregnant does not "severely constrain one's liberty," at least not in a way that would ground some moral prohibition on getting pregnant. Granted, parents have to make different choices than non-parents. But parents clearly retain the capacity to make such decisions. And, although the specific choices are different between parents and non-parents, they are no less valuable. So, if premise (A) is plausible, it is likely that premise (B) is not, because premise (B) is plausible only when we consider the value of liberty per se, qua capacity, and not the value of this or that specific choice, and vice versa if (B) is plausible.

The Argument for Diffidence

In the preface I outlined the skeleton of the argument from epistemic diffidence. What is important is to see the pattern of argumentation since the argument from epistemic diffidence makes reference to various justifications J, and J is subject to numerous substitution instances.

Starting at the very top of the dialectic, the belief in question is that abortion is permissible.

16 Belief (p) is subject to epistemic diffidence.
17 If belief (p) is subject to epistemic diffidence, it should not be acted upon.
18 Therefore, (p) should not be acted upon.

There are three features of beliefs that make it subject to diffidence: peer disagreement, undercutting defeaters, and failure to meet the burden of proof. As noted in Chapter 3, confronting peer disagreement should prompt us to question whether one has made a performance error on an issue that exercises the upper limit of human abilities. I shall assume that the practical issues discussed herein do so. Therefore, the hypothesis that one has committed a performance error is, for the intellectually conscientious, a plausible hypothesis. Chapter 2 explains in detail the various ways in which one's moral cognition can execute a performance error. So, in the setting of peer disagreement I have reason for thinking that my moral cognitive faculties are in a questioned source context. To the riposte that these reflections apply equally to the proponent of ~(p), the proponent of (p) is the one who bears the burden of proof. The moral costs for S in being wrong about ~(p), whether quantified or not, are not symmetrical as argued above. Thus, in the setting of high stakes, one's justification for (p) is more sensitive to defeaters.

The defense of premise (16) is distributed across the different strategies (I, IIa, and IIb) and key claims constituting them. Consider first the no-person strategy addressed in Chapter 4. One branch of the dialectic is something like the following: (a) the psychological view entails that there are two thinkers in one human being; (b) abortion is permissible only if the psychological view is true; (c) there are not two thinkers in one human being (the Unity Argument). Therefore the psychological view is not true. Therefore, abortion is not permissible. Of course, there are other branches of the dialectic, but, for the moment, I focus attention on (a) and (c) – abandoning (b) abandons the no-person strategy. Let J refer to any proposition that putatively justifies either ~(a) or ~(c). For example, I considered McMahan's part-whole distinction to justify ~(a). I argued, however, that his 'in-virtue-of' relation fails to satisfy his own desiderata for an explanans on either a causal or mereological interpretation. We can iterate this lesson such that for any substitution instance of J, there is a plausible rejoinder from an epistemic peer, or J does not, upon inspection, function as a justifier at all (see Chapter 4 on why BT experiments are under-motivating). Given the current dialectical state of the debate, therefore, the typical substitution instances for J are subject to peer disagreement, plausible rejoinder, or do not function as justifications at all.

An intellectual conscientious agent would see that the burden of proof for J is not met given the claims discussed so far. Therefore, premise (16) is true on the no-person strategy.

Turning to Thomson/Boonin's argument, a dialectic similar in form to the previous paragraph emerges. Consider premise (9) of the bodily rights argument. Let J be any proposition that would justify ~(9). Any substitution instance for J considered herein is subject to either peer disagreement, plausible rejoinder, or does not function as a justifier at all. Suppose J is the claim that the bodily rights argument still permits hysterotomies. But that argument met the counterexample from infant neglect.

Before concluding, it is important to observe that this argument avoids Boonin's objection to risk arguments,[25] since premise (16) is defended *by reviewing the justification for (p)*. Specific substitution instances for J are, on analysis, subject to peer disagreement, are implausible, or are irrelevant. The specific justifications for (p) do not meet the higher burden of proof for acting on (p).

Conclusion

Backing away from the details of practical arguments, there is a broader epistemic lesson in which the lessons of Chapter 2 are applicable. Both Boonin and McMahan (arguably the best defenders of abortion rights) endorse reflective equilibrium (RE) as a method for constructing moral justification. In a revealing passage, McMahan considers explanations for human worth and goodness distinct from his egoistic concern account. Other accounts, such as the Harm-Based Account, have the consequence that "it would be terribly bad if the fetus were to die instead" (McMahan, 2002, 78). He immediately observes that "most of us believe that the death of a human fetus is *not* a terrible tragedy" (2002, 78, emphasis added). McMahan reflects on the dialectic to this point and observes correctly that he is appealing to his own intuitions about the badness of fetal demise to defend his account of egoistic concern, and yet,

> [i]n the next chapter I will invoke this claim in order to defend these same intuitions. Although there is a certain circularity here, I do not believe that it vitiates either the defense of the claim or the defense of the intuitions. In epistemology, it is widely accepted that coherence among beliefs sometimes strengthens the case for thinking that each belief is justified.
>
> (McMahan, 2002, 78)

Boonin also observes correctly that RE begins by accepting our moral intuitions on certain action types, intuitions that may appear strong to the one who has them. We then construct moral principles to explain and collate our moral intuitions (Rawls, 1971, 20, 48–51). Considering counterarguments allow us to make various adjustments within our system of beliefs, thus the sobriquet equilibrium. But there is an important problem. When confronted with apparent counterexamples to our moral principles, we have two options. Boonin states, "[o]ne option is to revise our proposed theory so that it produces the 'correct' answers to some of the questions it initially got 'wrong.' . . . The other option is to abandon or revise some of our initial judgments" (Boonin, 2003, 11). But there is nothing other than the agent's own intuitions that dictates which option one takes. One's adjustment decision is arbitrary in this sense (Haslett, 1987). Furthermore, as pointed out by Depaul (1993), any coherence method in epistemology is subject to the no-contact-with-reality objection. One can have a widely coherent view that is morally wrong, as illustrated at the end of Chapter 2 with the example of Jay. These two problems, the arbitrariness of adjustment decisions and no-contact-with-reality, suggest that coherence is tenuous comfort to those who take seriously the risks in being wrong on issues that involve killing. The only way to break out of the circle is to take seriously peer disagreement. Considering the arguments canvased to this point, one should be epistemically diffident about (p).

In concluding this chapter, I extend some reflections from Sophie-Grace Chappell (2011). There are two distinct but mutually coherent ways in which inquirers approach the issue of abortion (Chappell discusses persons). We can either take an impersonal approach or an interpersonal one. For unborn human beings, we might think that this thing has no value yet and in order to have value it must be able to function in a sort of way. Or we might think that this thing is the beginning of a particular human life and this was what I looked like at that nascent stage of development. The former might look at early human beings as things, the latter as developing individuals. These approaches function like Jay's commitment to a romantic view of war, or Joan's empathic sensitivity to the suffering of others. Moral perception is not analogous to having an eye vis-à-vis visual perception, rather it is constituted by our fundamental moral commitments, emotional sensitivities, and motives that interpret and process moral information in a complex moral world. Not having the interpersonal orientation will mean not detecting the values having such an orientation disposes one to detect – similar to inattentional blindness in visual perception (see Chapter 2). In settings of peer disagreement, on difficult matters with a high risk in being wrong, the justification for abortion suffers epistemic diffidence.

Notes

1 For descriptions of various abortion procedures by a former abortionist, see Anthony Levatino, "Abortion Procedures: 1st, 2nd, 3rd Trimesters." Available at: www.youtube.com/watch?v=CFZDhM5Gwhk, accessed 2/15/2018.

2　See www.theabortionsurvivors.com, accessed 06/17/2019.

3　This point is confirmed by the narratives of those abortion doctors and clinic workers who leave the industry. See Johnson and Detrow, 2016; and numerous other shorter narratives compiled by Sarah Terzo at clinicquotes. com, available at: http://clinicquotes.com/category/former-abortionists-speak, accessed 5/31/2018.

4　The material presented in this section is heavily dependent upon the work of Condic (2008, 2013). There and Austriaco (2002).

5　By 'zygote' here I mean a human organism in the single-cell stage of development. Understood as a phase sortal, I effectively dodge Mills's reductio argument outlined on p. 335ff which considers the zygote simply as a single-cell. Mills's argument attempts to show that the zygote is not identical to the embryo. Understood as an organism in the single-cell *stage* dodges the reductio.

6　I put in quotation marks the 'egg' because Mills is right that on the view I endorse "Eggs never *become fertilized*" (2008, 328). They can *be* fertilized, but not *become* fertilized. By never "becoming" fertilized, Mills means that if a thing is an unfertilized egg, *that same thing* cannot survive to be a zygote. To *be* fertilized, however, merely acknowledges that the oocyte can receive spermatic contents. Once the increase in calcium occurs and cyclin-B is dissolved, the organism cannot be fertilized. It loses an essential property of being an egg. The egg, qua egg, does not survive the successful fertilization event.

7　Following Condic (2008), the language of fertilized egg commits a categorical error. If the egg is fertilized it is no longer an egg. It is correct however, albeit redundant, to say that the egg is unfertilized.

8　This argument follows the form offered by Patrick Lee (2010).

9　For what it is worth I do not see how this position avoids infanticide either. Born infants still require the behavior of one's parents to provide her or him with food, comfort, warmth, etc. In a sense, whether a person is dependent upon another's body versus her behavior does not seem to matter morally. So if dependence upon another's body justifies neglect, so does dependence on one's behavior.

10　Thanks to Mike Rota and Michael Degnan for various cases introduced in this section.

11　Boonin may think that, if there is a morally relevant difference, it is not a function of the killing–letting die distinction (2003, 199ff.). But, if Boonin grants that it is impermissible to neglect infants, and he appears to do so, he needs to explain why the features that make such neglect impermissible are not duplicated in the case of hysterotomy. Features such as personhood or interests might be candidates, but then it is no longer a bodily rights argument.

12　I do not consider S qua mother who mistakenly believes p (or ~p), because, as noted previously, mothers do not perform the act of abortion.

13　I am setting aside risks to the mother (Reardon, 2018) or the health care staff (Roe, 1989; and MacNair, 2009) who are performing or assisting in the abortion. Of course, adding such risks adds more weight to the risks in being wrong about (p).

14　Some do not respect conscience rights (Savulescu and Schuklenk, 2017). As noted in the text, the abortion rights arguments canvassed so far yield a judgment of permissibility. For discussion see Kaczor (2013) and my website for supplementary materials.

15　It is irrelevant to retort that in some cases it would have been better that this or that child had never been born. Such judgments are based on dubious quality of life judgments and are only justifiable, if at all, *after* a life has gone poorly.

16 One could modify the modality of the premises to 'an unwanted burden *can be* unjust.' This modification would render the premises much more plausible, but the conclusion would be innocuous, namely, 'an unwanted and burdensome pregnancy can be unjust.' It would be innocuous for two reasons. That it might be possible for an unwanted and burdensome pregnancy to be unjust does not argue for symmetry since being wrong about (p) *would* involve an unjust killing. Second, the mere possibility of an injustice occurring does not index a notable cost in being wrong for the reasons Boonin highlights, and I endorse, as discussed in Chapter 3 on pages 46–49.

17 Suppose, for instance, that the same type of labor is done but the laborer is compensated justly for it. The laborer may still be treated unjustly, but not because she or he is compensated justly.

18 Thanks to Matthew Braddock for urging me to consider this objection.

19 Specifically, it is a negative right, meaning that the state cannot preclude access, but it is not a positive right which would require the state to guarantee access. Thank you to an anonymous reviewer for further specification.

20 This point is made by Kelsey Hazzard in the documentary *The 40 Film.*

21 The cited reason closest in content was "physical problem with my health" (Finer et. al., 2005, 113). This was cited only by 12% of the respondents and we are not told which problems they were. For example, there is a difference in burden between experiencing headaches and having pulmonary hypertension which might become life-threatening in the setting of pregnancy.

22 Of note, my argument about costs in this section gains even more plausibility if the position at issue is merely that there should be stricter criteria for performing an abortion (relative to current US law), not abolition.

23 The change from 'not unreasonable in rejecting' to 'reasonable in rejecting,' or its cognates, is motivated by charity. Not being unreasonable is a weak epistemic state. Coherence is not even a requirement for 'not being unreasonable' in believing B since it only requires that B is not incompatible with my network of other beliefs N, but may also not be supported by them either – as would be involved if B were coherent with N. Not being unreasonable in believing B, then, is compatible with believing B for no reason whatsoever – just so long as one has no reasons against B. On this understanding, the dimwitted Nazi can be 'not unreasonable' in believing the stupid things she does. Such an epistemic state would render (B) initially implausible. In the interest of charity, then, Thomson must have in mind a stronger notion such as being reasonable in rejecting B which requires some support relation with a coherent network of other beliefs N. Thus, even if there are reasons for rejecting restrictive abortion policies, I still wish to argue that permissive abortion policies should not be presumed. As such, I am setting the bar higher for my argument not Thomson's.

24 I leave aside the implausibility of such a restriction counting as 'severe' when only one choice among several is being prevented. Consider how severely our field of choices is limited when obeying *jus in bello* criteria for just war. Consider how severely our field of choices is limited when conducting ethical research on human subjects. Severe restriction of one's choices is morally inert without a moral analysis of the choices in question.

25 The key idea behind Boonin's objection is that risk arguments require setting aside one's justification.

7   Human Embryonic Destructive Stem Cell Research

Stem cell research is best classified under the heading of regenerative medicine. Stem cells have the capacity to renew themselves and, under certain conditions, differentiate into specific cell types such as heart tissue or kidney tissue (NIH, 2016), thus regenerating organ function. Sources[1] of stem cells can be divided into two basic categories. The first comprises sources that involve destroying a human organism to extract the cells (e.g., 'leftover' embryos from IVF clinics or embryos purposely created by IVF or other technologies such as cloning). The other category comprises sources that do not involve the destruction of any human organism (e.g., reprogrammed somatic stem cells).[2] The medical promise behind stem cell research for either source is to repair organ dysfunction. On the assumption that disease or damage typically results in organ dysfunction due to cellular breakdown, injecting the right kind of stem cell into, for example, heart tissue, can rejuvenate the functioning of the heart (Patel et. al., 2016). Pluripotent stem cells can differentiate into most other types of cells such as neural, heart, liver, or kidney cells, etc. Research with cells from nondestructive sources (commonly but erroneously referred to as 'adult' stem cell research)[3] may use the patient's own stem cells to rejuvenate an organ that is not functioning optimally. Clinical applications using nondestructive sources of stem cells are quite common with over 75 diseases able to be treated or managed with such cells (Charlotte Lozier Institute, 2017). Furthermore, using such sources can bypass immune rejection issues that affect the use of embryo destructive sources. The reason is that nondestructive sources often use the patient's own stem cells, carefully-matched donors, or those whose compatibility appears not so essential: for example, umbilical cord blood stem cells (Laughlin et al., 2001; Ziegner et al., 2001).

What is the moral issue with using stem cells from destructive sources? A common understanding is to ask whether human beings at the embryonic stage may be included as "full members of the moral community" (Humber & Almeder, 2004, v), or whether they have full moral status which would afford them the "same rights, claims, and interests as ordinary adults" (Douglas & Savulescu, 2009, 307–308).

Both ways of understanding the issue are incorrect. Even if one does not consider all human lives as morally equal, it is a separate question whether it is permissible to perform lethal research on human subjects. The research ethics tradition was developed largely in response to serious ethical infractions that were committed in the name of advancing medical knowledge (LaFleur, Bohme, & Shimazono, 2008; Coleman et al., 2005). Consequently, human research subjects have enjoyed the focus of ethical protections even if we might think it is permissible to kill human beings for other reasons: for example, prisoners on death row.[4] This is not (necessarily) a case of schizophrenia in our moral tradition. The stricter conditions on research subjects follows in part from an honest recognition that our moral perception can be obfuscated when one is driven to find cures or significantly reduce suffering. The history of research ethics abuses is clear: dehumanizing research subjects is a distinct possibility in the setting of entrenched desires to make scientific advancements.[5] Even if one thinks that capital punishment is permissible, one could still consistently oppose killing prisoners for research purposes (Mitford, 1974; NCPHSBBR, 1975). This is also the case with pre-born human beings who may not be subjected to research known to be harmful (45 CFR Part 46. Sub-part B) even though abortion is legally permitted. The National Commission for the Protection of Human Subjects of Biomedical and Behavioral Research observes that "the woman's decision for abortion does not, in itself, change the status of the fetus for purposes of [research] protection. Thus, the same principles apply whether abortion is contemplated" (NCPHSBBR, 1975, 66; see also Napier, 2009). The idea is to treat equals equally. If we protect pre-born children who *are wanted* from harmful research, the same applies to those *not wanted*. Our choice does not affect the basic status that grounds their protection from research-related harms. So, the issue is not simply about full moral status and/or protection from harm in other contexts, but about whether all human beings should enjoy protection from destructive research.[6]

There are, however, certain facts about human development between conception and implantation that some argue would permit destroying nascent human beings. There are basically two categories of arguments. It can be claimed that nascent human beings are not individuals, at least not in the sense that you and I are individuals. It would follow that you and I cannot be identical to those human organisms that would be destroyed for research purposes – killing one of them would not be killing one of us. I address two tokens of such arguments, namely, the *twinning* and *totipotency* arguments. The second category of arguments challenges whether those human organisms that would be destroyed for research purposes are at all worthy, or have non-instrumental value. For these arguments, it may be the case that you and I are numerically identical to our existence at the embryonic stage, but we would not have acquired any worth yet – at least, not enough worth to protect us against being killed for potentially beneficial research. Arguments from *rescue cases* and *natural loss* are tokens of this strategy. Following the format of the previous chapter, I critically evaluate these four arguments in turn, and then canvas my argument from epistemic diffidence. I conclude that the judgment that young human beings may be killed for research purposes is subject to epistemic diffidence and therefore should not be acted upon.

The Twinning Argument

The twinning argument aims to show that the embryo is not an individual, and since only individuals can be proper subjects of protection, embryos may be killed for research purposes. Considered at its most generic level, the twinning argument comes in two steps (Khushf, 2006). The first step is a statement of empirical fact about human embryos, namely, that up to 14 days from conception, an embryo can divide into two embryos. This fact is referred to as twinning (or fission). The second step is a claim about what the possibility of twinning *means* concerning the ontological status of the pre-twinned embryo.

Let Z refer to a zygote and E to an embryo just prior to the twinning event at t1, and O1 and O2 refer to the embryos that result from twinning at t2. There are basically three options regarding the identity of E, O1, and O2. First, E is numerically identical to O2, and O1 is the result of asexual reproduction (or vice versa for E = O1). Second, E is an individual human being who dies at twinning and is not identical to either O1 or O2. Third, E is not an individual but is the matter out of which the individual organisms O1 and O2 arise.

With this picture in mind, consider the following formulation of the twinning argument from David DeGrazia:

> Until about two weeks after conception, an embryo can divide into two . . . Arguably, then, the [embryo] is not yet *uniquely individuated* in the sense that whether it, and it alone, will develop into a single human organism has not been determined.
>
> (DeGrazia, 2006, 51)

The conclusion of this argument is that E is not a "uniquely individuated" organism. The argument in outline seems to be as follows:

1 It is possible that E divide or twin resulting in two different organisms.
2 If it is possible that X divide or twin, then X is not an individual organism.
3 Therefore, E is not an individual organism.

Premise (2) is the key premise but it is false; for if X is not an individual organism prior to twinning, then what is *it* that undergoes twinning? Twinning presupposes *an organism* that undergoes twinning: it is certainly identifiable as *that organism which will undergo twinning*. As David Oderberg has noted,

> It is easy to show that it [the organism prior to twinning] would be an individual simpliciter. For an individual is definable as an entity which is a countably distinct instance of the kind of which it is a member. And an embryo younger than fourteen days, even if we know it is going to divide, is clearly a countable instance of the kind 'human embryo.' In respect of a woman only one of whose ova has been fertilized, the answer to the question posed within fourteen days of conception, "How many embryos is she carrying?," is "One".
>
> (Oderberg, 1997a, 274)

The human embryo, even prior to fission, is a countable organism of some sort. I can point to it and say 'that is a human embryo.'

One might suppose, however, that the pre-twinned embryo is constituted by numerous cells but is not itself an identifiable organism. Consider Robert Nozick's Vienna Circle example (1971, 32ff.) according to which different members of the Vienna circle fled to different countries during World War II but carried on their intellectual activities for the duration of the war. The example invites the question whether the pre-twinned embryo should be considered more like a group than an individual.[7]

Simply because something divides does not entail that that which divides is a group. Consider a contrast case for comparison. The nine-banded armadillo always has quadruplets, i.e., their embryos are *supposed* to twin. If one's development were like that, I harbor the intuition that the embryo prior to twinning is not an individual. But the human embryo is not supposed to twin, certainly not like the nine-banded armadillo.[8] The human embryo is oriented to maturity as an individual, and twinning is an anomaly.

Furthermore, this 'group' supposition fails to explain why we have the intuition that when the embryo develops past the 14-day point without twinning, one organism is 'doing' the developing. Based on a detailed review of embryogenesis, George and Tollefsen remark that,

> at fertilization, a new and complete organism comes into existence – a distinct, actively self developing human organism – for he or she exhibits internally directed, complex development between fertilization and the last point in time at which twinning may occur.
>
> (2011, 239)

Lastly, as discussed briefly in Chapter 6, early human development is a highly integrated activity that belies the supposition that the pre-twinned embryo is merely an unidentifiable mass of cells. So (2) is likely not true and the argument is unsound.

DeGrazia presents a second twinning argument that considers identical twin adults. If each adult came into being at conception, then each twin is identical to one zygote. DeGrazia rightly notes that this is incoherent. "For the two twins are numerically distinct, so they cannot *both* be identical to a single earlier zygote" (DeGrazia, 2005, 248). But from this observation he concludes that "*neither* identical twins nor chimeras could have come into existence at conception" (2005, 248). The only intervening premise DeGrazia mentions concerning twins is "and the twins were not individuated until twinning occurred" (2005, 248). This argument is slightly different than the one presented above because this one capitalizes on our intuitions concerning identity (specifically, the transitivity of identity), and not strictly on contentious biological claims about the pre-twinned embryo.

It is certainly correct to say that for identical twins, both did not come into being at conception. It is plausible to say, however, that one came into being at conception, and the other at the point of twinning through a form of asexual reproduction.[9] The twinning argument would be successful if its conclusion were limited to showing that not all human beings came into being at conception – some of us, namely twins, came into being at the point of twinning (George and Tollefsen, 2011, 54ff.). As to showing that *none* of us came into being at conception, the argument fails. For it is a logical fallacy to move from $\sim[(O1 = E) \,\&\, (O2 = E)]$ to $\sim[(O1 = E) \lor (O2 = E)]$. The intervening premise DeGrazia offers is really the conclusion of the argument (i.e., that the pre-twinned embryo is not individuated), but he does not supply the vinculum needed to establish that *neither* twin is identical to the parent zygote from the simple observation that *both* cannot be identical to it.

Some other comments are worth noting. First, in the many cases in which twinning does not occur, there is a strong intuition that one and the same organism develops beyond the 14-day point. We can identify it and point to it up to and through the 14-day point. DeGrazia wishes to argue, however, that the mere *possibility* of that one embryo dividing into O1 and O2 entails that the embryo is not an individual in the actual world (2005, 279ff.). DeGrazia has us consider a non-twin scenario with an adult human S and S's zygote Z in the actual world. He says,

> But that zygote [i.e., Z] could have split spontaneously, resulting in identical twins. If it had, presumably I [i.e., S] would not have existed, because it is implausible to identify me with either of the twins in that counterfactual scenario. If that is right . . . it follows that I am not numerically identical to that zygote.
>
> (DeGrazia, 2005, 248)

DeGrazia seems to be arguing as follows. Assume that S = Z. Now suppose that there exists a possible world W_i in which S has a twin.

DeGrazia supposes that in *that world*, it is not the case that S = Z. The necessity of identity, however, tells us that if S = Z, then necessarily, S = Z. Consequently, it follows that both ~(S = Z) and (S = Z). I share DeGrazia's sympathies with the necessity of identity. But this argument assumes that in W_i S is not identical to Z. As just argued above, the argument that S is not identical to Z involves a fallacy. At the very least, we cannot know whether S = Z in W_i.

What is more, the intuition that the organism maintains its identity in the non-twinning world cannot easily be ignored. To avoid the fallacy noted above, the proponent of the twinning argument would have to argue against the plausibility of asexual reproduction. But any argument for the implausibility of asexual reproduction must include premises whose intuitive plausibility overrides or outweighs the intuitive plausibility that in the non-twinning world the organism maintains its identity through development. None of the proponents surveyed here are successful in this regard.

These reflections apply equally to proponents of fusion. Cases of fusion are the mirror image of fission, in which two embryos fuse or coalesce early on at the morula or blastocyst stage of development resulting in one human being – they are called genetic chimeras, not to be confused with human–animal chimeras. One may have the intuition that prior to the possibility of fusion, there is no identifiable individual human organism. Two points are noteworthy in reply. First, the chimera results from the fusion of two distinct individuals: that's what makes it a chimera. When sodium is combined with chloride, one gets table salt; but sodium and chloride are individually identifiable prior to the fusion. Second, in cases in which fusion does not occur, the intuition is that two distinct organisms develop alongside each other. Cases of fusion are interesting but they do not challenge the individuality of the early human organism.

To conclude this sub-section, it may help to identify the loadbearing propositions. I have used the possibility of asexual reproduction as a riposte to the twinning argument. The proponent of the twinning argument would have to argue that organisms capable of asexual reproduction are not individuals or that the asexual-reproduction interpretation is false. The former way of saving the argument entails that every organism that can asexually reproduce is not an individual organism. But numerous organisms are capable of asexual reproduction at some point in their development and yet we consider such organisms *individual* organisms prior to the reproductive event (imagine brain fission cases, Parfit (1971, 4ff.), or cloning). It makes sense to ask what is *it* that reproduces? Any answer will refer to *an* organism of some sort. I am unaware of an argument for the second disjunct, but the prospects appear dim. Arguing against the asexual-reproduction interpretation must show not only that it is false, but that it *must* be false. The reason is as follows. Consider a possible world in which asexual reproduction occurs. In this world it is true that E = O2 for example (they are the same organism in that the asexual reproduction of O1 preserves the identity of the reproducer E →O2). So, assume ♦(E = O2). It follows from the necessity of identity[10] that ♦(E = O2). To defend the twinning argument then, the proponent needs to argue either that the necessity of identity is false or that it is not even possible for (E = O2). Both arguments would be tough to make out, and I am unaware of any plausible attempt to do so. There may be objections to the necessity of identity but it is used by proponents of the twinning argument (DeGrazia, 2005; Kuhse & Singer, 2009). Consequently, the proponent is saddled with the task of arguing that ~ ♦(E = O2). I conclude that there is nothing plausible about the twinning argument.[11]

The Totipotency Argument

Whereas the twinning argument aims to show that the pre-twinned embryo is not an individual human being in virtue of its divisibility, the argument from totipotency aims to argue for a similar conclusion based on slightly different empirical facts and ontological assumptions.[12] Both arguments argue that early human beings are not individuals; and both have a premise to the effect that the possibility of division precludes being an individual. But that premise is argued for on the basis of actual cases of twinning (which can take place up to 14 days), or by the totipotency of the cells (which is only characteristic of the zygote and morula, i.e., 5–7 days of development). Since twinning can take place after totipotency and the arguments are distinguished in terms of the empirical facts which putatively motivate a key premise, the two arguments are distinct.

As with the twinning argument, the totipotency argument begins with an empirical claim, namely, that the cells constituting the early embryo are each totipotent – each can form an individual human being. The second premise is some claim to the effect that being constituted by cells each of which can become an individual entails that the whole is not one organism but a cluster of collocated organisms or a heap. Whereas, for the twinning argument, the potential for divisibility blocks inferring that the pre-twinned embryo is an individual, the totipotency argument claims that the early embryo *is* a cluster of potential individuals. Another difference between the arguments is that the twinning argument focuses on the fact of twinning, whereas the totipotency argument depends on the nature of the cells that constitute the zygote and morula. The factual premises are distinct even if the conclusions and metaphysical premises are similar.

According to the totipotency argument, to be an individual organism one must be constituted by cells that are differentiated. Since the cells of the early embryo are undifferentiated, it cannot be an individual. Smith and Brogaard state the argument this way:

> At the stage of the multi-cellular zygote-bundle the zygote is most properly conceived of as a sticky assemblage of 8 or 16 entities rather than as a single entity. They are not one but many. Although they are surrounded by a thin permeable membrane, this membrane merely helps to keep the cells together in a spatial sense.
>
> (Smith & Brogaard, 2003, 60)

Each of the cells at this early stage is totipotent, meaning, roughly, that *each* can develop into a human being.[13] This seems to be why Smith and Brogaard say that the multi-cellular zygote is not one organism but many. They go so far as to say that the multi-cellular zygote "cannot even lay claim to the type of unity possessed by colonial organisms, such as certain forms of yeast, whose parts are connected via an exchange of fluids or signal molecules" (Smith & Brogaard, 2003, 60).

Helga Kuhse and Peter Singer endorse a similar argument, saying, "It is now believed that early embryonic cells are totipotent; that is . . . an early human embryo is not one particular individual, but rather has the potential to become one or more different individuals" (Kuhse & Singer, 2009, 342). The argument here refers to each cell's property of totipotency, and these cells constitute the multi-cellular embryo at an early stage of development. Kuhse and Singer (2009, 342) entertain what would happen if these cells were separated one from another. At the four-cell stage of human development, each of the cells is totipotent. Let's call the four-cell embryo Adam. Adam is constituted by cells A, B, C, and D. Suppose that the four cells are extracted and placed into distinct zonae pellucidae following which each has "the potential to develop into babies" (2009, 342). Call this scenario S1. After the extraction, we have Andy, Bill, Charles, and David. Kuhse and Singer conclude from this set-up that those who object to human embryo destructive research because it destroys an identifiable human being "would be on much safer ground were they to argue that a particular human life begins not at fertilization but at around day 14 after fertilization" (Kuhse & Singer, 2009, 343).

The totipotency argument appears to rest on one of two intuitions. It could rely on our intuitions regarding part–whole relations. A heap of undifferentiated cells whose role or function is not specified cannot be said to be a part of the whole. Parts are identified by their function vis-à-vis their contribution to the survival and growth of the whole; no differentiation suggests no function. This part–whole intuition as it is applied to early embryogenesis is inapposite. If totipotent cells were entirely undirected causes, generation of an individual would be an accident; but development is far too regular and ordered to be the result of chance (Henry, 2008, 48–49). Though totipotent cells are still undifferentiated when they separate into one of the three primary germ layers, one cannot conclude that they are without functions vis-à-vis the teleological development of the organism (Condic, 2013, 49ff.). A second intuition, invited by Kuhse and Singer's example of Adam, is that a thing which is constituted by potential individuals entails that the thing is not an individual.

The totipotency argument suffers from three main defects.[14] The early embryo is made up of either four actual individuals or four potential individuals. If they are four actual individuals then the totipotency argument cannot be used as a defense of embryo destructive research since doing so would kill four individuals at once. The totipotency argument must say that the four totipotent cells are each potential individuals. But that there are four potential individuals tells us nothing about the actual individuality of the early embryo. One can take each of my millions of cells and clone me. Each cell is potentially, in the same sense required by the totipotency argument, numerous individuals. But that hardly entails that I am not an individual.

A second defect is a misunderstanding of totipotency. Totipotency is a disposition like fragility. To say that a vase is fragile means that if it were dropped it would break apart (Contessa, 2013; Bonevac, Dever, & Sosa, 2011; Aimar, 2018).[15] But vases do not simply break apart willy-nilly without being in the conditions in which the disposition to break is actual. Totipotent cells are dispositions to form, by normal cell differentiation, whole organisms. Just as it is absurd to say that a vase is broken (when it clearly is not) simply on the basis that it has a disposition to break; so it is absurd to say that the four-cell embryo is really four individuals (or four cells that can enter into identity relations with individuals) simply on the basis that each cell has a disposition to form a human individual. Importantly, when the vase is broken it is no longer a vase. The vase has a disposition to *be* broken, but not to exist *as* broken. Likewise, when a totipotent cell comes to constitute a developing (and later, differentiating) human organism, it is no longer what it was, i.e., a totipotent *part*. Importantly, the totipotent cell does not survive long, but the organism it constitutes does. Understood as a disposition, the totipotent cell cannot be identical to an organism that develops from it since these are two different kinds of things. Having such a disposition is compatible with it being part of a whole.

The chief problem with the totipotency argument is the apparent inference from 'the embryo has the *potential* to develop into individuals' to 'the early embryo is *actually* not one human organism.' David Oderberg explains that,

> *potentiality is not actuality*. The potential of each cell in an embryo, early in its development, to become a distinct human individual is not the same as each cell's *being* a distinct human individual while it subserves the embryo of which it is a part.
>
> (Oderberg, 1997a, 280)

To avoid this modal fallacy, the proponent of the totipotency argument is forced to inject intervening premises such as 'the presence of totipotential cells impugns the *unity* sufficient to be an organism,' or 'it impugns the *coordinated activity* characteristic of an organism,' or 'it impugns the "unified causal interaction" (Smith and Brogaard, 2003, 49ff.) characteristic of individual organisms.' Whatever property the intervening premise points to as being absent, the claim remains that the mere potential to become an individual entails the actual absence of such properties. This just backs up the modal fallacy one more step. In what sense does the mere potential (of a cell) to form an individual entail the *actual* absence of whatever property the intervening premise references?

I conclude that the totipotency argument is either not an argument at all for the permissibility of embryo destructive research, since, on one understanding, it is an argument against the individuality of the morula, but not the cells constituting the morula; or it fails to understand totipotency as a mere disposition; or it commits a modal fallacy.

Rescue Cases

The next two arguments aim to rebut the claim that early human beings may not be killed because they have low moral status or worth. The conclusion of the arguments discussed in this section are that it is permissible to kill young human beings (even if they are living individuals) because they lack some feature of worth. The difference between the next two arguments and features of worth highlighted to justify abortion (e.g., interests) pertains to different moral intuitions: those concerning harm and those concerning saving. In relation to abortion, it is often argued that if a thing cannot be harmed (because it does not have interests or it does not yet exist), then no wrong can be occurring. But for the present issue, if a thing need not be *saved*, its moral status is diminished – even though that entity not only exists but may even have welfare interests. The arguments here aim to show that early human beings do not have moral status *sufficient to protect them from research harms*. As we shall see, the specific circumstances in which human embryos are stored, handled, and manipulated lend themselves to thought experiments which highlight our intuitions on who is worthy to be saved.

Suppose an IVF clinic catches fire. You have the choice to save a cryopreserved embryo or a six-year-old child. You only have time to save one. Which one do you choose? Most people would be inclined to save the child. Proponents of embryo destructive research then conclude that the embryo does not have the 'moral status' or 'moral worth' equal to that of a child, for otherwise we would not be so clearly inclined to save the child.

The case aims to justify an asymmetry between the moral worth of a child and the worth of a nascent human being. On closer inspection, such cases do not justify an asymmetry. There are important enthymemes in the argument which will emerge on inspection. The first premise is a statement of our intuitions on the rescue case:

4   Our intuitions tell us to save the child (all else being equal).
         To get the conclusion that the embryo lacks the same moral worth as the child, we need to import the following premise:
5   If our intuitions tell us to save the child instead of the embryo, then the embryo lacks the same moral worth as the child.
         From (4) and (5), it would follow that,
6   The embryo lacks the same moral worth as the child.
         Since the conclusion is that it is permissible to destroy the embryo for research purposes an additional premise is needed.
7   If an entity E (the embryo) does not have equal moral worth to another entity A (the child), then it is permissible to kill E for research purposes.
         Once (7) is made explicit, the proponent of the embryo rescue argument can draw the conclusion,
8   It is permissible to kill the embryo for research purposes (from (6) and (7)).

My own impression of this argument is that the premises on which it rests are clearly false. Premise (4) is a statement of fact about our intuitions regarding whom we would save (all else being equal). The argument appears valid, (6) and (8) follow from the stated premises. That leaves (5) and (7) open to dispute. Consider premise (5) for the moment.

This premise says that if our intuitions tell us to save x instead of y, then y does not have moral worth equal to x. Suppose, however, that x in this case is an embryo that is *yours*.[16] That is, suppose you and your spouse underwent an IVF procedure and the embryo you had the opportunity to save was your own. And next, suppose that instead of a child, you had the choice to save either your own embryo or someone else's embryo. Most of us in that situation would choose our own, hoping to have an opportunity to implant the embryo and subsequently rear our own child. But, given (5), your embryo has greater moral worth than the other embryos that are not your own. But this is an odd result, for if moral worth means anything, it must relate in some way to the embryo and not simply to your interests or desires or someone else's interests or desires. Therefore, the moral worth of the two embryos should be equal since they are similar, except for the fact that one is related to the rescuer and the other is not. Whom one chooses to save does not tell us much about the moral worth of the person who is not saved. This is no more apparent than in reasoning about pandemic-flu scenarios or any triage mechanism in the setting of scarce resources. Many state and hospital protocols concerning responses to a pandemic flu outbreak specify a triage or order of treatment preference.[17] But no one would say that those citizens that end up further down the list lack moral worth. These examples further undermine (5).

What about premise (7)? The important point is to observe that having an obligation to prevent the *suffering of the child* hardly entails that it is permissible *to kill an embryo*.[18] Likewise, an obligation not to kill an embryo is certainly consistent with having an obligation to prevent the unjust suffering of the child. Having unequal worth does not entail permission to kill the thing with lesser worth.

Of course, the way to avoid this inference is to explain one's intuitions outlined in (4) differently. One may explain such an intuition as being rooted in a belief that the embryo lacks moral worth because he or she lacks developmental maturity. On this story, the intuition outlined in (4) is based on a belief that one's moral worth increases as one develops. The problem with this story is that it recapitulates the *conclusion* drawn from the case. If one already believes that embryos lack moral worth compared with a further developed child, then the embryo rescue case can at best illustrate one's own beliefs, but not justify them.

Most of the critical points made so far coalesce around the same two ideas: x not having equal moral worth to y does not entail a permission to kill y (ad (7)); and preferring to save x instead of y does not entail either a diminution in worth or a permission to kill y (ad (5)).[19] The most the rescue argument shows is that it is permissible to forego saving the embryo given the exclusive choice between child and embryo with all else being equal. Not much else can be derived from it.

There is more to consider here in that another version of the embryo rescue case does not rely on the enthymemes outlined above. This second version is fleshed out in sufficient detail by Charles Hinckley II. I will call the example 'Sophie's choice' as it is a permutation of the popular case outlined in William Styron's eponymous novel. Styron tells the story of a Nazi soldier who captures a Polish woman Sophie and her two children. In an insidious exchange, the soldier demands that Sophie choose between the lives of her two children in that she has to choose which one is to be killed. If she refuses to choose, both will be killed. Of course, the point is that Sophie's choice between her children is a bitter one she initially refuses to make, but facing the death of both, she chooses her daughter with dire emotive consequences. The permutation Hinckley adds is that instead of choosing between one of her two children, she is given a choice between an embryo and her daughter. Hinckley observes, "If Sophie had to choose between one of her children and a blastocyst, embryo, or fetus, her choice ought to be much easier" (Hinckley, 2005, 129). The suggestion is that, if we agree, we are committed to the idea that the embryo bears lesser value. This latter version is what I will refer to as Sophie's choice.

Sophie's choice is a case where the choice is not whom to save, but whom one allows to be killed even if one does not intend this. The example works best assuming Sophie's complicity in the killing. The choice is easier when it is between the embryo and the mother's grade-school-aged daughter. This example purports to show that embryos do not bear moral worth sufficient to protect them from being killed. Hinckley concludes, "But we have reason to think the level of biological and cognitive development of embryos makes them expendable whereas children are not" (Hinckley, 2005, 130). The argument seems to be as follows:

9 We do not feel the same remorse or similar emotional state in response to the embryo being killed versus the daughter being killed.
10 Our having no remorse or similar emotive response to x being killed indicates that x does not have moral worth.
11 Therefore, the embryo does not have moral worth.

This argument rests on the fact that it would be 'easier' to make the choice. And this ease of conscience is taken to indicate that the embryo is 'expendable.' Though more interesting than the previous version of the rescue argument, I do not find it any more plausible.[20]

My first criticism is that there are clear counterexamples to (10):

I One life is lost in an earthquake on some obscure island in the South Pacific.

Our response to this is not remorse, or a similar emotional state, but may even be relief: we may say 'at least only one was killed.' Clearly, though, that one life has full moral worth in spite of our lackluster emotional response to the case.

It may be objected that (I) is not analogous to Sophie's choice because there is no act of killing on anyone's part, and no reference to a choice that is comparatively easier. This is not a plausible reply because it would seem to undermine the purpose of the embryo rescue case, which is to justify embryo destructive research.[21] Sophie's choice itself is not analogous to embryo destructive research where there is nothing comparable to a soldier threatening the lives of all of those closest to you (the disease/illness might be threatening, but the embryo certainly isn't). Any counterexample to (10) is permitted, then, so long as the disanalogies are not greater than the disanalogies between Sophie's choice and embryo destructive research. In any case, a more analogous case can be generated.

II A madman goes on a rampage in a mall in China but miraculously ends up killing only one person.

Here, there is deliberate killing by human agency, just as in Sophie's choice. Our emotive response to this case may be one of relief again: 'only one person was killed.' No remorse or similar emotive state is invoked in us, and yet we would all have to admit that this one *adult* person is a proper bearer of moral worth, even intrinsic moral worth.

These counterexamples aim only to show that our emotional response to some cases is not an accurate indicator of someone's moral worth because in many cases remorse or a similar emotive state is never invoked. Reflecting on these cases illustrates that our intuitions track not the intrinsic moral worth of the persons/objects involved, but rather our *attachment* to the persons/objects involved. Even so, we may consider a more analogous counterexample to (10),

III   A commandant offers Sophie a choice between two people: (i) her daughter or (ii) the Nazi soldier who arrested her, but who is scheduled to be killed by a firing squad because he later conscientiously objects.

This case is analogous in many respects to the original except that instead of Sophie's embryo and her daughter, the choice is between the man who arrested her and her daughter. Intuitively, Sophie has an 'easy choice' in (III) in the sense that her daughter is clearly more precious to her than the very soldier who arrested her. But granting this in no way defends the unjust killing of the conscientious objector or entails that he bears any less moral worth than her daughter.

There is, however, a disanalogy between Sophie's choice and case (III). (III) has us take the perspective of Sophie herself. Once we put ourselves in her shoes, it is obvious that we would not think twice about choosing to save our daughter. From *our* perspective, however, we can empathize with the soldier's plight in being unjustly killed, since he is trying to escape the Nazi system and not be part of its atrocities. We would still choose to save the daughter, but the choice would not be as easy as Sophie's choice to save her daughter. But this disanalogy is a backhanded confirmation that our intuitive responses to the cases suggest that our intuitions track our social attachments, and not someone's intrinsic moral worth.

The basic lesson learned from this critique is that the arguments infer from whom we choose to save (or allow to be killed in a tragic dilemma) a conclusion as to whom we may intentionally kill for research purposes. But our basic moral obligations governing whom we save are certainly different from our moral obligations not to kill. Inferring from our intuitions on such cases to the case of embryo-destructive research commits a categorical error and, therefore, the arguments are invalid. Moreover, in tragic dilemmas, it is unclear what our moral obligations are at all.

Concluding this sub-section, I have argued against a widely utilized argument for there being a moral asymmetry (sufficient to justify killing) between the worth of a born person and an incipient human being. The arguments constructed from rescue cases fail to show either that human embryos lack moral worth, or that, even if they did, such a diminution in worth would be a sufficient reason to permit killing them for research purposes.

Natural Loss Arguments

The basic structure of natural loss arguments is to point to commonly known facts about how embryos can die due to natural causes. But if embryos matter morally, then incidences of natural loss should be considered tragic, and health care resources should be devoted to preventing such loss. But no one, not even pro-lifers, thinks this. Therefore the embryo does not matter morally. To my knowledge there are two main academic versions of this argument, one from Toby Ord (2008) and another from Jeff McMahan (2007). I consider McMahan for two reasons: Ord's argument has already been subjected to criticisms,[22] and McMahan's argument seems to be more intuitively persuasive. I will explain why after presenting his case.

McMahan begins his argument with a description of twinning. He then moves to the conclusion that in the typical case, twinning results in the 'parent' embryo dying:

> What the phenomenon of twinning shows is that some of us begin to exist at a different time and in a different way. Monozygotic twins, on this view, begin to exist not at conception but when an embryo divides . . . [W]hen an embryo divides to form twins, if the division is symmetrical, the original embryo also ceases to exist.
>
> (McMahan, 2007, 177)

McMahan concludes,

> when symmetrical twinning occurs and an embryo ceases to exist, this should be tragic. . . . [W]e should ensure that all instances of twinning are asymmetrical division [take place at different times], so that no one ceases to exist. But these suggestions are absurd.
>
> (McMahan, 2007, 178)

The conclusion of the argument is that the embryo does not matter as you and I do. Properly understood, this is not a version of the twinning argument that concludes that the pre-twinned embryo is not an individual. McMahan's presentation of the twinning argument aims to show that the pre-twinned embryo has little moral worth.[23] If the embryo dies in cases of twinning, we should mourn the fact that there are twins. But we do not, much less do we think that such events ought to be prevented from happening and that health care resources should be devoted to preventing twinning.

This argument has more purchase than Ord's presentation since McMahan's argument only requires us to admit that twinning is something that we need not stop or try to prevent through health care resources. This is an intuitively plausible concession; twinning is not something we *ought* to stop. In contrast, Ord's argument requires us to accept that health care resources need not be devoted to preventing spontaneous abortions (this is what we need to accept to find his 'conclusion' absurd). The problem is that many of us do not accept that claim, and, factually speaking, there are important resources devoted to prevent spontaneous abortion (Marino, 2008, 26).

There are two routes by which one could attack this natural loss argument. The first is to resist the conclusion that the embryo dies. The second is to accept the interpretation that the embryo dies, but resist the moral lesson McMahan would have us learn from it. I have already critiqued twinning arguments above. Interpreting twinning as a case in which the originating embryo dies requires assuming that a necessary condition for survival is the existence of an ostensible closest continuer.[24] Such a view is problematic for a number of reasons (Hawley, 2005; Wiggins, 2001, 57ff.), the chief of which is that it violates the 'only a and b' rule. David Wiggins states the idea this way:

> In notionally pursuing object a in order to ascertain its coincidence or non-coincidence with b, or in retracing the past history of b to ascertain its identity link with a, I ought not to need to concern myself with things that are other than a or other than b . . . But the identity of a with a, of b with b, and of a with b, once we are clear which things a and b are, ought to be a matter strictly between a and b themselves.
>
> (Wiggins, 2001, 96)

The basic idea is that whether or not a is identical to b depends on what a and b are and the relevant relations between *them*. Katherine Hawley further observes that there is "something especially objectionable about making identity through time contingent upon the (non) existence of a rival" (Hawley, 2005, 605). Therefore, I focus my comments on the moral lesson McMahan intends.

First, the premise of the argument against human embryo destructive research is that nascent human beings are vulnerable human subjects (Napier, 2009) with, at least, a modicum of moral 'status' or 'value' that protects them from being intentionally killed as part of scientific research. Human beings in the context of research enjoy an initial stance of protection according to which the researcher must justify why she wants or needs to conduct this research (Jonas, 1969, 245; Emanuel, Wendler, & Grady, 2000). McMahan's moral lesson though is that we would have an obligation *to save* the pre-twinned embryo if it matters "in the way you and I do." Properly understood, my argument aims only to show that the embryo may not be killed as part of a research project, because he or she is vulnerable. An obligation to save, however, may require more in terms of moral worth or status (i.e., for those who view human beings as having unequal status) and at any rate, it will require opportune circumstances. I cannot be expected to save a drowning victim if I am wheelchair-bound. While there may not be an obligation to save everyone, there is an obligation not to kill anyone. We have an obligation not to kill embryos in virtue of the vulnerability they have qua research subjects. As such, I think that the embryo 'matters in *similar ways* as you and I do' to the extent that neither embryos nor adult persons may be killed as research subjects. Because of the limited scope of my argument against killing nascent human beings for research purposes, a proponent of it can be unperturbed by the fact that the embryo dies in the course of a natural and quite uncommon event.

Furthermore, even if twinning involves the demise of the parent zygote who matters in the way you and I do, it does not follow that this is 'tragic;' nor does it ground a 'serious moral reason' to try to stop twinning from occurring. Twinning is a natural event that is rare. It is not known what causes twinning; much less could it be reliably predicted in each individual case. What kind of monitoring device would be used to predict twinning? How could such predictions be empirically grounded given the size of the zygote, its location, and the complex internal workings of the zygote which may generate twinning? The point is that a serious moral reason to prevent the death of X may not exist even if X matters "like you and I do." Consider the use of proportionate or disproportionate means of sustaining life (Panicola et al., 2011, 277ff.). Such means are not morally required even if they forestall death, and even if the patient is the proper bearer of moral worth. Devoting health care resources to a rare and largely inscrutable event is not a just allocation of those resources, given other pressing needs for such resources, even if the pre-twinned embryo matters "like you and I do."

Perhaps McMahan intends by the use of the term 'tragic' that we ought to mourn or be horrified upon discovering that twinning has occurred. But this does not follow either in that mourning makes sense when it is a loved one who dies, someone for whom we have built up an emotional bond. But a pre-twinned embryo does not enjoy such bonds with others except perhaps for particular situations such as IVF where parents are aware of their embryos' existence, very much wanted them to live, and can indeed mourn their deaths. We should expect, then, that our emotive response to a pre-twinned embryo dying will normally be less even if he or she matters as a vulnerable human subject who ought not to be killed.

The Argument from Epistemic Diffidence

Indexing the Burden of Proof

The structure of the argument is like that outlined in the previous chapter. Moral risk indexes the burden of proof. Specifying what the moral risks are gives us a sense of whether the risks are asymmetrical or not. So in this section I outline the respective risks. For simplicity and coherence, (p) represents the proposition that it is permissible to destroy human beings at the embryonic stage of life *for research purposes* – thus distinguishing it from the abortion issue. Not-(p) will simply be the claim that such an action is not permissible.

As with the abortion issue, if a researcher believes (p) and is wrong, then that researcher would be destroying nascent human life. The putative justification that the embryo will die anyway does not avoid this cost. Many patients in the ICU will die anyway, but it would still not be justifiable to kill them for research purposes (hereafter, every instance of 'killing' is understood as for research purposes unless otherwise noted). The 'they will die anyway' argument only works if one implicitly assumes that nascent human beings have little moral status. Assuming that they do have moral status, the argument becomes inert.

What are the costs in being wrong that not-(p)? The answer requires specifying what the benefits are in the setting of alternative ways to procure those same benefits without killing. As remarked in the introduction to this chapter, the benefits are clinical effectiveness in regenerating organ function. There are many sources of pluripotent stem cells, however, which can be utilized to realize these benefits that do not involve intentionally destroying nascent human beings. Blastomeres are already removed from human embryos in the setting of preimplantation genetic diagnosis (PGD) – though in saying this, I do not endorse PGD for a number of reasons separate from issues of killing. Presumably, individual cells at the blastocyst stage of human development could be extracted without significant risk or harm to the human being, and the cells would be pluripotent stem cells. Human embryos in IVF clinics that are thawed and are organismically dead might have viable individual stem cells remaining.[25] In a process called altered nuclear transfer, one might do what would otherwise amount to cloning a human being but modify the nucleus prior to insertion into the mitochondria such that a headless entity would be developed (Mosteller, 2005). Stem cells from hydatidiform moles would not involve the destruction of the human being since such moles are better described as clusters of human tissue but not a human organism. Again, stem cells from miscarried embryos/fetuses and human embryos removed by salpingectomy for ethically legitimate reasons (e.g., resolving an ectopic pregnancy) would yield pluripotent stem cells without the intentional destruction of those human beings. Certain sources of stem cells in the developed adult body show pluripotent characteristics as well, as do umbilical cord blood stem cells (Chen et al., 2001; Carlin et al., 2006; Xiao et al., 2005). Final mention should be made of induced pluripotent stem cells (iPSCs), though this list is not exhaustive (Kwak et al., 2018). Not all would agree that all of these options are morally acceptable, but certainly some are, and some are in clinical use.

Since there is not much appeal in extending the functionality of one's bodily organs without also regenerating brain function if one suffers from severe dementia, one of the more important aspects of regenerative medicine is finding sources of stem cells that are able to differentiate into neural tissue. Sources of multipotent neurological cells (Martinez-Morales et al., 2013) include neural crest stem cells (from human hair/ teeth), olfactory cells (Murrell et al., 2005), and adult dental pulp stem cells (Arthur et al., 2008; Kiraly et al., 2009). Mesenchymal stem cells from bone marrow (Crain, Tran, & Mezey, 2005; Jiang et al., 2002), adipose tissue (Sun et al., 2009),[26] and umbilical cord blood show pluripotent properties. Cells from these 'adult' sources demonstrate abilities to differentiate into neural cells and have been used successfully in stroke patients (Chen et al., 2001; Tang et al., 2007). Neural stem cells exist in the adult brain, particularly in the sub-granular and sub-ventrical regions (Gage, 2000). Finally, ventral mesoencephalic stem cells for the treatment of Parkinson's (Kim & de Vellis, 2009) can be derived from fetuses without intentionally killing them in cases of spontaneous abortions, or salpingectomies to resolve ectopic pregnancies, etc. (Ishii & Eto, 2014).

What about the potential for clinical effectiveness? The iPSCs and multipotent adult-derived stem cells largely bypass immune rejection issues (Condic & Rao, 2010, 1124) because they are considered autologous (from the patient's own body) stem cell sources.[27] Furthermore, autologous hematopoietic stem cells are "standard practice" (Rao, Ahrlund-Richter, & Kaufman, 2012, 55) for a variety of hematologic disorders, thus undercutting a significant need to explore other types of cell transplantation therapies. Of the trials listed on Clinicaltrials.gov that involve stem cell transplantation "all . . . were dominated by use of adult SCs [stem cells], primarily hematopoietic SCs, with some trials using umbilical cord blood derived SCs. There were an increasing number of trials using mesenchymal stem cells (MSCs) from 2007" (Bubela et al., 2012, 138). Bubela et al. go on to note that "[n]ewspaper articles focused mainly on human embryonic SCs and neurological conditions . . ." (Bubela et al., 2012, 5) inferring that the promise the media presented to the public about embryonic derived stem cell sources was significantly inflated. All in all, clinically usable stem cells are almost entirely from non-destructive sources. And since there exist sources of pluripotent stem cells that do not suffer from immune rejection issues (iPSCs) and can be modified without genetic change (Warren et al., 2010), there is no clinical reason for thinking that barring human destructive research would at all compromise the development of regenerative therapies.

What are the moral costs in being wrong about (p)? Answering this question requires specifying the source of wrongdoing. One could object to scientific research because it is not valuable (Emanuel, Wendler, & Grady, 2000). In explaining value, Emanuel, Wendler, and Grady note that non-valuable research would be research that has "non-generalizable results, a trifling hypothesis, or substantial or total overlap with proven results" (Emanuel, Wendler, & Grady, 2000, 2703). If human embryonic stem cell research were to be translated into the clinic, the cellular transplantation would be allographic and would be subject to typical immune rejection issues; whereas using the patient's own cells, as with adult sources or via direct reprogramming, is theoretically more relevant for transplantation (and, indeed, this happens already). As such one could argue that human destructive stem cell research is not scientifically valuable in that other more stable and 'proven results' exist. Bonnie Steinbock (2005, 26) appears to endorse the same idea saying, "if it were easy to come up with an alternative source of ES [embryonic stem] cells, there would be no question that this should be done." If we understand her conditional to require the creation of pluripotent stem cells – embryonic stem cells are not necessary – then we have numerous alternatives already, as canvassed above. Furthermore, the National Bioethics Advisory Commission (NBAC) says that human embryo destructive research "*is justifiable only if no less morally problematic alternatives are available for advancing the research*" (NBAC, 1999, 53, emphasis original).

   The other moral costs to being wrong about (p) can simply be that human destructive stem cell research involves the destruction of nascent human beings for research purposes, where such research also holds out little hope of benefiting people more than what is available already. The burden of proof is entirely on the side of defending (p).

The Argument from Epistemic Diffidence

The Preface introduced the bare outline of the argument that is duplicated in most every chapter of this volume. Starting at the very top of the dialectic we can substitute for (p) the belief that human embryo destructive research is permissible.

12   Belief (p) is subject to epistemic diffidence.
13   If belief (p) is subject to epistemic diffidence, it should not be acted upon.
14   Therefore, (p) should not be acted upon.

The defense of premise (12) is that none of the arguments typically offered for the permissibility of such research meets the burden of proof. Arguments for either the no-individual or the non-valuable conclusions suffered from severe defects. To take only one example, at best, twinning arguments have to say that we do not know which one of the continuers is the same individual as the original embryo. Given that the burden of proof is on the proponent of destructive research, an argument from ignorance is insufficient. Each of the four arguments can be thought of as a justification J for (p). Descending down the dialectic, we discover sub-justifications for J; for example, to make valid the totipotency argument, one must understand a totipotent cell as a potential individual. But understanding totipotency as a dispositional power undercuts claims that the cell is identical in kind to the individual to which it may give rise. A vase is able to be broken, but it goes out of existence when it is broken. If a totipotent cell were to develop and differentiate qua separate organism, it would go out of existence (Burke, 1996). Claims, then, that totipotent cell B can be identical to a human being in some possible world misunderstand what totipotency is. So, to defend the totipotency argument, one would have to understand totipotency *not* as a dispositional property. But that would be arbitrary and would depart from a common-sensical understanding of the term. Since the proposition 'totipotency is not a dispositional property' is being used to defend the totipotency argument, which is used to defend acting on (p), it is a load-bearing proposition the justification of which hardly meets the burden of proof. Because there exist viable alternatives to human destructive research, and the arguments I have canvassed here prove tenuous or fallacious, belief in (p) should not be acted upon.

Notes

1 Stem cells can also be distinguished in terms of their potential to become other cells. The normal pathway to cellular differentiation is: totipotent ⇨ pluripotent ⇨ multipotent ⇨ fully differentiated. A totipotent stem cell is a cell capable of becoming any cell in the body, or of becoming a new individual of that species. A pluripotent stem cell is a cell capable of becoming any tissue or organ within specific organ systems of the body. A multipotent stem cell is a cell within an organ system capable of becoming any tissue or organ within that system. Fully differentiated cells are the cells that form the specific tissues and organs of our body; these are the cells that actually carry out the metabolism of the body. Only the cells of the zygote and morula are totipotent. The cells of the blastocyst and gastrula are pluripotent (the trophoblast and inner cell mass of the blastocyst, and the three primary germ layers of the gastrula). Then, from these three germ layers (ectoderm, mesoderm, and endoderm), all the organ systems of the body will form (multipotent cells). Multipotent cells can differentiate into cell types within the cells' generic kind, e.g., mesenchymal stem cells can differentiate into heart tissue or blood cells but not liver tissue which is endodermal.
2 See the dated but relevant analysis of alternatives (President's Council on Bioethics, 2005) and an updated commentary (Condic & Rao, 2010).
3 Adult stem cell research is an erroneous designation because umbilical cord blood stem cells have been used to treat various diseases, and fetal stem cells from miscarriage do not involve an intentional killing but can be used to treat various diseases as well.
4 I do not think that such an action is permissible. My aim is merely to show the independence of the research ethics issue.
5 For the Nazi experiments, an additional source of dehumanization was, of course, Nazi ideology itself. See Vetlesen (1994).
6 For more clarifications, see Napier (2016, 79).
7 Nozick's use of the example is slightly different than the one I make here. His use is to motivate discussion of the closest continuer theory.

8 I owe this example to Helen Watt.

9 This explanation was first posed to me in conversation by Rev. Alfred Cioffi PhD (Genetics) – per request.

10 (x) (y) [(x = y) → □ (x = y)]. A proof of this is offered by David Wiggins (2001, 114–116). See also, Wiggins (1974, 343ff.) Following Wiggins in this regard, E and O2 (and O1) refer to members of a substance-sortal, in this case, human being. Thus, E = O2 is simply saying that E and O2 are the same human being considered at t1 and t2 respectively.

11 For more see the exchange between Oderberg (2008b), Persson (2009), and Oderberg (unpublished).

12 Since my chief goal is to articulate the argument from epistemic diffidence I proceed in a summary fashion here. For more detailed discussion of both twinning and totipotency arguments, see Oderberg (1997a), George and Tollefsen (2011), and Napier (2010).

13 Another interpretation of Smith and Brogaard is that they think that the multi-cellular zygote is not one organism not because of totipotency, but because of the non-differentiated character of the cells that constitute the zygote. This interpretation may or may not be correct, and I think my criticisms below are apt even allowing for this distinction. But I would caution against this interpretation anyway. The standard definitions of totipotency make essential reference to non-differentiation. *Merriam-Webster* defines totipotent as "capable of developing into a complete organism or differentiating into any of its cells or tissues," *Merriam-Webster Online Dictionary* 11th ed., s.v. "Totipotent." Available at: www.merriam-webster.com/dictionary/totipotency (accessed April 15, 2010). Consequently, the non-differentiated character of the cells cannot be considered a problem separate from them being totipotent.

14 One defect not discussed here is the description of the early embryo as a mere cluster (Smith & Brogaard, 2003, 55). For a more accurate description, consult Condic (2008, 2013). If the early embryo were *merely* a collection of totipotent cells with no communication and coordination of activity, it is a sheer miracle that only one human being develops in most cases. Advocates of the totipotency argument owe us an explanation as to why a mere cluster of cells consistently and almost invariably develops into one human being without prior coordination and communication. Their argument could be understood to involve the claim that the coordination is not *enough* to be considered an organism. As Condic points out, however, the coordination is teleologically ordered in that the organism is preparing for developmental events that occur later and these events are crucial for the growth and survival of the organism. (See, for example, Condic's discussion of meiosis, 2008, 3ff., and fns 14 and 26).

15 Simona Aimar (2018, 3–5) proposes a possibility view which departs from the simple counterfactual account I endorse in the text. For the possibility view, X is fragile if and only if there is a possible world in which X breaks. I do not find this view plausible enough to supplant the more commonsensical counterfactual view. When I say that Bill is irascible, I mean more than that in some possible world Bill gets angry. I mean to say that Bill has a tendency to get angry – he gets angry easily in this or that circumstance. The possibility view does not capture this meaning. Furthermore, the possibility view does not appear informative since it does not distinguish commonsensical differences. I might say that a class A chess player and a master level player have a disposition to defeat a grandmaster on Aimar's account since, in some possible world, either scenario obtains. But clearly, I do not mean merely that in some possible world or other a master level player defeats a grandmaster

player. The distinction is more than the frequency of possible worlds in which the master beats the grandmaster for it is the likeness of ability that explains the increased frequency. Lastly, the possibility view does not account for some teleological orientations that are towards very unlikely events (e.g., each sperm is very unlikely to fertilize an ovum; nonetheless, that is what sperm are for). It appears that on the possibility view, each sperm does not have the disposition to fertilize since it would fertilize in only a few possible worlds.

16 I owe this counterexample to Matthew Liao (2006, 142) but I draw different conclusions from it.

17 See, for example, State of Tennessee Department of Health *Pandemic Influenza Response Plan: April 2009.* Available at: http://health.state.tn.us/CEDS/PDFs/2006_PanFlu_Plan.pdf, 143ff.

18 Here I might be conceding too much. I do not think that one is obligated to save the child, but it is certainly permissible to prefer the child over the embryo. If the embryo is my own, implantation and gestation is *guaranteed*, and normal development is certain, etc., I am inclined to think that I am permitted to save my own embryonic child. My intuitions here are not unorthodox either, since they show up in triage discussions when, for instance, triage protocols favor those patients that stand the best chance of surviving the longest (White et al., 2009). In any case, no one concludes that those who are in a more serious condition may be intentionally killed for research purposes.

19 Sandel (2005) is sensitive to the idea that the embryo need not be equal in moral worth to the child in order to be a proper object of respect or "awe." Sandel fails, however, to explain how the rescue case suggests that the embryo may be killed for research purposes and how this is consistent with the embryo being a proper object of respect and awe.

20 One might see similar intuitions highlighted by McMahan's frozen child case (2007) but with a few differences. McMahan supposes that if we were to come across a civilization in which they had frozen their children, we would make the sacrifices required to unfreeze them and raise them. The fact that we don't do that for human beings frozen in IVF clinics indicates the lower moral status we think they have compared with children. In reply, there are people who adopt human beings from IVF clinics – though the practice is controversial for reasons independent of moral status. Furthermore, there is an implicit inference being made by McMahan in drawing out the lessons of the frozen child case. I think that all Iraqi citizens have equal inherent dignity and that their country should not be invaded. But I did not have an obligation to ward off the United States' military actions in 2002. Prisoners have inherent dignity and I believe they should not be killed, but I do not thereby have an obligation to save someone from death row. Obligations to save are context specific, such that the absence of an obligation to save S can be compatible with S having full moral status. Saving nearly 500K frozen embryos is a practically impossible task, and moreover, many of those who believe the embryos have full moral status would see the genetic mother as the only person with the moral right or duty to gestate them (Watt, 2006).

21 Researchers using human embryonic-derived stem cells often use them from existing cell lines. The argument I endorse in this chapter is limited to the conclusion that no new lines should be created. An argument that one is appropriating evil (Kaveny, 2000) is the only but plausible prospect for arguing against all use of human embryonic-derived stem cells.

22 See the articles following Ord's article on the same issue, especially Sarah-Vaughan Brakman (2008) and Dodson, Toth-Fejel, and Stangebye (2008).

23 McMahan explicitly rejects the typical conclusion drawn from the twinning argument saying that the fact an embryo can undergo division "is no reason

to think that it is not a unique individual. It is no reason to think that an ameba is not an individual ameba, that it can divide, or that any other cell is not a unique individual object because it can undergo fission" (McMahan, 2007, 177).

24 For a discussion see Parfit (1971); Nozick (1981, 29–70); Noonan (1985); Shoemaker (1984).

25 Here too, I do not endorse the use of such sources for a number of reasons. The embryos here would die 'naturally' only as a result of being treated inhumanely by freezing them. Moreover, it is too easy to justify *deliberately* thawing them so that they die; and if they are viable, they would have to be transferred to a mother. For more discussion see President's Commission on Bioethics (2005).

26 The reference here is to adipose cells being reprogrammed into a pluripotent state and thus are better classified as iPSCs. However, this deserves separate mention because cells from adipose tissue are more easily reprogrammed than somatic cells – though they might also count as 'somatic' insofar as they are cells easily accessible in the human body. Further, the reprogramming was done in the absence of a feeder culture, thus bypassing likely sources of contamination.

27 For cells sourced from an adult, this is not a controversial claim. For iPSCs, there is some debate (Zhao et al., 2011; Okita, Nagata, & Yamanaka, 2011; Condic & Rao, 2010). Whereas all pluripotent stem cells can form teratomas when transplanted, this effect is lessened when differentiation of the cells is done prior to transplant (Okita et al., 2011). Furthermore, the teratomas formed from iPSCs are typically less complex than those formed from embryo-derived stem cells (Condic & Rao, 2010, 1123).

8 Euthanasia

For the previous two issues discussed, the personhood of that which is killed (Warren, 1973, 1992) is one key issue. For the euthanasia debates, however, the personhood of those killed by voluntary euthanasia is not in question. Even some candidates for non-voluntary euthanasia, such as infants and the demented elderly, are persons on McMahan's (2002) and Baker's (2000) accounts. Furthermore, numerous moral traditions tolerate very narrow criteria for permissibly killing persons such as killing in self-defense, just war, or an insane gunman – all of which involve an aggressor.[1] Yet those killed by euthanasia are not threatening the lives of others so the justification for killing someone in self-defense, etc., is not applicable. These two opening observations suggest that the issue of euthanasia is whether it is permissible intentionally to kill someone who is not threatening the life of another (hereafter, the innocent).

The issue is whether the scope of permissible killing extends beyond only killing those who are unjust aggressors. Whatever that argument may be, it cannot entail that killing an innocent patient is obligatory. The reason why is because we have the intuition that physicians may conscientiously object to participation in euthanasia. As such euthanasia proponents (e.g., Young, 2018) argue that euthanasia is permissible but not obligatory. So, whatever it is that makes euthanasia permissible, it cannot be that a patient has a *claim* right[2] to it, but a right that others not intentionally interfere with one's choice.

If euthanasia is permissible, the killing involved might count as an *exception* to the prima facie prohibition against killing innocent persons. Understood as an exception to a right not to be killed (like Feinberg's notion of waiving my rights (1978, 114ff.)), the issue of euthanasia is whether there are reasons sufficiently weighty to offset the prima facie prohibition on killing innocent persons. Are there good reasons for the exception (hereafter, I refer to this simply as 'the exception')?[3]

The format of this chapter is different from the previous ones in that the argument from epistemic diffidence spans the entire chapter. Crucial premises in that argument are motivated along the way, particularly in defining the issue. The next section canvases the requisite definitions such as means, ends, intentions, etc. In the third section I aim to define the issue and comment briefly on what values can be presumed at the front end of the discourse. The fourth section outlines the relevant arguments. And the fifth section critically evaluates the arguments for an exception.

Definitions and Clarifications[4]

Euthanasia is the intentional killing of a patient by a health care professional because death is thought to benefit the patient.[5] Euthanasia is distinguished from murder in so far as death in the former case is thought to benefit or be good for the patient. Even involuntary euthanasia will be a case where death is thought to be in the objective interests of the patient, and therefore does not necessarily count as murder.

Passive and Active

Euthanasia is typically divided into passive and active to distinguish between how the doctor accomplishes the end of killing the patient. For passive euthanasia, a doctor intends to have a patient die by withholding or withdrawing a means of sustaining the patient's life. If the patient lives after withdrawing treatment, such as a respirator, the doctor's action plan is considered unsuccessful. For active euthanasia, a doctor intends to have a patient die by injecting lethal drugs, typically those that cause cardiac cessation. For both passive and active, the intention is the same, i.e., the death of the patient. The aim/target/plan is to render the patient dead.

Intention, Means, Side Effects

It is important to be clear that, by intention, I mean one's reason for acting (Shaw, 2006, 2015), which includes one's beliefs about the goodness of a certain state of affairs and the means to achieve it. But intention also specifies that towards which one's will is oriented. I may have any number of reasons for acting in any number of ways. But doing *this* action on *this* occasion involves a reason for doing so and my "will is set on achieving it" (Pilsner, 2006, 12). Intention includes both an intellectual and volitional component. As part of the intellectual component, it includes both one's *chosen* means and end.[6] Intention is one's plan of action that requires beliefs about cause–effect relations (i.e., that this means brings about this end) and what states of affairs are good – one sets out to obtain an end one apprehends as good. At the same time, intentions should be distinguished from cause–effect relations themselves, from what an agent may know, and from the agent's desires and motivations (Pellegrino, 1996). Lastly, chosen means should be distinguished from accepted or tolerated side effects. I explain such distinctions presently.

If I pound a nail I am bringing about two states of affairs: making a noise and securing two objects. I cause both, but only intend the latter. I may know that both effects will occur, but I intend only one of them. The next two examples illustrate how desire and intention are distinguished. If I have a social phobia, I may not desire to be around crowds of people, but I would intend to do so as part of what I believe is beneficial psychotherapy. I may desire to watch lowbrow television programming in the evening, but instead I intend to read and study for an upcoming exam. The action I do in cases of conflicting desires must be intended.[7] With regard to the distinction between intention and motivation (Masek, 2009), one's actions may be motivated out of fear, altruism, and hatred, etc., but the actions partly informed by such motivations may include lying, stealing, and murder. Intentions partly specify or define *actions*; fear, hatred, and altruism are species of *motivations*. Hatred, for example, is not an action, but murder is. Murder is an act of intending someone's death to deprive the victim of a good (i.e., life). Explaining why I have the intentions I have may involve appeal to one's motivations. But the explanans and explanandum cannot be conflated.

Lastly, one's chosen means cannot overlap with accepted or tolerated side effects. Suppose I stand to earn a lot of money from my uncle Charlie's life insurance policy. In one scenario I choose to kill him in order to obtain that money; in another scenario I do not intend his death but he dies of natural causes and I inherit the money. In the first case his death is a means to my intended end, but in the second it is clearly not a chosen means. (Strictly speaking, it is not a side effect either since it is not an effect of my actions.) Suppose I have cancer and ingest chemotherapy which causes both the destruction of cancer cells and hyperemesis. Hyperemesis is a side effect of my action plan even if it occurs before my healing. Side effects are those effects of my actions that occur outside of what I specifically intend. The spatial metaphor of 'outside' is meant to capture the idea of aiming at states of affairs I apprehend as good. Side effects might be accepted, tolerated, or downright repudiated, but in neither of these options do I intend a side effect. This is not to say that I cannot be held morally responsible for any evil side effects of my actions. A scientific researcher doing a phase I first-in-human trial might intend to find a cure for a rare disease and choose appropriate means for doing so, but because of negligence in reviewing preclinical evidence she can be held morally responsible for serious adverse events that were not intended.

Even so, there are very good reasons to believe that intentions figure prominently in a moral analysis. Garcia (1997, 171ff.) observes that the applicability of terms in our moral vocabulary such as 'lie,' 'rape,' or 'kidnap,' require that the agent has certain intentions such as to deceive, to coerce, etc. Intentions partly fix what moral action-types there are. More importantly, intentions matter morally because they are a "form of morally significant favoring, a form of response to something – such as life or death – that has positive or negative value" (Garcia, 1997, 174). Similarly, Lynn A. Jansen (2010) comments that since intentions are one's reasons for acting, they infuse one's actions with reason. The intentions of an agent "condition the meaning of his action . . . The reason that guides his action conditions the meaning of what he does . . . And the meaning of his action, both to himself and to others, is an ethically significant factor in assessing his conduct" (Jansen, 2010, 28).

Dworkin et al. (2013) appear to agree when they say

> it is morally permissible for a doctor to deny an organ to one patient, even though he will die without it . . . But it is certainly not permissible for a doctor to kill one patient in order to use his organs to save another.
>
> (Dworkin et al., 2013, 664)

They go on to observe correctly that the distinction here is not between act and omission. Given Garcia's and Jansen's reflections, the reason is that the second doctor takes a stance against the worth of the person. Dworkin et al., however, locate the difference in whether the patient wants to be killed. They say "[w]hen a competent patient does want to die, the moral situation is obviously different" (Dworkin et al., 2013, 665). The Meiwes-Brandes case – discussed in more detail in Chapter 10 – rebuts the plausibility of this claim. Armin Meiwes posted an advertisement on a website devoted to cannibalism that said he was looking for someone to slaughter and be consumed. A few months later Bernd Brandes consented to being slaughtered and eaten. Jonathan Haidt comments on this case that "if your moral matrix is limited to the ethic of autonomy, you're at high risk of being dumbfounded by this case" (Haidt, 2012, 146). If our commitment to the value of autonomy is *exclusive*, we have no grounds for opposing Meiwes's actions. Our opposition to consensual slavery, slaughter, or cannibalism cannot be chalked up to "squeamishness" (Brandt, 1975, 110) or conservative alimentary restrictions, but to the fact that someone intentionally destroyed someone's life.

The chief reason for thinking that intentions figure prominently in a moral analysis is that they fix what our response to a good is. If I intend to speak falsely, that flags how little I value knowledge for the person to whom I lie. If I intend to save another person's life (knowing certain risks in doing so to my own life), that flags how much I value that person's life. Intentions signal how I value certain states of affairs. So, if I were to intend someone's death, that intention signals how much I value that person's existence. In lying, I am setting out to keep my hearer from acquiring knowledge. But if knowledge is a good thing for my hearer to have, I am doing something wrong by lying – likewise for intending death. Because intention involves an intellectual and volitional component, intending death entails taking a stance against another's existence – I must will the person's non-existence. If it turns out that the patient's life is intrinsically worthwhile, setting out to destroy it would be doing something wrong. Having such an intention signals a disordered will and false apprehension of the true worth at stake.[8]

Finally, intentions are morally important because we can control them, but we cannot necessarily control every foreseen side effect of our actions. John Keown notes that "we can always avoid intending bad consequences, [but] we cannot always avoid foreseeably bringing them about" (Jackson & Keown, 2012, 105). Since we should be held morally responsible only for what we can control (Fischer & Ravizza, 1998), intentions index that for which we are morally responsible.

Understood as both involving an intention that the patient be dead, passive and active euthanasia are identical in this respect. Hence, much of the discussion on euthanasia – which assesses whether a moral distinction between active and passive euthanasia exists (Foot, 1967; Rachels, 1986) – is misguided. Suppose I intend to kill uncle Charlie for his inheritance. Upon entering his house I notice that he is drowning in his bathtub. I do nothing. I have intended an omission, and my omission is subject to moral appraisal. Christopher Tollefsen comments that,

> when I see my rich uncle drowning in the tub, if I fail to go to his aid in order that he drown, so that I might collect the inheritance, my action is one of willful murder, regardless of the fact that it is partly constituted by an omission. It is no less an action than anything else that is performed intentionally.
>
> (Tollefsen, 2006, 456)

Conversely, not all forms of withholding or withdrawing life-sustaining treatment can be understood as passive euthanasia since the intention can be restricted to 'relieving the patient of futile or overly burdensome treatments' (see Cavanaugh, 2006). Henceforth, 'killing' or 'to kill' should be understood as intentional.

Voluntary, Non-Voluntary, Involuntary

Whereas the passive–active distinction applies to how the doctor accomplishes his/her end, the next set of distinctions apply to how things look from the patient's viewpoint. Euthanasia may be 'voluntary,' 'non-voluntary,' or 'involuntary.' Voluntary euthanasia is defined as an act of euthanasia (whether passive or active) on a competent patient who has requested it, which includes requests through a valid advance directive.

Because voluntariness comes in degrees,[9] there appears to be a problem. Being voluntary in a *strong sense* means, at least, being free from undue influence (think back to Sophie's choice; she clearly did not voluntarily choose to have her daughter killed). Since pain and suffering are likely undue influences, requests for euthanasia because one is suffering unbearably are likely not voluntary requests in this strong sense. Alfonso Gómez-Lobo observes that terminally ill patients "may be depressed and under various forms of psychological pressure, especially if the view that the terminally ill should die and thus stop wasting medical resources . . . becomes socially accepted" (2002, 108). An autonomous decision in this strong sense is unlikely in such circumstances. Take away the pain or depression, and patients withdraw their requests for dying in 98%–99% of cases (Royal College of Psychiatrists, 2006, 2.4).

A request to be killed may be voluntary in a weak sense, which requires an understanding of the consequences, an ability to reason (Appelbaum, 2007), and being free of "external" influences (Appelbaum, Lidz, & Klitzman, 2009, 33ff.). But not all weakly voluntary requests for euthanasia should be honored, as when I request euthanasia because I have a headache or am moderately depressed – i.e., not enough to exert undue influence. In such cases I understand the consequences and can reason. Because I am not subject to excruciating suffering or an unbearable condition, my choice would be less influenced by external factors. But because such conditions are *bearable*, by hypothesis, my request loses its moral urgency.

Non-voluntary euthanasia is defined as an act of euthanasia (whether passive or active) on a patient who is not able to request it (such as a baby or demented patient). And involuntary euthanasia is defined as an act of euthanasia (whether passive or active) performed on a competent patient who does not want to be killed, but the medical staff thinks it is in the best interest of the patient to be dead. Involuntary euthanasia is still conceptually distinct from murder, but most people agree that it is a form of wrongdoing nonetheless.

Physician-assisted suicide (PAS) is defined as an act whereby a physician intentionally assists a patient to commit suicide by providing a prescription of lethal drugs. Unlike euthanasia, the final act which causes the patient's death is performed by the patient rather than the doctor. It is widely agreed that assisting in an evil act with the intention to see the evil act performed is itself an evil action. Planning and facilitating an immoral act is also an immoral act. So, if killing someone were wrong, PAS would be wrong as well. Conversely, if killing someone were permissible, aiding in the patient's death would be as well. Although euthanasia and PAS are conceptually distinct, their moral status is correlative.

What Can Be Presumed

As with any dialogical context, answers to the question 'is euthanasia an exception to the general prohibition on intentional killing?' make use of presumptions. As discussed in Chapter 2, presumptions are defined with reference to a point in a dialectical exchange and in relation to a specific challenger such that P is presumed if and only if the challenger is obliged to concede P at that point in the exchange. Presumptions in moral discourse are a function of what values may be taken for granted. On the issue in question, Joel Feinberg grants that prior to encountering arguments for voluntary euthanasia, all innocent human beings, in virtue of being human, have a right not to be killed. He remarks that, "it is hard to shed the intuitive conviction that there is somehow *something* that is 'absolute' in the natural or human right to life" (Feinberg, 1978, 98).[10] It is safe to presume that killing innocent persons is impermissible, especially when it is not necessary to save others. So, the ethical question for euthanasia is not whether suffering can have redemptive value. The question is simply whether euthanasia is an exception to the prohibition on killing innocent persons.

The apparent anodyne quality of this presumption is belied by the discourse on euthanasia. A predominant feature in this discourse is to *construct criteria* that makes it *impermissible to kill* another person. The background assumption for this discourse to make sense is that permissible killing is the default position. Richard Brandt appears to endorse this understanding of the dialectic when he asks "can this view that all killing of innocent human beings is morally wrong *be defended*, and if not, what alternative principle can be?" (Brandt, 1975, 106; emphasis added). Brandt thinks that the onus of proof is on the claim that killing an innocent human being is sufficient for wronging that person. One must *argue* that one's criteria for impermissible killing is a necessary condition; one must find that property or feature that *makes it* wrong to kill someone. The implication is that failing these projects, killing is permissible. Once these assumptions are made apparent, it is clear that they get things backwards. We do not need a reason *not* to kill, we need a reason *to* kill.

There are serious doubts, therefore, that the permissibility of killing innocents – even those who want to die – can be presumed. Although more is said below about the putative value of autonomous choices, specifically the choice to die, I note here that there are numerous values on offer which help to index presumptions. They include the values of life, health, and the healing ends of medicine.

Before proceeding, let us consider two objections to the claim that life and health function as presumptive values. Alan Goldman (2010) mentions that we do not place life and health as having "top priority." He states that, "if our primary goals were always to minimize risk to health and life, we should spend our entire federal budget in health-related areas. Certainly such a suggestion would be ludicrous" (Goldman, 2010, 76). Suitably circumscribed, his point is correct; but the claim that life and health have presumptive value in moral discourse avoids his objection. It would follow that we should spend our entire federal budget on health-related areas if health were the *only* value. But it is not part of one's understanding of the ends of medicine, or one's opposition to euthanasia for that matter, that health and life are the only values. Rather, they are values that we cannot *aim* to eliminate, destroy, or diminish. This latter claim is compatible with there being any number of important values for which it would also be impermissible to will against, and the promotion of which is justifiably weighed against the promotion of health given the resources at hand.

Furthermore, Goldman's observation cannot be used to illuminate the issue of euthanasia. An absolute prohibition on torture does not entail having to spend the federal budget promoting or defending bodily health and integrity. Likewise, an absolute prohibition on euthanasia does not entail any privileging of values in our fiscal decisions. The position only states which values cannot be acted against; as to which values should be promoted, it remains open.

Further on, Goldman claims that there is no difference between existing in an irreversible coma and death. He concludes that our lives have no intrinsic value. "It is plausible to maintain that life itself is not of intrinsic value, since surviving in an irreversible coma seems no better than death" (Goldman, 2010, 77). It is true that being permanently unconscious rules out having good experiences and engaging in worthwhile life projects. In relation to having good experiences, the irreversibly comatose person and the dead person are alike. But it does not follow that there is no intrinsic value to one's life. The 'no better than' relation is flanked by the relata of having good experiences: not having good experiences in a comatose state is no better than not having good experiences while dead. One cannot infer the absence of intrinsic value from this jejune observation because, if life has intrinsic worth at all, it is going to have that kind of worth independent of good or bad experiences. So, observing that there is no difference between the comatose and the dead person along one axis of evaluation does not tell us much about intrinsic worth. There is no reason, then, not to presume the values of life and health. Arguably, the healing profession cannot make sense without understanding these values as remaining, if you will, even in the setting of disease and disability (Sulmasy, 2008).

The Arguments

Arguments Against

The basic argument against euthanasia can be understood as follows. Euthanasia is the intentional killing of an innocent human being. It is impermissible to kill an innocent human being – certainly in contexts where such killing does not involve saving the lives of others.[11] Therefore euthanasia is impermissible. To the question 'can life itself be so good that it cannot be rational or moral to end it?' the opponent to euthanasia can answer that if 'life itself' refers to you, or me, or Ladmaker then it cannot be rational ever to intentionally kill us. But if the 'it' in that question refers to one's bad experiences, the opponent to euthanasia can consistently hold that it would be rational to end those experiences. The distinction between my life and my experiences is discussed in more detail below and was addressed in Chapter 5.

Additionally, arguments against euthanasia emphasize the equality of all human lives, from which it follows that no one should be discriminated against. However, in legalizing assisted suicide, one

> sets up a double standard: some people get suicide prevention while others get suicide assistance, and the difference between the two groups is the health status of the individual, leading to a two-tiered system that results in death to the socially devalued group. This is blatant discrimination.
>
> (Not Dead Yet, 2018)

When the most frequent reason for requesting euthanasia is loss of autonomy or independence (Jones, 2015, 8) – i.e., one is disabled in some way – and the fundamental justification for euthanasia is that death will benefit the person, one cannot but conclude that being disabled is a reason for killing someone; they are better off dead. This conclusion is contrary to our ethical commitment to equality and to numerous commentators in the disability rights literature. Kittay (1999, 150), for example, offers the following reflection on discovering her daughter's intellectual disabilities. "Sesha would never live a normal life . . . Yet throughout this time it never even occurred to me to give Sesha up, to institutionalize her . . . She was my daughter. I was her mother. That was fundamental." The point is that disability does not detract from someone's worth. She concludes, "[t]hat which we believed we valued . . . the capacity for thought, for reason, was not it, not it at all" (1999, 150).

Might the cost in being wrong in accepting these arguments be that patients would be left to writhe in pain and suffer? The opponent to euthanasia does not see the issue as involving the choice between, on the one hand, opposing the killing of patients while letting them writhe in pain or, on the other hand, permitting the killing of patients while risking abuses – such as granting the request for euthanasia of a clinically depressed 80-year-old who could have a quality life were he to be treated (Arras, 2010, 575). Dworkin et al. (2013, 665) appear to endorse this dichotomy when they motivate their position by discussing patients who feel "anguish . . . at remaining alive, but intubated, helpless, and often sedated near oblivion." This understanding of the issue is embarrassing. If they are intubated and the respirator is not conferring a reasonable hope of benefit, one can do a palliative wean without intending the patient's death. Depending on the circumstances and wishes of the patient, such an action would not necessarily involve an intentional killing of the patient. If they are "sedated near oblivion," then in what sense can they feel anguish?

Part of their misunderstanding can be attributed to a misunderstanding of palliative care. The root meaning of the term 'palliative' stems from the Latin term *palliare* which means to cover over something – a *pallium* is a noun and refers to a cloak. Palliative care aims to cover over symptoms of disease and illness. Understood as such, it can begin as soon as the first responders arrive and can span someone's entire hospital stay. It can begin on a newborn as well as the elderly. When palliative care is understood not as a last resort or as synonymous with hospice or end-of-life care, but rather as distributed throughout someone's entire exposure to health care delivery, symptom management and quality of life significantly improve.[12] It does so because palliative care focuses on pain and symptom management, setting goals of care, prospective care planning, and emotional and spiritual support.

Viewing palliative care as distributed throughout one's care improves that care. Casarett et al. (2008) followed 524 patients, 296 of whom received palliative consultation plus usual care and 228 who received just usual care. On a 32-item survey (i.e., FATE), those receiving palliative care showed significantly better scores (typically by a factor of 10+ points) with the greatest discrepancy on "Care around the time of death" in which the scores were 63 vs 45 respectively. In terms of receiving adequate symptom management, a four-point Likert scale was used: 0 = always, 1 = often, 2 = sometimes, 3 = never (thus, higher scores equaled better outcomes). Those receiving palliative care showed a mean of 2.15, versus 1.88 for usual. The biggest difference pertained to the incidence of PTSD, with 1.92 and 0.77 respectively. The highest satisfaction for the palliative care group concerned the absence of unwanted treatment and being admitted/residing in the facility of the patient's choice.

Palliative care improves quality of life, lowers depressive symptoms and incidences of PTSD, and reduces the use of burdensome and pointless treatments. It can also improve survival from a mean of 8.9 months for usual care, to 11.6 months for palliative plus usual care (Temel et al., 2010). Lastly, inpatient palliative care requests frequently identify prior unrecognized problems and unmet needs (Manfredi et al., 2000), and they result in lowering the following: length of stay in ICUs (Norton et al., 2007), likelihood of dying in an ICU (Elsayem et al., 2006), and costs of care (Penrod et al., 2006). How often is it that patients are receiving intensive care, chemotherapy, or some other high dose treatment in their last week of life, with all the side effects associated with that level of care? Given the empirical evidence on the effectiveness of palliative care, and the personal testimony that many physicians are not adequately trained to meet a patient's goals of palliation, opting for euthanasia does not solve the underlying problem. Better medicine, not easier killing, appears to be the more parsimonious prescription (Keown, 2009).

So, there are principally two justifications for prohibiting euthanasia. The first is that the prohibition against killing innocents does not admit of exceptions; and the second is a commitment to the equality of all human lives.

Arguments For

Dan Brock (1992) is typically cited as providing the most straightforward justification for euthanasia. Brock presents an argument for the permissibility of euthanasia based on two fundamental values: self-determination and individual well-being. His argument can be read as providing two arguments – one based on each value – or as one argument where well-being is understood to morally justify the key premise in the argument from self-determination. I interpret the argument in the latter way for reasons of charity – motivating euthanasia based on *one* value or *another* strikes me as handcuffing the proponent's case by letting one value bear the burden of proof.

Consider first the value of self-determination. Brock rightly considers self-determination a value and asks whether this value extends to include choosing the "time and manner" (1992, 11) of one's death. In answering this question, he appeals to the inherent variability in people's thresholds for what counts as a meaningful life. Brock states that "there is no single, objectively correct answer for everyone as to when, if at all, one's life becomes all things considered a burden and unwanted" (1992, 11). Because there is no single objectively correct understanding of when one's life becomes "a burden and unwanted" Brock moves to conclude the following: "If self-determination is a fundamental value, then the great variability among people on this question makes it especially important that individuals control the manner, circumstances, and timing of their dying and death" (Brock, 1992, 11).

The value of self-determination – or its cognates such as autonomy or personal interest – functions as a principal value in arguments for the permissibility of euthanasia. Dworkin et al., for example, say that,

> A person's interest in following his own convictions at the end of life is so central a part of the more general right to make "intimate and personal choices" for himself that a failure to protect that particular interest would undermine the general right altogether.
> (Dworkin et al., 2013, 662)

From these quotations, we can piece together the argument that euthanasia is permissible because self-determination is a value.

1 Self-determination/autonomy is a fundamental ethical value.
2 The value of self-determination 'extends' (or includes) choosing the time and manner of one's death.
3 Euthanasia involves choosing the time and manner of one's death.
4 Therefore, euthanasia is consistent with a fundamental ethical value.

To derive the conclusion that euthanasia is permissible requires a few more premises to the effect that choices consistent with a fundamental value are permissible *and* there are no other values that might be impugned by the choice for euthanasia. A choice to die might be rational from the perspective of the sufferer, but euthanasia might remain inconsistent with, for example, the healing ends of medicine. So, even if an autonomously made choice to die has value, the permissibility of euthanasia does not necessarily follow.

One could avoid additional premises by understanding the value of self-determination in premise (1) strongly such that an autonomous choice to die is a sufficient condition for that choice being permissible. There are two issues with this understanding. First, the stated value is the value of a specific autonomous *choice* not autonomy understood as a power or an ability to make decisions. But for any given choice, it is not obvious that the choice is valuable, even if being autonomous is a presumptive value. Simply choosing x does not itself morally justify doing x; we have to know what x involves (Keown, 2009; Oderberg, 1997b, 239ff.). That I autonomously choose voluntary slavery or to be killed and eaten hardly justifies such choices.

Second, the strong interpretation would force proponents of an exception to hold that autonomy is the *only* relevant value. Proponents could claim that other values, such as the healing ends of medicine, are not sufficiently weighty to offset the value of one's autonomous choice to die. But how would one *argue* for this claim? Suppose for simplicity that there are two values at stake, the value of protecting medical practice as a healing art on one hand (Pellegrino and Thomasma, 1988, chs 5 and 10) and the value of respecting one's autonomous choice to die on the other. On this strong understanding of (1), the latter value is weightier. The argument as to why, however, cannot appeal to the value of an autonomous choice to die itself since that would be viciously circular. And it cannot appeal to the value of a choice to die in other contexts since that value would no longer be incompatible with the healing ends *of medicine*. The prospects are dim, then, for defending a strong understanding of premise (1) in a way that avoids dogmatism or irrelevance.

Therefore, the argument for euthanasia being permissible needs to include a separate premise. I suggest the following, or something trivially different.

5   There are no other fundamental values impugned by euthanasia and any action consistent with fundamental values is permissible, all things considered.

It follows that,

6   Euthanasia is permissible.

Premises (2) and (5) are the premises needing further justification. Opponents to euthanasia could accept premise (1) but reject the conclusion since self-determination might not be the *only* value, but rather, a value along with the inherent and irreplaceable worth of the person. That observation alone puts pressure on premises (2) and (5).

The value of well-being, as Brock understands it, is meant to motivate premise (2). By well-being, Brock wants to accept that life can go well for some people, but poorly for others. He says that "continued life is seen by the patient as no longer a benefit, but now a burden" (Brock, 1992, 11). And this may be especially true in the terminally ill or dying patient. The notion of well-being is, then, one's own subjective assessment of how one's life is going in terms of its worth and quality. If life can become burdensome, one's well-being is low. If a patient judges that nonexistence is better than terminal and intractable suffering,[13] then choosing to be killed is rational.

Why think that it would be rational? Brock argues that this is what we do already, when we honor a patient's request to forego means of life-sustaining treatment.

> But when a competent patient decides to forgo all further life-sustaining treatment then the patient, either explicitly or implicitly, commonly decides that the best life possible for him or her with treatment is of sufficiently poor quality that it is worse than no further life at all.
>
> (Brock, 1992, 11)

The same type of reasoning is present in requests for euthanasia. If a patient judges that her life can be "of sufficiently poor quality," intentionally ending that life is no different than what we do now – *if* forgoing life-sustaining treatment is permissible for the reason that the patient's life is of sufficient poor quality. The key is to understand that the patient must make this judgment. So, in the settings in which the patient is suffering in ways she or he deems unbearable, it appears consistent with the value of autonomy to desire ending one's life. Therefore, the value of self-determination extends or includes choosing the time and manner of one's death.

The defense of premise (5) appeals to similar ideas. In rebutting claims that life has inherent worth, arguably a value incompatible with the value of choosing to be killed, proponents typically make a distinction between biological life and biographical life (see Chapter 5). The basic idea is that life 'itself' is not inherently or intrinsically worthwhile, only one's overall experiences are. Shelly Kagan (2018) helpfully refers to this view of life's worth as the "neutral container view." Biological life itself merely enables me to have a good (or bad) life (experiences).

How do these distinctions work to support (5)? Brandt says that the "person who is contemplating suicide is obviously making a choice between future world-courses; the world course that includes his demise, say, an hour from now, and several possible ones that contain his demise at a later point" (2006, 391). Further on he says that

> the basic question a person must answer, in order to determine which world course is best or rational for him to choose, is which [one] he *would* choose under conditions of optimal use of information, when *all* of his desires are taken into account.
>
> (2006, 391)

To the objection that few people can know with certainty future world courses, the situations in which we can be certain are those facing a terminally ill patient. Furthermore, we should understand these world courses to include principally experiences; and whether these world courses are good or bad depends upon whether these experiences satisfy one's desires and preferences overall (Brandt, 2006, 392). Consequently, a neutral container view of life's worth justifies there being 'no other fundamental values.'

In an interesting twist to the development of pro-euthanasia arguments, Emily Jackson (Jackson & Keown, 2012, 38–39) appears to reject the neutral container view (though critical analysis below suggests that this cannot be the case). She observes that such a theory "involves making a quality of life judgment that some believe to be irreconcilable with the principle that all lives are of equal value" (2012, 38). If my experiences are incongruent with my preferences and desires, then my world course is going poorly. On the neutral container view, my life has lower worth. Someone else whose desires and preferences are being satisfied appears to have a more worthwhile life. Such a result violates the principle that all human lives are of equal worth.[14] Her response is to accept that her view involves a judgment that someone's life has ceased to benefit him, but she rejects inferring from this that the person has no worth. Instead she holds that wanting

> to be there when someone we love dies and to be able to comfort them in their final days and hours, is prompted by love and compassion, and does not entail subscribing to the view that the person's life has become worthless.
>
> (Jackson & Keown, 2012, 39)

But this concession cannot be a plausible feature of a pro-euthanasia argument. First, the scene Jackson describes in the second quotation is that respect for the person's worth is compatible with allowing someone to die *sans* intentional killing; but she has not argued that such respect is compatible with euthanasia. It may be, but it is unclear how the argument would go. If I respect knowledge, that is, if I think that knowledge is worthwhile to have in myself or others, I am not going to lie to others, and I will be wary of self-deception. If I think that someone's reputation is worthwhile, I am not going to calumniate that person. If I think that someone has inherent worth, I am not going to eliminate him or her – consider my reflections on the Charles–Ladmaker narrative (Chapter 5).[15] Henceforth, I take the more canonical route and understand the defense of (5) as requiring something like a neutral container view of life's worth. What makes life valuable is having valuable experiences; valuable world-courses in Brandt's terminology.

Appraisal of the Arguments

We began the penultimate section with an outline of what can be presumed, namely, the prima facie prohibition on killing an innocent human person. If there are any exceptions to this prima facie prohibition, there must be positive reasons in favor of them. I address in this section whether the arguments in favor of an exception are plausible. I also address whether the values appealed to in such arguments could plausibly function as presumptions. The argument that follows can be understood as two-tiered. The first tier argues that the values proponents of an exception appeal to cannot be presumed. Having leveled the dialectical exchange, the second tier argues that the standard arguments in favor of euthanasia are not good arguments.[16] If there are no good arguments for that exception the prohibition against killing innocent human persons stands.

Ad Premise (5)

The first critical point is that the distinction between biological and biographical life is not exhaustive. It ignores the idea defended in Chapter 5 that you and I have inherent and irreplaceable worth. In that chapter I did not argue against interest or biographical accounts of life's worth. What I argued is that these accounts are not comprehensive; they do not capture the many vectors by which we can assess the worth of a human being. What needs ending in certain clinical circumstances is the suffering, and what morally justifies ending that suffering is that it is bad. What is decidedly not bad is the person him- or herself. Ladmaker never becomes bad, even though his experiences are horrible. Just as intelligence remains good even if I come to know horrible events or come to hold false beliefs; so life itself remains good even if I experience suffering (Gómez-Lobo & Keown, 2015, 70). One cannot move from someone's suffering being bad to the life of the person him- or herself being bad.

Observing that there are other views of life's worth does not argue against the container view. The argument against the neutral container view is, however, simple and conclusive. We need merely to ask who is it that judges whether one's biographical life is good or not? The answer of course is that the person is judging the quality of his or her experiences. The experienc*er* and the experiences cannot be the same. The chief idea reached in the previous chapter on dignity was that the experienc*er* has inherent worth; the evaluat*or* of one's quality of life has inherent worth. I am not a mere container for experiences, and yet, it is impermissible to kill *me*. Furthermore, there is the point already noted that the neutral container view violates our commitment to the equality of all human life. So, even if S is suffering and suffering is bad, and it is permissible to end bad things, it still does not follow that it is permissible to kill S.

Some proponents of an exception might claim that suffering is undignified, or that having a low quality of life renders one's life not worth living. In response, if suffering compromises or lessens our dignity then by killing the person we are not 'respecting' or 'upholding' their dignity. By hypothesis, they do not have dignity and therefore such worth cannot be upheld or respected. If all that makes one's life good is one's biographical life and one's biography is poor, killing that person would be inconsequential because what is killed has little value. Furthermore, if suffering makes us lose value, why try to save a person or restore her to health? Health care is a proper moral response to illness and disease because the people who are ill are valuable. Daniel Sulmasy captures this point the following way.

> It is in recognition of that [intrinsic] worth that we have established the healing professions as our moral response to those of our kind who are suffering from disease and injury. The plight of the sick has little instrumental value, rarely serving the purposes, beliefs, desires, interests, expectations of any of us as individuals. Rather, it is because of the intrinsic value of the sick that healthcare professionals serve them.
>
> (Sulmasy, 2008, 478)

Providing health care to disabled and diseased human beings *makes sense* only if those human beings have intrinsic dignity. If one loses her value because she is suffering, then her claim on our moral response to that suffering diminishes. Instead of taking one's suffering as a reason for thinking that the sufferer's worth is lowered, I am suggesting that the suffering cannot be viewed as bad unless we first view the sufferer as inherently good. It is because the sufferer has inherent and undiminished worth in the setting of suffering that we abhor *the suffering* so much. Suffering does not lessen one's dignity but shines a light on it.

Ad Premise (2)

Regarding the value of self-determination and autonomy, it is common to all commentators on the debate that autonomy qua power or ability is a value. Whereas my ability to choose is valuable, each of my choices do not necessarily have value. When we think of what choices are valuable, everyone agrees that choices about our associates, our career, our life plans and projects, are valuable. I shall refer to this class of choices as 'intra-life choices.' But there is the class of choices concerned with killing oneself. This action class I will refer to as 'contra-life choices.' What is uncontroversial is the value of making intra-life choices; what is controversial is whether the value of contra-life choices, if they have any, is sufficient to displace the presumption against killing innocent people.

Premise (1) tells us that autonomy is a fundamental value. If by autonomy one means the *ability* to make choices, the argument to (6) does not follow since the latter references a specific choice. If by autonomy one means to refer to intra-life choices the argument to (6) again does not follow since the latter refers to a contra-life choice. I might add that (1) is quite plausible if it is referring to the value of one's intra-life choices. If the value of autonomy in premise (1) is meant to include the value of contra-life choices it is begging the question. Premise (2) is true only if the choice is contra-life. What this means is that the success of the argument depends upon arguing that the value of one's intra-life choices 'extends' in some way to include contra-life choices in a way that is neither question-begging nor equivocating.

As noted above, the first tier of my procedure assesses whether the value of a contra-life choice can be presumed. The importance of doing so can be appreciated by the following argument. If the value of a contra-life choice is presumed, the value of ending one's life would function as a value we can take for granted. On such a scenario, one would not need to argue for an extension.

The value of a contra-life choice, however, cannot be presumed. Even on the neutral container view of life's worth, life needs to be going badly before one is justified in ending it. If contra-life choices have presumptive value one would not *need* to have a bad biography, to use Rachel's term, before one is justified in ending one's life. What we need is an argument *for* an exception, not a presumption in favor of it.

What can be presumed is that bad experiences are not valuable. As argued above, it would not follow from this that I am worthless, nor would it follow that ending my life is valuable. So, the value of choosing to end my life cannot be a presumed value. (It certainly is not on an epistemic par with other presumptions such as that a person missing for more than eight years is dead, or that a child under eight has no criminal intent (Rescher, 2006)).

We can now turn to the second tier of my procedure and argue that premise (2) is likely false. At this point in the dialectic the question is whether choosing to end one's life is a value sufficient to motivate an exception. To avoid circularity, one would need to argue that such choices are valuable. But one cannot use the value of intra-life choices to argue that contra-life choices have value, or even that they have presumed value. One cannot, for example, infer that determining the time and manner of one's death is valuable because choosing to be a professor is a value. The choices are categorically different. Furthermore, since premise (2) is true only if contra-life choices have value, the argument also risks equivocation if premise (1) is interpreted as referring to the value of intra-life choices – unless that which makes intra-life choices valuable is the same feature that makes contra-life choices valuable. Given the difference in content between these two choice types, the only feature common to both might be that they issue from the same autonomous will. But again, what one wills does not morally justify what one wills. So, the 'extension' that premise (2) claims is not only not likely, but categorically false.

These reflections provide a riposte to Dworkin et al. (2013, 662ff., quoted above) where they make two claims. One claim is that the choice to have one's life ended is a personal choice. The second is that we have a right to make personal choices. It follows that we have a right to choose euthanasia. With the distinction between intra- and contra-life choices in mind, we can understand the dialectical burden this argument inherits. The argument that we have a right to make *all* personal choices must be argued for on one of two grounds. The first ground is to suggest that we have a right to make personal choices that are intra-life and infer from the value of intra-life choices the value (and right) to make contra-life choices. (As already noted, one cannot just assume that contra-life choices have value since that is exactly what is at stake). The other ground is to suggest that we should be allowed to make personal choices because we are the only ones who bear the effects of those choices.

We have already considered the first ground and there are at least two ripostes to the second. Daniel Callahan observes that this notion of autonomy is one among many values since we can easily "imagine a good for others beyond that which they imagine for themselves" (1984, 41) and we can persuade them that their moral choices are wrong. More importantly, the notion that my autonomy and personal choices are hermetically sealed is a notion corrosive of friendship and community. Callahan states,

> This understanding of autonomy is hazardous to moral relationships and moral community. It buys our freedom to be ourselves, and to be free of undue influence by others, at too high a price. It establishes contractual relationships as the principal and highest form of relationships. It elevates isolation and separation as the necessary starting point of human commitments.
>
> (Callahan, 1984, 41)

If my friend is considering killing himself, an act with which I disagree, the notion of personal choice appealed to by Dworkin et al. suggests that I lack any philosophical justification for intervening in his choice to die. It is his choice and he is the sole bearer of its effects. To be sure, the intuitions that inform pro-euthanasia arguments can be made consistent with the good of friendship (i.e., compassion in alleviating the suffering of another). My point is only that in arguing for the permissibility of euthanasia, *the notion of autonomy* appealed to is not obviously consistent with the good of friendship. It is entirely too strong, and I doubt whether it is at all relevant (compassion for the sufferer seems more dominant).

The second riposte is to observe that the moral permissibility of one's choice does not immediately follow from the fact that the chooser is the only bearer of the choice's effects.[17] Such a view would entail that I cannot do wrong to myself. But of course, I can treat myself poorly, such as making choices that frustrate my objective interests.

The Groundless Objection

I suspect that compassion for the sufferer is the principal idea that motivates the permissibility of euthanasia. If we focus on the good of ending suffering, without entirely abandoning the relevance of self-determination, we can understand the pro-euthanasia argument as follows. First, we can define the circumstances in which one might entertain killing an innocent person.

(Cir):   S is suffering *in a way* such that S is neither harmed by nor deprived of overall good experiences by the killing.

And the conclusion of the argument is,

(Perm):   It is permissible to kill S in (Cir).

With this initial set-up, we can ask what substitution instance for justification J permits inferring from (Cir) and J to (Perm)? The defense of premise (5) suggests the following.

Jnec: It is impermissible to kill S *only if* (i) S is harmed by or (ii) deprived of overall good future experiences.
Jsuff: If S is neither (i) harmed by nor (ii) deprived of future overall good experiences, then it is permissible to kill S.

(Jnec and Jsuff are equivalent by transposition.) The relevant notion of harm is acting against one's considered interests. So, if killing the person is not against the person's considered interests, killing would not harm the person. Beauchamp and Childress write, "if a person freely elects and authorizes death . . . active aid in dying at the person's request involves no harm or moral wrong" (2001, 148). The relevant notion of deprivation is the absence of future overall valuable experiences. Emily Jackson remarks

> [i]f someone was [sic] to ask me what is valuable about my life, I would talk about my friends, my family, my work and the things I enjoy doing . . . There is nothing independently valuable about being alive, other than that it enables me to live a life.
>
> (Jackson & Keown, 2012, 42)[18]

The derivation to (Perm) can take one of two routes. (Cir) paired with Jnec entails (Perm) by *modus tollens*; and (Cir) paired with Jsuff entails (Perm) by *modus ponens*. The permissibility of euthanasia is simply (Perm), according to which it is permissible to kill S when S is neither harmed by nor deprived of future good experiences by the killing.

What is the argument for excluding a third condition, namely, (iii) S is innocent, as a necessary condition for impermissible killing? Suitably added, Jnec reads,

Jnec+: It is impermissible to kill S only if (i) S is harmed by or (ii) deprived of overall good future experiences, or (iii) S is innocent. (And by transposition, Jsuff+).

One can see that if Jnec+ is true, (Perm) is not since those killed by euthanasia are innocent. The easiest way to rebut Jnec+ is to assert that euthanasia *is* permissible (i.e., Perm) as a premise and derive ~(Jnec+) by *modus tollens*. Of course, the easiest way is also the most obviously question-begging way.

Suppose we try a more inductive route. At issue is whether condition (iii) functions as a necessary condition for impermissibility. Consider cases involving innocents who are killed, for example, killing the POW, the concentration camp victim, or the depressed patient, all of whom might be suffering and they might want to die (call these 'the alternatives'). These cases provide intuitive inductive evidence for condition (iii) – assuming that killing the alternatives is impermissible. Yet, they putatively satisfy the negations of (i) and (ii) as do patients for whom euthanasia proponents think it is permissible to kill. It looks as if Jnec or Jsuff entails that killing one of the alternatives is permissible.

Either killing the alternatives is permissible or it is not. If not, a proponent of euthanasia has an adjustment decision to make – discussed in Chapter 3. She may reject the permissibility of euthanasia or not. If she continues to accept (Perm), she must reject (iii) to preserve (Perm), and add other conditions to Jnec/Jsuff to ground or justify the impermissibility of killing the alternatives. The goal of the latter conjunct is to find a feature that is present in the alternatives but is not present for those in euthanasia-permitting circumstances (or vice versa). Justifying this distinction is to ground a reason for dividing the class of innocents into those for whom it is permissible to kill, and those for whom it is not.

How is one to proceed? Before answering this question, it is necessary to understand an elementary epistemological distinction

Beliefs are divided broadly into basic beliefs and non-basic beliefs.[19] Non-basic beliefs are justified on the basis of other beliefs. Basic beliefs can either be justified or not, but not on the basis of other beliefs. If they are justified, then they are justified on the basis of non-doxastic states, such as an experience or intuition. Whether the experience or intuition is veridical, e.g., produced by a reliable faculty, will dictate whether the non-doxastic state in question can justify the basic belief. Though the following examples are controversial, they illustrate the point behind this technical language. Perceptual beliefs based on visual sensing at medium distances in good lighting are examples of justified basic beliefs since they are justified on the basis of perceptual experiences which are not other beliefs. My belief that the piano I see has fewer than 88 keys is justified, however, on another belief, namely, that I am at a concert purporting to use period instruments.

We can now answer what justifies the distinction between killing a terminally ill patient and killing one of the alternatives. Either the distinction is a basic belief or it is inferred from another belief. If the distinction is basic, this would amount to saying that it is permissible to kill the terminally ill patient, but not permissible to kill the concentration camp victim or the POW, full stop, no reason. If the distinction is a basic belief, (Perm) *just is* true with an additional conjunct that the killing of the alternatives is impermissible.[20] This disjunct is clearly unsatisfactory.

If it is a non-basic belief, it must be justified on the basis of other beliefs. What other beliefs? One feature that is different between the two classes of innocents might be that the cause of suffering for the terminally ill patient is internal (i.e., disease), and for the POW it is external (i.e., captors). Why think that the internal/external distinction provides a sufficient reason for distinguishing between permissible and impermissible killing? Again, this is either a basic belief or a non-basic one. If it is basic, it is wholly unconvincing. There is nothing apparent about causes of suffering that are internal that would justify killing me; likewise, causes of suffering that are external is hardly *the* reason for not killing me. If the defense of euthanasia depends on making it, the argument from epistemic diffidence follows easily given the cost in being wrong in the setting of peer disagreement. If it is non-basic, it must be justified by another belief. Again, we can ask what other beliefs? If that other belief just is the conjunction of (Perm) with the belief that it is impermissible to kill the alternatives, this would be circular reasoning.

Must the rejection of Jnec+ be justified by circular reasoning? That S is innocent is either a sufficient reason for making it impermissible to kill S or it is not. If it is a sufficient reason, then ~(Perm) follows. If it is not a sufficient reason, then the category of permissible killing explodes. The default position or presumption is that if S is innocent, it is impermissible to kill S. Therefore, the reasons for denying condition (iii) as a sufficient condition must have started with certain privileged beliefs about which innocents it is permissible to kill. The previous paragraph argued that any reason for thinking that killing S is permissible either reduces to unconvincing grounds, or circularity threatens. My point here is that a likely scenario is this: an intuition that suffering patients may receive aid in dying comes first and reasoning second (Haidt, 2001), namely, Jnec. Putative counterexamples to Jnec, such as cases of killing the alternatives, are absorbed in a way that preserves the starting intuition. Given the psychology of moral belief formation outlined in Chapter 2, the only motive for rejecting condition (iii) is an intuitive conviction that (Perm) is true. After all, why not simply reject (Perm) when confronted with an inductive case for Jnec+? The answer is simple: (Perm) is held with a greater intuitive conviction. As argued in Chapter 2, that fact is tenuous epistemic comfort. Given the cost in being wrong, and the presence of peer disagreement, one should hold (Perm) with epistemic diffidence.

One can do this exercise for any dialectical encounter on euthanasia. The recipe is straightforward. Identify the conditions under which it is permissible to kill P. Next, show that those conditions entail that it is permissible to kill S when it clearly is not. One can either reject the necessity of the original conditions (and thereby reject (Perm)), find a further specifying feature that distinguishes the two cases, or reject the intuition that killing S is impermissible in the counterexample. Choosing one of the latter two options *instead of* the first option must be a function of one's starting intuition that it is permissible to kill P. What must ground this adjustment decision in a commitment *prior to the adjustment decision itself*, that it is permissible to kill P. Hence my suspicion that (Perm) is groundless.

Does this recipe apply equally to arguments opposing euthanasia? It does not since the presumption is that no innocent person may be killed; and this was argued for in Chapter 5. Even so, anomalies to Jnec+ can be constructed; the spelunker case might be one of them in which it may be permissible to kill a very small subset of innocents. But the dialectical burden is not merely to point out anomalies. One must say that such anomalies invalidate Jnec+ in circumstances that patients face. It is simply a quantificational fallacy to infer from 'it is permissible to blow the big man to bits' to 'euthanasia is permissible.'[21] I have argued that there can be either no argument at all or no good argument for why innocent patients count as an exception to Jnec+.

At the beginning of the dialectic, what we wanted was a reason for thinking that there is an exception to the prima facie prohibition against killing innocent persons. We have canvassed two principal arguments for thinking that there should be such an exception specific to circumstances (Cir). I have argued that both arguments are inert in terms of motivating such an exception. The self-determination argument is inert principally because it either assumes that contra-life choices are valuable, or such choices are valuable because intra-life choices are. The former route begs the very question at stake, and the latter commits a categorical error. The argument from suffering is inert principally because the neutral container view is not an exhaustive appreciation for the worth of persons. And, grounds for accepting a moral principle that permits inferring the permissibility of killing in euthanasia is epistemically circular. The ground for making adjustment decisions in the setting of putative counterexamples is to maintain coherence of one's beliefs with the permissibility of euthanasia. So far, we have no good argument for an exception to the prohibition against killing innocents. Since that prohibition functions as a presumption in the argument, we have no reason for displacing it.

It will not do for the critic to respond by pointing out that the opponent to euthanasia does the same thing; she has her own stock set of assumptions and the potential counterexamples are absorbed in such a way as to preserve the belief that killing innocent patients is wrong. The example that I have in mind are putative counterexamples to the intention/foresight distinction. As noted above, such examples are either unilluminating, or they confuse the intention/foresight distinction with its causal cousin, viz., the active/passive distinction (Hershenov, 2008b). The justifications I have surveyed for why there should be an exception have themselves proved inert or are non sequiturs. Even if my interlocutor disagrees about my assessment of the strength of such justifications or their logical relevance, the epistemic significance of disagreement, especially in the setting of epistemic circularity, strongly suggests moderating the strength of one's belief that euthanasia is permissible.

Conclusion

In a large-scale study on patients who requested assisted suicide, all suffered from depression or hopelessness (Breitbart et al., 2000). Add to this evidence from Herbert Hendin's work according to which, "No group of suicidal patients has been more ignored than those who become suicidal in response to serious or terminal illness" (Hendin, 1999, 558). To understand the problem of ignoring seriously ill patients, Gregory Hamilton and Catherine Hamilton point out that there are basically two approaches to the suffering of terminally ill patients: the treatment model and the competency model.

The treatment model aims to treat what has gone wrong. In the context of euthanasia, what needs 'treating' are the feelings that give rise to requests for suicide. Hendin states that the goal of the treatment model is to "understand and relieve the desperation that underlies the request for assisted suicide" (Hendin, 1999, 553). On this model, suicidality is seen as a disturbance in the normal mental functioning of a patient. Hamilton and Hamilton note that such patients often suffer from feelings of worthlessness, demoralization, or guilt and may be making a plea for reassurance . . . Exploring such feelings and fantasies and whatever other concerns arise can be reassuring and validating for the patient and can go a long way toward dispelling feelings of demoralization and worthlessness.

(Hamilton & Hamilton, 2004, 3)

So, the treatment model sees behind the requests to the underlying pathology or problem. If the request for euthanasia or PAS is animated by depression and fear, the treatment model focuses on treating depression and fear. Think of the treatment model this way: it recommends loving patients the way Charles loved Ladmaker, by seeing through Ladmaker's suffering to his undiminished humanity.

In contrast to the treatment model, the competency model is the dominant model employed in settings where euthanasia or PAS is legal. On this model, the goal is not to treat an underlying pathology or mental condition, but to test for competency. And competency is present if the patient understands the consequences of his or her choice to receive euthanasia or a lethal medication. The guidelines for health care professionals who receive requests for PAS in Oregon state that "[i]f the mental health professional finds the patient competent, refusal of mental health treatment by the patient does *not constitute a legal barrier to receiving a prescription for a lethal dose of medication*" (Ganzini & Farrenkopf, 1998, 31, emphasis added). Since the competency model focuses narrowly on whether the patient understands the consequences of his/her decision, few patients (only 5%) are referred for a psychiatric evaluation prior to receiving a lethal prescription (Oregon Health Division, 2004). Clearly, this is not treatment but rather is *ignoring* the clinically significant problems that patients encounter when they get seriously ill. As noted above, when patients who request euthanasia/PAS are treated for their depression, 98%–99% revoke their request (Royal College of Psychiatrists, 2006).

The debate on euthanasia takes place within the following context. Patients already have access to technical and competent palliative care, and they can withhold or withdraw treatments that they deem to be burdensome. What is being refused in these cases is the treatment, i.e., the treatment is judged worthless not the patient's life (Keown, 2006, 110ff.).[22] Furthermore, for the euthanasia debate both sides agree that the potential subjects of euthanasia are unqualifiedly persons – at least for those who defend voluntary euthanasia. And the patients whom proponents of euthanasia think it is permissible to kill are not threatening the lives of anyone. Considering the arguments addressed above, there is not a sufficiently persuasive reason to offset the presumption against killing innocent and likely vulnerable people. The proposition that euthanasia is permissible should be held with diffidence and, therefore, should not be acted upon.

Notes

1 For the moral tradition I find most plausible, even here the killing cannot be intentional (Rhonheimer, 2011; and Cavanaugh, 2006, ch. 1).

2 A claim right to x generates *duties* on the part of others to provide x, or for others not to interfere with one obtaining x. See Feinberg (1978, 95ff.). If S has a claim right to life, we incur an obligation not to kill S and not to let him die if we can easily save him. So, a claim right to euthanasia would obligate a doctor to perform it. Feinberg prefers to understand the right to die (which includes the right to euthanasia or physician-assisted suicide) as a discretionary right. Feinberg states, "just as my right to live imposes a duty on others not to kill me, so my right to die . . . imposes a duty on others not to prevent me from implementing my choice of death" (1978, 121).

3 The issue is not whether there is a class of actions that count as an exception, but whether euthanasia is a member of that class. One could construct a logically possible scenario in which our moral intuitions suggest that killing the innocent person is permissible (for what it is worth I cannot think of any); but to function as a reason for the permissibility of euthanasia, there must be a reason for why euthanasia counts as one of those scenarios.

4 The form and content in this section follow closely Keown (2009).

5 By specifying a health care professional, I am requiring that the act of euthanizing the patient must be a voluntary act so as to rule out zombies killing patients on a euthanasia ward (Wreen, 1988).

6 For further discussion on these opening points, see Michael Bratman (1981, 2000), Robert Audi (2001, Part II), Elizabeth Anscombe (2000), Cavanaugh (2006), and an under-appreciated though informative work by Eric D'Arcy (1963).

7 There might be cases of knowingly performing action A but without intent to do A. Consider cases involving duress where it is clear the agent does not desire to do X, but does X under threat. My own intuitions are hazy on whether acting under duress to do X must involve intending X. Fortunately, this complication does not affect the doctor's action in euthanasia (except in cases where a conscientious objection is overridden).

8 This is not the place to defend the existence of moral absolutes (see Shafer-Landau, 2005 and Kramer, 2009), or to specify their content (see Rhonheimer, 2011, Part III). As can be gleaned from the text, I consider moral absolutes as action-types which are specified in part by one's first-person intentions. Putative counterexamples might describe a case in which one intentionally kills but does so permissibly. The big man in the cave example (Foot, 1967) is one such case according to which spelunkers are trapped in a cave and it is filling with water. A big man makes a run for the only aperture and gets stuck. The only option of getting out is to light one of the sticks of dynamite and blow the big man to bits, effectively reopening the aperture. Cases like this are unilluminating because they invite intuitions on at least four different issues at once: (1) Is the action of blowing up the big man permissible? (2) Is that action best specified by one's intentions to blow *him* up? (3) What could be one's intended end versus the merely foreseen side effects? (4) Is there an absolute prohibition on intentionally killing innocents? If one answers 'yes' to (4), she will likely answer (1) in the negative. Or, if one answers 'yes' to (1) *and* (4), she will say about (2) and (3) that the intention is something like 'removing an obstruction so that the spelunkers are saved.' These answers are all consistent with the case description. I can go on, but my point is to illustrate that the case description cannot adjudicate our different intuitive responses to it.

9 Because inducements come in degrees, financial, emotional, degree of pain, or suffering, and because inducements affect the voluntariness of one's choices (Appelbaum, Lidz, & Klitzman, 2009, 34), voluntariness comes in degrees.

10 By a human right, Feinberg (1978, 97) understands it as one of the rights we have "in virtue of their fundamentally important, indeed essential, connection with human well-being" and belong equally to all human beings in virtue of being human. By a right to life, Feinberg understands it as a right not to be intentionally killed (1978, 94)

11 I reserve the right to say that is not permissible in these contexts either, but that is a context different from the one in which euthanasia might be entertained. In any case, the context as described refutes Brandt's (1975, 108ff.) understanding of the issue. Brandt thinks that it is sufficient to set aside the strong prima facie obligation not to kill innocents by entertaining the famous spelunker example noted above. Brandt thinks that it is permissible to blow up the big man. In addition to the problems highlighted by this example and others like it, this is clearly a duress situation in which the killing could only be justified, if justified at all, with reference to saving the many spelunkers. No proponent of euthanasia argues for the permissibility of euthanasia, however, because it would save the lives of others. So, Brandt's exception to our obligation not to kill would still not at all justify euthanasia.

12 Sean Morrison, the director of the National Palliative Care Research Center, notes that in his entire medical education, including medical school and residency, he received a 30-minute lecture on pain management (Morrison, 2010, at 17:50ff.), and even then, it only focused on how the opioids are metabolized in the kidney!

13 The condition that the suffering be intractable is morally required since, if it were manageable, resolving it by eliminating the patient is a killing that no longer obviously benefits the patient. If modern palliative care can mollify one's suffering – thereby providing a benefit the lack of which putatively justifies euthanasia – but I kill the patient instead, I must take a stance on the patient's life that looks more like malice than mercy. Suppose two options X and Y lead just as well to an end E, and that I know this. If I choose X instead of Y, there must be something about X itself or its other effects that I am willing.

14 Jeff McMahan observes correctly that most of us have the intuition that killing innocent persons is equally wrong. He also observes that his time-relative interest account for the wrongness of killing delivers a different result thus clashing "with most people's intuitions" (McMahan, 2002, 238). It is interesting to point out that instead of rejecting the time-relative interest account, McMahan rejects these "common intuitions as errors of moral phenomenology" (2002, 238). But this is a tenuous strategy since the arguments for questioning our equality intuitions may also apply to McMahan's intuitions that motivate his time-relative interest account.

15 Brett Wilmot (in conversation) has suggested to me that recognition of something's worth and ending that thing's life are compatible as can be appreciated when we euthanize our beloved pets. The analogy with pets is not meant to say that we euthanize pets, therefore we may euthanize people. His point is to show the compatibility between loving something and intending to end its life. Care should be exercised in exploiting this analogy nonetheless. I think Wilmot is correct to point out that one can have the *psychic state* of loving x, and at the same time the psychic state of intending to end x's life. Understood as motivating the compatibility of two psychological states, Wilmot is correct. But a moral claim to the effect that it would be permissible to kill x does not necessarily follow. Wilmot does not want to exploit the pet analogy to derive moral conclusions on how to treat humans – since doing so would

be subject to a number of disanalogies. To take just one disanalogy, dogs are euthanized if they have attacked human beings on multiple occasions. But persons guilty of battery are not candidates for the death penalty. Here's another, we undress in front of our pets but not generally in front of others! So, if the pet analogy is limited to motivating a psychological claim, no moral conclusions follow. If the analogy is meant to derive moral conclusions, it becomes a bad analogical argument.

16 The standard of a good argument I accept here is that the argument is valid, and that the premises are more plausible than their negations.

17 Factually speaking, unless one is a hermit, all of one's choices have effects on others. I entertain this claim only because it shows up when defending both legally permitting euthanasia and allowing for conscientious objection.

18 Here we see Jackson's endorsement of the neutral container view rendering her treatment implicitly inconsistent.

19 See Audi (2001, 32ff.).

20 This appears to be Lachs's position when he considers aiding in the suicide of a lovelorn teenager and a terminally ill patient. He says, "Many observers of no more than average sensitivity . . ." (2010, 562) can see the difference and "Even people of ordinary sensitivity understand that . . ." (2010, 565) there is a difference. No reasons are offered for why we should prevent the lovelorn teenager's suicide and yet aid in the terminally ill patient's suicide.

21 For an instance of this fallacy see Brandt (1975, 108).

22 Commenting on his clinical experience, Baruch Brody (1996, 99) thinks that the common refrain of "Mama wouldn't have wanted to live this way" should be taken to mean that death is the intended means to avoid continued suffering. His interpretation does not follow the logic of such refusals. If the treatment does not correct the patient's condition, it is not doing what was expected; viz., it fails to confer a benefit. Ineffective treatment is futile. Refusing it need not require judging the worth of the one who is doing the refusing. This is not gerrymandering intentions. Consider the treatment being effective and the refusal no longer makes sense. When it is ineffective, it is refused. The difference maker is the effectiveness of the treatment. The logic of such refusals, then, refer to the worthlessness of the treatment.

Part III

Balancing Dignity and Autonomy

9 Decision-Making for Patients with Suppressed Consciousness

The previous two parts aimed to argue that one ought to have epistemic diffidence towards *acting* on the belief that intentionally killing a human being is permissible. This diffidence applies to abortion, human embryo destructive research, and euthanasia. In this part I explore whether the argument can be extended to cases that are not obvious cases of intentional killing but are intentional omissions so that the patient will die. In this chapter and the next, I argue that the same epistemic diffidence applies to certain cases of removing life-sustaining means. The judgment about which we should hold epistemic diffidence is that the patient's wishes (in the cases addressed) are morally *sufficient* for the clinician to act on them. The cases I have in mind in this chapter are patients in a minimally conscious state (MCS) who have refused tube feeding in an advance directive. In the next chapter I consider patients who are apparently lucid and competent but have refused therapy that could obviously benefit them with clearly manageable burdens. And the final chapter considers whether a research subject's consent is enough to justify doing more than minimal-risk research on him or her. More broadly understood, the argument over the next three chapters aims to rebut the trend in contemporary bioethics that takes the autonomous patient's wishes or a research subject's consent as morally sufficient for acting on them.

In the present chapter, I proceed as follows. In the first section I explain what the condition MCS involves and the specific clinical circumstances to which my argument applies. There are basically two morally sufficient reasons to justify withholding means of sustaining life from the patient: (a) the patient's applicable advance directive (whether written or oral), and/or (b) the patient's best interest. The second section explains and defends the first part of my argument according to which neither (a) nor (b) function as a morally sufficient reason to withhold tube feeding from MCS patients. The third section intercalates between the two parts of my argument a rebuttal to the first part: in arguing that advance directives are not morally sufficient, I may be accused of unjustified paternalism. The third section rebuts this and related objections. The fourth section initiates the second part of my argument according to which

MCS patients should not have tube feeding withheld. Dialectically, it is one task to argue against arguments for W (section two), but quite another to argue for not-W (section four).

The Minimally Conscious State

The minimally conscious state is a "condition of severely altered consciousness in which minimal but definite behavioral evidence of self or environmental awareness is demonstrated" (Giacino et al., 2002, 350–351). Patients in MCS are conscious and aware. They retain some or all of the following abilities: (a) being able to follow simple commands, (b) being able to respond to yes/no questions, (c) intelligent verbalization, and (d) purposeful behavior such as responding appropriately to the semantic content of a question (Giacino et al., 2002, 351). Large-scale neural activity in the 'higher-cortices' is a feature of MCS that distinguishes it from the vegetative state. Through various neuro-imaging techniques, we know that MCS patients show neuroanatomical activity strongly indicating conscious awareness and higher-order cognition including semantic and emotional processing (Laureys et al., 2005a; and Schiff et al., 2005). Specifically, Laureys et al. observed that "cortico-cortical functional connectivity between auditory cortex and a large network of temporal and prefrontal cortices was more efficient in 15 MCS patients than in 15 vegetative state patients" (Laureys et al., 2005a, 730–731). The importance of these findings is that MCS patients evince functional *integration* between different processing centers, which suggests higher-order cognition, but they lack the ability to *express* such processing fully or consistently. These results were confirmed via metabolic studies using FDG-PET (fluorodeoxyglucose with positron emission tomography) in which brain regions associated with language processing and possibly volition were notably active (Bruno et al., 2012, 1096). On the basis of these studies and in particular imaging studies of cortical activity, MCS patients should not be viewed as lacking a 'self'; they are conscious, by behavioral criteria, and *likely* retain reasoning abilities on the basis of neuroimaging data (Braddock, 2017).[1]

I emphasize 'likely' here because of a concern about the reverse inference fallacy (Nachev & Hacker, 2010). The reverse inference fallacy occurs when one reasons as follows: if subject S is given a task T under fMRI, for example, we may see that brain region r shows activity. From this observation, one may infer that brain region r grounds/causes cognitive function for task T, namely, if brain region r shows activity, then S is engaged in task T. Reverse inference is a fallacy because it is an instance of affirming the consequent of a conditional to infer the antecedent. If I am in Chicago, then I am in Illinois. But, if I am in Illinois, it is not necessarily the case that I am in Chicago, I could be in East St. Louis. So, the reverse inference fallacy is a fallacy if one is constructing a deductive argument. If, however, one understands the consequent as *evidence* for the antecedent being true, there is no fallacy (Nachev & Hacker, 2010, 71). Being in Illinois is evidence for being in Chicago, even if it is not strong evidence. Maybe a better example is to contrast the following inferences. If I am in Chicago, then I am in Cook County. I am in Chicago. Therefore I am in Cook County. This much is deductively valid. Conversely, if I am in Cook County, that *is evidence* – stronger evidence than simply being in Illinois – that I am in Chicago. I interpret neuroimaging studies to say that certain brain region activation is evidence for, not a deductive proof of, certain cognitive functioning. Therefore, I am not committing the reverse inference fallacy.

Several therapeutic modalities are effective for improving MCS patients' cognitive abilities. Deep-brain stimulation (DBS) has been effective for increasing arousal, limb control, and oral feeding (Giacino et al., 2012; Chudy et al., 2018). Notably, the subjects in Giacino et al.'s study were chronic MCS patients with no signs of improvement in the two months preceding enrollment. Dopaminergic agents, specifically amantadine, have improved acute MCS patients significantly (Whyte et al., 2005). Recently, transcranial direct current stimulation (tDCS) has been used with some evidence of benefit (Bai et al., 2017). Bai et al., though, only measured cortical excitability and not behavioral effects. Clinical response to tDCS was noted in a subgroup of MCS patients who had grey matter preservation and metabolic activity in the dorsal-lateral and medial pre-frontal cortexes, precuneus, and the thalamus (Thibaut et al., 2015). Additionally, the following modalities have shown some benefit in subjects satisfying the vegetative state criteria: zolpidem, median nerve stimulation, extradural cortical stimulation, spinal cord stimulation, and intrathecal baclofen (Georgiopoulos et al., 2010). Lastly, outcomes of patients in MCS show a positive trend that is not temporally restrained – the length of time being minimally conscious is not correlated with lower outcomes (Voss et al., 2006). Nakase-Richardson et al. (2012) followed traumatic brain injury patients who had a Glasgow Coma Score (GCS) of 3 on ED admission (3 is the lowest score compatible with life). Sixty-eight percent regained consciousness, 19.6% achieved functional independence, and 18.7% demonstrated employment potential. It is important to emphasize that the inclusion criteria were also unconsciousness and a GCS of less than 6 (worse than MCS) upon admission to a rehabilitation center. Of course, more evidence and research would be illuminating, but part of the tendency my argument aims to resist is what Joseph Fins refers to as the "societal neglect syndrome" (Fins, 2015). The point is to resist the urge to assume a static picture of the patients on whom one provides ethical commentary. Any ethical commentary on a specific MCS patient should *at least* tell us whether therapeutic interventions were attempted.

Lastly, most MCS patients require artificially delivered nutrition and hydration – typically, PEG tube feeding. The clinical circumstances to which my argument applies include MCS patients who require tube feeding to survive. I focus on tube feeding since its purpose is merely to nourish and hydrate, i.e., to provide basic necessities.[2] Whether one is sick or healthy, we need nutrition and hydration. Furthermore, tube feeding (via PEG) is typically quite easy to administer, once placed. Further acuminating the scope of my argument, I focus on MCS patients whose refusals of tube feeding are based on a judgment that MCS involves a low quality of life (QoL).[3] My argument assumes these features of a patient's setting. If the critic imports into this setting other complicating features,[4] such as other pathologies, that would not be a criticism of my argument.

Undercutting the Argument from Advance Directives

End-of-life decision-making should focus on the question of whether *a clinician* is morally justified to withdraw a means of sustaining life from the patient in the actual clinical circumstances the clinician faces. The reason for this emphasis is that the clinician is the agent of the action. The key question I answer in this section is whether a clinician is morally justified in withdrawing tube feeding from a patient who is in MCS. Broadly construed, there are two ways in which this judgment can be justified. The first is if the clinician is justified in believing that S *would want* PEG feeding withheld or withdrawn in the present circumstances. The second is if the clinician is justified in believing that it would be in S's *best interest* to have PEG feeding withheld in the present circumstances. I address only the former justification presently.

Consider the following train of thought (Davis, 2009). Suppose S decides at some point in the past that she would not want PEG feeding if she were in MCS because that would involve what, in her assessment, is a low quality of life. Suppose also that S is no longer competent to make decisions for herself. Advance directives are morally sufficient to act upon only if[5] those directives are applicable; and to count as applicable there must be justification for moving from 'S decided to refuse PEG feeding' to 'S would decide to refuse PEG feeding.' The argument from advance directives would hold, then, that a clinician is justified in withdrawing PEG feeding from S only if the clinician is justified in believing that S *would* not want it. And the clinician's evidence for believing this comes from what S had decided in the past (when she was competent).

My task in this section is to argue that this line of reasoning suffers from an undercutting defeater. In particular, I argue that one cannot move from

> (Past) S decides at some time in the past to refuse PEG feeding in MCS because this would involve a low quality of life.

to

> (Present) S *would* decide to refuse PEG feeding in MCS because this involves a low quality of life.

In a typical clinical scenario, (Past) supplies sufficient evidence for (Present).[6] I shall argue that it does not for patients in MCS. There are basically two empirically informed reasons for blocking this inference in the case of MCS patients. The first is what I refer to here as the 'disability bias.' The disability bias is the trend by third parties to devalue or rate the quality of life of those who are disabled as being significantly lower than how the disabled themselves judge their lives. I argue that the evidence for the disability bias applies as well to MCS patients. The second reason comes from research by Sehgal et al. (1992) showing that, for certain classes of patients, a significant percentage of them would not want their advance directives followed.

The Disability Bias

The present task is to argue that third-person QoL judgments are unreliable. The reason for focusing on third-person judgments is because we issue *advance* directives from that very standpoint. The *future* patient does not know what it *is* like to be disabled. The argument herein does not argue that being minimally conscious is a quality way to live. I do not know whether it is or is not. Thus, my argument aims only to block the inference from a third-person QoL judgment to one's actual first-person QoL judgment.

Quality of life studies performed on those with severe motor disabilities show that the patient's own assessment is at or slightly below the quality of life scores of normal controls. What is more, when non-disabled controls are asked what the disabled think of their own quality of life, the non-disabled rate it significantly lower than the disabled actually do. This serves as evidence for a disability bias. The disability bias is a judgment about a disabled person's quality of life and it counts as a *bias* because it does not reflect what such persons actually judge about their own quality of life. After presenting this evidence, I address why the evidence, which focuses on those with severe motor disabilities, is applicable also to those with cognitive disabilities, such as MCS.

Consider first patients with locked-in syndrome (LIS). Locked-in syndrome is a disorder typically caused by a stroke to a portion of the brainstem, commonly the pons. We can think of the brainstem like a two-way highway with multiple lanes. For LIS patients, all lanes are open going *into* the brain; they can see, think, hear, and understand. All lanes going *from* the brain are closed. They are completely paralyzed but, in classical LIS, retain voluntary control over blinking and eye movement.

What is it like to be fully conscious and fully paralyzed? Apparently, it is not as bad as one might think. Steven Laureys et al. (2005b) summarize much of the literature on this topic considering quality-of-life measures, end-of-life decision-making, and suicidal ideation. In all three areas, the conclusions may strike some as surprising. Ghorbel (2002; see also Doble et al., 2003) administered self-reports on mental and physical well-being.

Self-scored perception of mental and physical health were not significantly different than age-matched normal controls. Leon-Carrion, van Eeckhout, and Dominguez-Morales Mdel (2002) discovered that, of 44 subjects, 48% regarded their mood as good whereas only 5% regarded it as bad. Thirteen percent noted that they were depressed, 73% enjoyed going out and 81% met with friends at least two times a month. Of note, suicidal ideation was correlated with perception of pain, indicating that proper pain management might decrease the incidence of depression generally and suicidal ideation specifically. A subset of patients in the Ghorbel (2002) study suffered total LIS, but very few had suicidal ideation even after being locked-in for six years. On a scale from 0–10 (never to constantly), only four patients experienced suicidal ideation more than 3 on the scale, compared with eight who *never* had suicidal ideation and only four who rarely had it. Regarding treatment choice, 80% wished to receive antibiotics if they were to contract pneumonia and 62% elected to be full codes.

Bruno et al. (2011) explored QoL assessments with 91 LIS patients. Of these, 47 patients expressed happiness, with only 18 expressing unhappiness. Unhappiness was associated with lack of integration into social life, anarthrea, and lack of recreational activities. Bruno et al. conclude:

> Our data stress the need for extra palliative efforts directed at mobility and recreational activities in LIS and the importance of anxiolytic therapy. *Recently affected LIS patients who wish to die should be assured that there is a high chance they will regain a happy meaningful life.*
>
> (Bruno, 2011, 1, emphasis added)

Lulé et al. (2009) discuss the "disability paradox" that this evidence suggests. Severely disabled patients, like those in LIS and amyotrophic lateral sclerosis (ALS), adapt to their disabilities as indicated in higher QoL scores the longer they have experienced the disability. Important for my purposes is the following observation, "Preliminary results from our study on clinicians' perception of LIS show that in 97 interviewed healthcare workers the majority (66%) considered that 'being LIS is worse than being in a vegetative or minimally conscious state'" (Lulé et al., 2009, 347). This assessment is clearly incongruent with what LIS patients themselves think.

Research involving ALS (a motor degenerative disease leading to progressive paralysis) patients shows the same mismatch between clinicians' and patients' QoL judgment. A common sequelae of ALS is ventilator dependence. On the Life Satisfaction Index (using a Likert scale 1–7), ventilator users reported a mean score of 4.98. For perspective, normal controls reported a mean LSI of 5.33. The remarkable finding in this study was not only that ventilator users had near equivalent LSI scores as normal controls but also that health care professionals' assessment *of the ventilator users'* life satisfaction was 2.42 – far below the patients' own assessment of their life satisfaction (Bach, 2003, S25).

Similar findings on quadriplegics secondary to high-spinal cord injury (SCI) were reported by Gerhart et al. (1994). Quality of life measures were administered to SCI patients and their health providers for comparison. Ninety-two percent of patients reported that they were glad to be alive; whereas only 18% of the health professionals imagined that they themselves would be glad to be alive if they were quadriplegic. Eighty-six percent of the patients rated their QoL as average or better (than pre-SCI). Only 17% of their medical staff thought that SCI patients could have an average or better QoL.

Amyotrophic lateral sclerosis patients themselves seem to experience the same mismatch between their pre-paralysis/vent dependence period and when they need respiratory support on a regular basis. Again, Bach notes that, when queried early on in the development of ALS, patients refuse respiratory support if they were in need of it. However, their minds change when they become dyspneic and non-invasive respiratory aids prove effective. (In many cases, general QoL judgments by ALS patients match normal controls *throughout* the illness. This again illustrates adaptation, see Lulé et al., 2012.) Notably the "patient's attitude toward the use of ventilatory aids seems *to reflect his/her physician's attitude and the nature of the treatment options being presented rather than his/her own informed rational decision*" (Bach, 2003, S26–S27, emphasis added). Bach's research on ALS patients shows rather vividly the mismatch between clinicians' and patients' QoL judgments and even QoL judgments between healthy and disabled patients.

Laureys et al. (2005b) comment that the results here run contrary to what many health professionals think. Many clinicians are involved with the patient populations discussed here only on a short-term basis when the patient is at his or her worst. Because of this, clinicians may simply assume that the patient would refuse further support and would want to die.

> As a result, debates about cost, daily management, quality of life, withdrawal or withholding of care, end-of-life decisions and euthanasia often go on with prejudice and without input from the conscious but mute and immobile patient. . . . Clinicians should realize that quality of life often equates with social rather than physical interaction and that the will to live is strong when struck by an acute devastating disease.
>
> (Laureys et al., 2005b, 506–507)

Several themes emerge from considering these studies. First, clinicians' assessments of their patients' quality of life are typically *much lower* than what the patients themselves judge. Second, lower QoL assessments by patients do *not* correlate with the level of disability, and higher QoL assessments are associated with higher integration into the patient's social network. They are taken on walks, read to, etc. Third, there is usually a period in the early stages of severe disability with acute onset that patients report unhappiness. After a period of adaptation and re-integration, patients return to QoL judgments on par with or slightly below normal controls. Because of this, Bach (2003, S23) notes that, for ALS patients, advance directives are inappropriate because such patients are typically ill-informed about non-invasive respiratory aids, and they suffer from a bias against being disabled inherited from their physician.

The conclusion I wish to draw from these studies is that our assess-ment of what it is like to be disabled is radically incongruent with that of those who experience the disability first hand.[7] Consequently, we should be skeptical of our quality of life judgments from the third-person stand-point. But it is just from this standpoint that we issue *advance* directives. So the distortion that infects the third-person standpoint applies to one issuing an advance directive that will be applicable to their future disa-bled self. *We* think LIS would be a bad way to live, LIS patients do not think so. *We* think MCS would be a bad way to live. It may be the case that they do not think so (to the extent that they can understand).

The Lability of Advance Directives

Sehgal and colleagues (1992) studied whether and to what extent patients want their advance directives followed. Sehgal et al. chose dialysis patients since they are already receiving a form of life-sustaining treatment and therefore are more informed of what that involves. Subjects were given a hypothetical scenario in which they envision suc-cumbing to Alzheimer's disease. They were asked several questions two of which are pertinent for my purposes. First, they were asked whether they would want dialysis continued or stopped in the context of Alzheimer's disease. Second, subjects were asked how much *leeway* they would give their physician and surrogate to disregard their stated wishes if their physician or surrogate thought that disregarding those wishes would be in the subject's best interests. Leeway was defined on a four-point scale ranging from no leeway, a little leeway, a lot of leeway, and complete leeway.

Overall, 52% of the subjects want dialysis continued in the context of Alzheimer's disease. For all subjects, 39% of them elected no leeway to their decision, followed by 19%, a little leeway, 11%, a lot of lee-way, and 31%, complete leeway. That is to say, more than 42% gave at least a lot of leeway to their own advance directive. Sixty percent of the subjects with prior written directives wanted their advance directives fol-lowed strictly (no leeway). Only 33% of those with no written directive elected no leeway. Other demographics of those who elected no leeway include 44% of those under 65 years of age compared with only 28% over 65 years of age. Only one of 11 subjects with a history of cancer wanted their directive followed strictly. And only one of 12 with a history of stroke wanted their directive followed strictly. These last two trends indicate that those familiar with health care delivery were either more amenable to best interest judgments than their own preferences, or they simply did not have strong preferences to refuse dialysis. The authors conclude that "following all advance directives strictly may not reflect patient preferences" (Sehgal et al., 1992, 62). And, more importantly, "over half the subjects [61%] would allow very specific advance directives to be overridden. Thus, even very specific advance directives do not provide physicians with a complete understanding of patient preferences" (Sehgal et al., 1992, 62).

In concluding the previous two subsections, it is important to understand the epistemic work this evidence is meant to do. Suppose we want to know whether a particular drug is toxic and that there is a theoretical reason for thinking that it is lethal (for example, it has a molecular composition similar to known lethal drugs). There is, yet, no evidence for its actual safety. So, we perform experiments on some macaque monkeys and they all survive. That all the monkeys survive is evidence (though not sufficient evidence) that the drug is safe for humans. But suppose also that the monkeys all survived high doses of other drugs known to be lethal to humans. This evidence clearly undercuts the initial, albeit paucious, evidence we had for thinking that the drug is safe. If we bring the drug to market anyway, we would be doing something careless and irresponsible – even if, by luck, no one dies from the drug. Why? The cost of being wrong is high (numerous human lives might be killed by the drug), and our original reason is no longer a reason (the drug may be lethal and our evidence base would look just the same). An undercutting defeater (Pollock & Cruz, 1999) is a reason for thinking that the evidence for a proposition no longer functions as evidence for it (Chapter 1 considered the example of the widgets looking red even if they were not).

The evidence canvassed so far functions as an undercutting defeater to the judgment that MCS patients would not want PEG feeding. The reasons upon which such a judgment is based are undercut. The evidence for the disability bias tells us that third-person QoL assessments about the disabled are not evidence for the claim that the disabled patients themselves would judge their life as having a low quality; just as 'the widgets are under red lamps' undercuts the evidence that the widgets are red, and 'the monkeys did not die from known lethal drugs' undercuts the evidence that the drug is safe for humans. The evidence from Sehgal and colleagues suggests that a patient's own specific preferences are not held strictly. Having a *written* directive appears to be associated with 'no-leeway' but only for 60% of those subjects. If we make the choices binary (follow strictly (no-leeway) versus not strictly (a little, a lot, complete)), having a written directive predicts no-leeway only slightly above chance since 40% of those with written directives elected to have their preferences followed with at least some scope of leeway.

What Follows from this Evidence?

It is important to say why the disability bias for motor disabilities applies to those suffering a disorder of consciousness. The inference from 'the disability bias infects QoL judgments for patients with motor disabilities' to 'the disability bias infects QoL judgments for those with disordered consciousness' is mediated by three interrelated points.

a   We do not know what it's like to be compromised in the way MCS patients are. This lack of knowing 'what it's like' is present in any third-party assessment of a disabled person's quality of life. Certainly, one reason why the QoL judgments by the non-disabled and the disabled diverge is because the non-disabled lack the 'what it's like' aspect about living with a disability. In fact, skepticism about what it's like to be minimally conscious is irremediable since MCS patients typically cannot communicate to us what it's like to be disabled as they are.

b   Another feature of third-party QoL judgments about the disabled is that they likely issue from an 'I wouldn't want to live like that' sentiment. The skeptical effect of this sentiment is the plausibility of change. On this point, Michael Wreen is entirely correct when he says, "a clear-thinking and rational person . . . realizes that, however certain he may be of his values and desires now, they could change radically under desperate, life-threatening circumstances, and some provision should be made for the possibility of such a change" (2004, 328). Sehgal and colleagues demonstrate the likelihood of this lability.

Furthermore, this sentiment is not indexed to a type of disability. Any severe disability falls under the sentiment when issued from a third-person standpoint. The evidence canvassed in this section indicates that such a sentiment changes in the case of motor disability, and there is no positive reason to think that it does not change for cognitive disabilities. Arguing that being in a minimally conscious state is *objectively* worthless fairs no better. Any justification for such a judgment must fall back on a third-party assessment of an MCS patient's experiences, but it is just these judgments of which we should be suspicious. The empirical evidence indicates that being disabled is not correlated with a lower quality of life judgment.

An analogy may help understand the skeptical effects to which I'm drawing attention. Suppose I discover that the drug I have taken can affect one's vision such that one conflates similar objects – I see what looks like a dog, but it really is a fox, or a raccoon for a cat, etc. Suppose I come to see what looks to me like a dog. Knowing that I have taken this drug, I should be skeptical of this judgment. Evidence of the disability bias functions as a reason for being skeptical of one's third-person quality of life judgments similar to how knowing the drug's effects functions as a reason for being skeptical of my perceptions of putative canines.

Continuing with the example, the scope of skepticism extends to any judgment where the object shares similarities to other objects within a similarity; if I see what looks to me like a hyena, I should also be skeptical. Conversely, if I see what appears to be a dog, I know that what I am really looking at cannot be an anaconda. But if I come to see what appears to me as a platypus which really is a platypus, knowing that the drug confuses *similar* images but *not by how much* – I should still be skeptical that what I see is a platypus. It might be a beaver or otter even though the differences here are more pronounced than between a dog and a fox. We know that the 'I wouldn't want to live like that' sentiment and 'not knowing what it's like' are reasons for being skeptical of third-person QoL judgments for severe motor disability and they may likely extend to ground a similar skepticism for MCS patients.

c   The functional abilities of MCS patients may be underestimated since it is likely that treatment modalities (amantadine or DBS) are not even tried before withdrawal decisions are made, often due to prejudices (Fins, 2015). Neuroimaging studies have taught us at least one thing about MCS patients, they are more cognitively active than what can be demonstrated through spoken communication (see page 190). A general epistemological dictum is apropos here: absence of evidence does not entail evidence of absence. In general, whether someone is conscious and to what degree of consciousness the person attains is a different question from whether he can *demonstrate* that he is conscious or the degree to which he is conscious. We cannot infer from 'patient M cannot *demonstrate* that she is conscious and aware through spoken communication' to 'patient M is not conscious or aware'. Consequently, the inference from 'the disability bias infects QoL judgments for motor disabilities' to 'it infects QoL judgments for cognitive disabilities' is more continuous if we take seriously the neurobiological evidence that minimally conscious patients retain cognitive function and that the disability bias issues from a feature common to both QoL judgments for motor and cognitive disabilities, i.e., a third-person assessment informed by either a lack of knowing what it's like or an 'I wouldn't want that' sentiment.

My argument against the advance directive argument aims to ground the disparity between first- and third-person judgments when those judgments pertain to one's quality of life. A third-person judgment that MCS involves a low quality of life is not a strong enough reason for thinking that the first-person judgment would involve the same assessment. *The evidence would look just the same even if the first-person judgment did not correlate with the third-person judgment.* The reason is that the evidence in this case just is the third-person judgment, and we have seen that it is not discriminating evidence for what the first-person judgment would look like.[8] The widgets may really be red, the drug really safe, and MCS patients may really not want PEG feeding. But because the evidence upon which we base these judgments is compatible with the widgets not being red, the drug not being safe, etc., we cannot rely on it.

Furthermore, the typical reason for thinking that an advance directive of an MCS patient should be respected is that it is an informed refusal by the patient when she was decisional. But the disability bias tells us that it may *not* have been informed insofar as it was rendered from the third-person standpoint with no knowledge of what it's like to be in a minimally conscious state. Add to this the evidence that quite a few patients view advance directives not as irrefragable commands (Sehgal et al., 1992) but as guides to their general value commitments, and the argument from advance directives is effectively undercut. Rudner's guidance (Chapter 3) suggests further that if there is a high cost to being *wrong* that an MCS patient *would want* tube feeding withheld, an undercutting defeater is sufficient – with no other justification – for continuing tube feeding.

The cost in being wrong in thinking that (Past) provides sufficient evidence for (Present) in an MCS patient is that one lets a conscious patient dehydrate to death, plausibly going against what the patient's actual wishes may be and withholding an easy means of sustaining his or her life. The burden of proof is on those who would argue to remove PEG feeding. To say that the disability bias is not ubiquitous is not sufficient to override the burden. The evidence for the disability bias is strong enough to undercut the inference from (Past) to (Present) in any given case.

The following is a summary of my argument in this third section. The scope of 'disabled populations' in the premises should be interpreted to include MCS patients as well as LIS, SCI, etc.

1   Advance directives (specifically, refusals based on quality of life judgments) are issued from the third-person perspective.
2   For certain disabled patient populations, third-person quality of life judgments (including best-interest judgments) do not provide evidence for what the patient's actual quality of life judgment might be. (Disability bias and lability of advance directives premise.)

3   Therefore, for certain disabled populations, advance directives do not provide evidence for what the patient's actual wishes might be.
4   If an advance directive does not provide evidence for the patient's actual wishes, it is not applicable.
5   Therefore, for certain disabled populations, advance directives are not applicable.

Objections

Because my argument says that it is impermissible to act on a patient's previous refusal when she or he was decisional, an obvious moral concern is that I am ignoring the presumption in favor of advance directives having moral authority. The purpose of this section is to deflect this and related concerns.

One practical consequence of my argument may be that a minority of MCS patients would have their wishes not fulfilled. Some commentators might take that to be a symmetrical cost. But, again, this would ignore the clinical scenario my argument is indexed to, namely, PEG feeding is a fairly easy means to deliver and receive,[9] and – per the lesson learned from QoL studies on LIS patients – treating disabled patients as the persons they (still) are is imperative (see my concluding remarks below). In point of fact, far from ignoring a minority of patient's wishes, my argument is that, in the absence of evidence to the contrary, the evidence of disability bias is strong enough to undercut the inference from (Past) to (Present) in most cases. All of what I have argued for is to act *in accordance with* what the patient *presently* wants. A patient's wishes retain moral authority on my view. Here is how to see the point. The reason why past wishes are important is because they are supposed to provide evidence for what the patient would or presently wants (but cannot communicate it). This fact is normatively relevant only because what the patient presently wants (or would want) is morally important. My argument is compatible with this line of thought. I wish only to say that, in the case of disability, past wishes are likely not indicative.

A few other parries are sufficient to deflect concerns about paternalism. The first is that the conclusion of my argument is technically not paternalistic at all. The bad kind of paternalism requires one agent A going against another *fully autonomous* agent's choice and A justifies the act on the basis that the agent is benefited (Wreen, 2004). Since MCS patients are likely not fully autonomous, the bad form of paternalism does not even apply.

Is going against a *precedent* fully autonomous choice so bad? The badness of paternalism correlates with the goodness of the choice being impugned. And it is unclear what normative weight a precedent autonomous choice bears, especially when it may be subject to a bias. That I have chosen X does not by itself justify doing X. To justify a choice, one needs to cite the goods realized by the choice. And in the case at hand, one of the goods at stake is keeping a conscious patient alive through simple means and the choice might be biased anyway. Autonomy considered qua ability strikes me as extremely valuable. Autonomy qua discrete choice is valuable only as a function of the goods such a choice realizes.

Some other important objections may now be addressed. Walter Glannon (2013) takes the position that tube feeding should not be given to MCS patients. Specifically, he discusses patient M who was minimally conscious and the English Court of Protection ruled that it would be impermissible to withhold tube feeding from her. Glannon thinks that the English court erred in its reasoning and in its conclusion. Glannon summarizes his reasoning as follows, "[t]he poor prognosis for MCS patients, the fact that M was regularly in pain and likely suffering from it, her complete dependence on others, and the lack of restorative therapies made the burdens outweigh the benefits for her" (Glannon, 2013, 2). Glannon seems to think that tube feeding would *only* be worthwhile in conjunction with effective therapies aimed to restore cognition and physical mobility "to beneficial levels" (Glannon, 2013, 2). On some points I tentatively agree with Glannon, and so properly understanding the borders of my argument requires limning where Glannon and I agree and where it appears we disagree.

I tentatively agree on the following items: (1) Glannon notes that patient M was in intractable pain. If true, this might be a reason for withholding tube feeding. My agreement is cautious since it is unclear what kind of palliative care the patient was receiving. If it were known that the patient was in pain, proper pain management should address the issue. In any case, truly *intractable* pain is typically a sign that some other pathology is inflicting the patient (e.g., stomach cancer), in which case my argument does not apply. (2) Glannon notes that death does not always harm the one who dies. Technically speaking, if harm is understood as violating someone's interests and it is not in someone's interest to continue living, then death is not a harm – on this definition of harm.[10] My agreement is cautious since it would be a mistake to think that the category of harm *exhausts* the category of wrongdoing. It would be wrong, for instance, to push a suicidal teenager off a tall bridge but that would not be violating his interests. Consider raping a patient in a persistent vegetative state (PVS), or using PVS patients for car safety testing (Watt, 2000) or for orthopedic surgical practice. All of these actions would be seriously wronging the patient, but arguably not harming the patient (if harm is indexed to interests).[11] (3) Glannon notes that, if the clinicians improve the conscious awareness of an MCS patient "without a corresponding improvement in pain management" (2013, 2), one would be doing more harm than good. My agreement is cautious because it hardly seems relevant. No one would argue for improving cognition without improving pain control. In fact, improving cognitive function could improve pain management because we could then ask the patient if she or he were comfortable.

As for the likely disagreements, Glannon notes that "a reasonable level of quality of life implies a sufficient degree of pain control and a sufficient degree of functional recovery, such that the patient is not *completely dependent on others*." And he repeats the point a few lines later, claiming that a source of suffering is not only from physical pain but "[t]hey could also suffer from the experience of being completely dependent on others" (Glannon, 2013, 2, emphasis mine). These comments clearly demonstrate the disability bias articulated above. On Glannon's reasoning, LIS patients, quadriplegics, and advanced ALS patients do not have a "reasonable level of quality of life" since they are completely dependent upon others and they lack a "sufficient degree" of functional recovery – whatever that can mean. Would Glannon hold that we should dehydrate them to death even if they indicate that they want to live (as most do)? If he answers 'no,' then what exactly is this notion of a "reasonable level of quality of life" doing in his argument? Is not such a notion endorsing a particular conception of the good which might not be congruent with the patient's own conception? Furthermore, what is to count as a "sufficient degree" of functional recovery? Answering these questions appears difficult if one wants to avoid the disability bias.

Lastly, one might say that my argument proves too much. It entails that it is impermissible to withhold or withdraw any means of sustaining life that is minimally burdensome (objectively considered). My position is that a patient may refuse a means of sustaining life even if she or he were perfectly functional. What is required before honoring such a wish, however, is that the patient give us a reason for doing so, and that reason has to be something more than just citing the patient's own condition. Suppose a patient refuses dialysis simply because she is in renal failure. That does not give us a reason to *withhold* dialysis. If anything, it *explains* why she *needs* dialysis. If she says that dialysis is too burdensome for her (e.g., she lives three hours away from the center) or is too expensive on her insurer, she has given a reason. Likewise, refusing tube feeding because one would be minimally conscious and cannot swallow is not a reason to withhold tube feeding. That would simply be an *explanation* for why the patient *needs* tube feeding.

The conclusion reached after the first argument is merely that an argument for respecting a patient's advance directive suffers from empirically informed undercutting defeaters. Showing that there is insufficient evidence *for* P is not itself an argument *against* P. In this case, P represents the clinician's judgment that she may *act on* the belief that S would want some means of sustaining life withdrawn at present. The second task of this chapter is to argue that the clinician may not act on the belief that S would want some means of sustaining life withdrawn at present.

Epistemic Diffidence and the Argument for Not Removing PEG Feeding

The argument I defend in this section is that a clinician should have epistemic diffidence toward the belief that it is permissible to withhold tube feeding from an MCS patient – in the circumstances I described in the first section. Consistent with the thread of argument in this book, if a belief is subject to epistemic diffidence, it should not be acted upon.

Let's assume that a reason for withholding tube feeding from an MCS patient, in the circumstances I defined in the second section, are either that the patient in question has issued a precedent refusal, or it is judged to be in the patient's best interest not to receive tube feeding. In the third section I argued that both reasons suffer from undercutting defeaters. As the drug case illustrates, however, *pairing an undercutting defeater with a judgment that has a high cost to being wrong suggests that one should not act on that judgment.*

To formulate the question I aim to answer in this section as succinctly as I can, the following nomenclature is necessary. Let R stand for

R = A patient S's precedent refusal of tube feeding, in the context of MCS, should be respected.[12]

And let not-R simply be the negation of R according to which S's precedent refusal should not be respected. We can now ask whether there is a higher cost to being wrong about R compared with not-R. In this section, I argue that there is. Specifically, the form of the argument in this section may be summarized as follows:

6 If the cost of being wrong about R is higher than not-R, one may *act on* R only if R enjoys stronger justification than not-R.
7 The justification for R is not stronger than not-R, and the cost of being wrong about R is higher than not-R.
8 Therefore, one may not act on R.
    On the assumption that the precedent refusal is based on a quality of life judgment, (8) entails,
9 It is impermissible to withhold tube feeding from an MCS patient who has refused it based on a quality of life judgment.

The key premise in this argument is (7). The third section argued for the first conjunct of (7). The second conjunct of (7) might be defended along the following lines. A patient who is in MCS, in the clinical scenario I am assuming, can be kept alive easily through PEG feedings, and they are consciously aware of their surroundings. Furthermore, some therapeutic modalities are successful in improving functionality. The cost here is letting a consciously aware patient dehydrate to death when we could improve her functionality. And if we cannot improve her functionality, she is still minimally conscious and able to experience her environment. We could still include her in social activities and recreation. A cost for being wrong about not-R is that we go against what the patient *had* wanted; and if my argument in the third section is plausible, the precedent refusal is likely biased anyway.

In arguing that the costs in being wrong about R are high, however, it appears I am relying on an implicit premise according to which living while in MCS can still involve a quality life. This is not the way to argue for premise (7). I harbor a third-person quality of life judgment that being in MCS would involve a severe diminution in my current quality of life. Rather, I prefer to defend (7) from the standpoint of how clinicians should *treat* such patients; not whether such patients are really living quality lives. It is rather admirable, and quite virtuous, to love and care for someone whose experiences and circumstances involve a very low quality of life. The admirability of our moral actions is not solely a function of whether the beneficiaries of our actions have a high quality of life; but is more so a function of our own disposition towards the weak and vulnerable. I can argue for (7), then, by citing the cost to the clinician if she were to discharge opportunities to love and care for patients who are particularly vulnerable and disabled.

In Chapter 5, I related the story of Charles and Ladmaker per Primo Levi. Narratives like the one Levi bequeaths are revealing on two accounts. The first is that Charles's actions are clearly admirable. What accounts for our admiration is that Charles's love went so deep. Our admiration is parasitic on Ladmaker's immense vulnerability and need. We can see the value of Charles's actions in virtue of the fact that he loved and cared for someone who is particularly decrepit, malodorous, and woebegone. The admirability of his actions are in proportion to the suffering and vulnerability of Ladmaker. (Though Charles's actions are not condescending – see the second point.) With this first point, I am suggesting that we flip the traditional way of assessing moral actions in the clinical setting. Charles's love and care for Ladmaker was admirable precisely *because* Ladmaker had a low quality of life. Rather than undercutting one's reasons for engaging in sacrificial acts of love, a low quality of life calls for them with a more stentorian tone.

The second lesson is orthogonal to the first – understanding quality of life on the horizontal plane of one's experiences, and inherent dignity as 'vertical.' The admirability of Charles's actions invite us to see through affliction and disability to the irreplaceable worth of the sufferer. What did Charles see; to what did he respond? A plausible explanation is that he saw clearly that the suffering of Ladmaker was bad; but with greater acuity he saw that Ladmaker retained inherent worth.[13] I argued in

Chapter 5 that we should look more closely at the *irreplaceable* person as being animated with inherent value, which is consistent with being immersed in affliction or disability.

For MCS patients, their quality of life might be low in our opinion, and possibly in theirs. But there is something admirable about loving and caring for them and seeing them as Charles cared for and saw Ladmaker. Their irreplaceable value remains despite their suppressed consciousness. In fact, it would be surprising if one's irreplaceable (and ineffaceable) value waxed and waned depending on whether the person is *able to demonstrate* to others that she can think. The proper response to MCS patients is to love them without condescension, and this point places the onus of proof on those who wish to withhold an easy means of sustaining life.

To summarize, the cost in being wrong about R is that the clinician in acting on R would be discharging an opportunity to engage in admirable care and love for the patient whose quality of life might be particularly low. Rather than seeing a low quality of life as a reason to withhold easy means of sustaining life, we should see it as a reason to care more deeply, as illustrated in the exchange between Charles and Ladmaker. A further cost is that the clinician would be ignoring the irreplaceable and inherent worth that remains in an MCS patient, obscured as it is by a low quality of life. The cost in being wrong about not-R might be the existential suffering an MCS patient might experience in not having his wishes honored. But this risk is one for which we have no evidence; I have taken pains above to argue that a low quality of life is evidentially inert to justify believing that the patient would not want to live. Considering all moral costs, the cost in being wrong about R is higher than the cost of being wrong about not-R.

Conclusion

What is the scope of my conclusions in this chapter? Does my argument entail that advance directives for demented or Alzheimer's patients are not applicable? At the risk of a frustrating response the answers are both yes and no. My principal concern is to challenge the prevailing orthodoxy that makes two questionable assumptions. The first is that advance directives are accurate portraits of the patient's mind; the second is that our prospective quality of life judgments are accurate. I have provided evidence here that both assumptions are empirically unsupportable. What follows from my argument is that advance directives that are based on third-person QoL judgments are a precarious source of information on what the patient might really want. It does not follow that advance directives are useless sources of information. Hence, they can be used for cognitively challenged patients, but only very carefully (Wreen, 2004, 322ff.).

We would do better to do two things that would redeem the relevance of advance directives. The first is for clinicians who work with disabled populations to check their own potential prejudices on how valuable their patients' lives could be. In their work on deep brain stimulation, Giacino et al. (2012) have received criticisms, not for the fact that they are doing neurosurgery on the non-consenting, but that they are even trying to develop therapeutic interventions for MCS patients. Their colleagues complain that MCS would be a state worse than death. To which they reply that such comments,

> [r]eflect . . . the aforementioned biases that . . . nothing can or should be done to them. However, this stance immediately becomes problematic if one considers that these patients are conscious and that some of them might have degrees of awareness that suggests that they are cognizant of the isolation that our collective societal neglect has imposed upon them. In our view, there are moral and fiduciary obligations to intercede and attempt to remediate their potential sense of isolation.
>
> (Giacino et al., 2012, 346)

The proper response to severe disability and dependency is a deeper and more involved care, i.e., love without condescension. A state that would be worse than death is to be disabled, dependent, *and* ignored or treated with the disability bias.

The second is for more efforts at advance care planning, especially with diseases that have fairly predictable courses and timelines, such as Alzheimer's and certain causes of dementia. If we do at least those two things my conclusions in this chapter become much more circumscribed around a small set of patients; and possibly much more palatable to otherwise critical readers.

Notes

1 Error rates in diagnosing patients as in a vegetative state (VS), when they are really minimally conscious or locked-in, are quite common (see Andrews et al. (1996) where 43% were misdiagnosed, and Gill-Thwaites (2006) where 45% were misdiagnosed). And some in VS modulate brain activity in light of external stimuli (Monti et al., 2010). Because of these facts, my argument should be understood to include patients who appear in VS, but are really covertly conscious (Owen, 2013); they cannot demonstrate (to us) that they are conscious, but they likely retain cognitive and volitional abilities.
2 See Meilaender (1984).
3 I disagree with the language of 'quality of life' judgment for the simple reason that it is not theory neutral. It invites the idea that one's value is determined solely by how that person sees her value. This language endorses subjectivism without arguing for it. A second reason is that even proponents of this language really do not mean to refer to the quality of someone's *life*. They mean

the quality of one's experiences or circumstances. With these confusions in mind, I capitulate and use such language throughout.

4 One such feature might be that the patient has refused tube feeding if in MCS based on the burdens, financial or otherwise, to their family. I have no principled objection to honoring *that* wish, but I am suspicious of the anti-communitarian assumptions informing it.

5 For advance directives to count as applicable other necessary conditions that together may be sufficient are that the patient was informed (the patient has considered the relevant medical information), voluntary (is not being coerced), and rational (has made inferences based on the relevant information). And that the specific decision fits the actual clinical circumstances. My argument, however, is only to challenge whether the applicability condition is satisfied.

6 This assumption is problematic mainly because patients for whom advance directives are needed typically do not have present wishes since they might be unconscious or unable to process any relevant information. But this is a problem for all advance directives no matter what their content is. For a host of other philosophical problems affecting advance directives, see Vogelstein (2017), Dresser and Robertson (1989), Kuczewski (1997, 125ff.), and May (1998). I assume in this chapter that advance directives are morally relevant without explaining why (see Davis, 2009, sect. 4.4).

7 See Goering (2008) for an effective response to those who wish to contest the veracity of these QoL judgments by the disabled.

8 Justifying the removal of tube feeding from MCS patients with reference to best interest does not fare any better. The reason is that best interest judgments are, by definition, made from the third-person perspective. For best interest judgments we are no longer asking 'what would the patient decide?' but 'what should we decide given our knowledge of the patient's clinical circumstances?'

9 Potack and Chokhavatia (2008) observe certain complications. Most of the major complications occur in fewer than 2.5% of cases, and some complications are with the surgical procedure itself. Once placed, it is usually tolerated. Peristomal wound infection appears highest but is also manageable and occurs in patient populations other than the MCS population.

10 Beauchamp and Childress appear to hold such a view. "These arguments [for what counts as wrongdoing] suggest that causing a person's death is morally wrong, when it is wrong, because an unauthorized intervention thwarted or set back a person's interests" (2001, 148).

11 To accommodate these examples, one would have to understand interests more objectively. But then it is questionable whether not existing can be in a living thing's objective interests.

12 I set aside considering best interests since, if there is a high cost to being wrong about R (where the patient's wishes are known), so much more is it the case when the patient's wishes are not known.

13 This is part of the reason why I object to quality-of-life language. Such language does not encompass what is most essential about our worth.

10 Decision-Making for Patients with Apparent Competency

In the previous chapter I argued that a patient's previously stated wishes are not applicable to cases involving severe disability partly because those wishes are issued from the third-person standpoint. In this chapter I focus on patients whose first-person wishes are clearly known, but we should still be epistemically diffident in following them. Specifically, I'm concerned about patients who refuse a life-sustaining/saving measure that promises to work and does not present obviously onerous burdens to the patient. Refusals of low burden/high benefit treatments require a more fastidious analysis of whether the patient is rendering a competent refusal. Absent reasons for thinking the patient is offering a competent refusal, one should be epistemically diffident about honoring such refusals.

Consider the following case. A 30-year-old female is admitted with a chief complaint of lower extremity immobility with an unremarkable past medical history. She is diagnosed with lower-leg compartment syndrome with onset of gangrene. The patient had been sitting in a yoga-type position – sitting on her heels – and she fell asleep. Although a fasciotomy was considered, it would not arrest the infection. The patient required a bilateral below-knee amputation (BKA) to save her life. The patient was alert and oriented and refused a BKA after having this option explained to her. A psychiatric assessment was done in which the consultant indicated that she retained competency to make health care decisions. Her social history includes being single, and her mother and father lived in the region. Her employment history included some theatre work, modeling, and she is pursuing a career in singing.

It is common in clinical ethics to frame this type of case as a question of competency: is the patient competent to refuse or not? If she is, then the physicians should respect her refusal. Although I find this reasoning sufficient for many cases, it fails to handle the complexities of this particular case. In this case, I was consulted by an attending physician who was confused about what to do even after a psychiatrist declared the patient competent. What makes this case ethically difficult is that the procedure in question promises a significant benefit, not just objectively speaking in terms of medical probability and magnitude, but from the patient's perspective as well – she had well-developed life plans and aspirations. Although a BKA can be considered burdensome, the burdens can be compensated for by prostheses and supportive rehabilitation. Situations in which the procedure is life-saving (or life-preserving) and does not excessively compromise the patient's quality of life, and yet the patient refuses it, are what I call 'high-stakes cases.'[1]

Such cases are high stakes for both the patient *and* the clinicians. The stakes for the patient are obvious. The stakes for the clinicians are that rendering a judgment that 'the patient is making a competent and autonomous decision' morally entails respecting that decision – at least, I will assume this principle here. Respecting a refusal of a life-saving/preserving procedure typically involves the patient's death; and the other option involves saving the patient's life with little to no diminution in her quality of life or it subjects the patient to manageable burdens.[2] Consequently, the cost of being wrong that the patient is competent is high and, correlatively, the justification for that assessment must be strong. Therefore, epistemic pressure is placed on the judgment that 'the patient is making a competent and autonomous decision.' This chapter concerns, chiefly, the epistemic stakes as they pertain to the *clinicians' assessment* that the patient is rendering a refusal that should be respected. Specifically, I outline features of a patient's decision that supply adequate justification for the clinician to judge that a patient's refusal in a high-stakes context may be respected. Absent such justification, the judgment that the refusal is a competent one should be held with epistemic diffidence.

There are two basic routes by which clinicians have addressed cases like this one.[3] The first route is to have the patient declared incompetent simply in virtue of rendering the 'wrong' decision; and what counts as wrong is determined by the clinicians. This option would involve doing the BKA. A second option is to follow the wishes of any patient who demonstrates certain intellectual abilities. This option would involve discharging the patient to hospice. The former option is too paternalistic; the latter option ignores the moral gravity of the situation. The route I canvas here aims to countenance the moral gravity of such cases, but also allows for respecting a high-stakes refusal.

What is original about my analysis is twofold. (i) It is typical to assess competency with reference to the patient evincing certain intellectual abilities (Appelbaum, 2007, 1836). But, as the case above illustrates, such an analysis is not 'deep enough' to tell clinicians what to do in high-stakes cases – for the patient was clearly competent. We need more than merely an assessment of the patient's abilities; we also need to know whether those abilities are being *exercised* by the patient in the token instance of rendering the refusal. In this regard, I exploit the distinction between *being competent* (which asks whether the patient retains certain abilities) and rendering a *competent refusal* (which asks whether the *judgment* the patient makes in refusing a life-saving/preserving procedure is informed by good reasons). (ii) My focus is on the *clinicians' judgment* that the patient has offered a refusal that may be respected. Specifically, I address the question, 'what epistemic features of the clinician's judgment that "P's refusal is a competent one" must be present before he or she *acts on* that judgment?' Since the focus is on the quality of the clinician's judgment, a discussion of certain epistemic properties that judgment must evince is relevant.

The outline of the chapter is as follows: I begin with a brief description of the epistemic principles relevant to justification in high-stakes contexts. I then describe current standards for assessing competency and argue that stricter standards are necessary in those contexts. I end with some clarifications and application to cases.

The Basing Condition

I believe a lot of things: I believe that Bigfoot does not exist, that it is currently sunny outside, that it will be sunny outside tomorrow – given the testimony of a meteorologist – etc. The basing relation is the relation between my beliefs on one hand (it will be sunny tomorrow) and my reasons for those beliefs on the other (the meteorologist is reliable and she said it will be sunny). More specifically, it is not enough that I *have* other beliefs that may support or provide reasons for the target belief, but that the target belief is *based* on these other beliefs. Consider some examples.

> The detective believes that Jones is the murderer. He accepts the contents of a forensic report indicating that DNA evidence strongly points to Jones. But the detective believes that Jones is the murderer not on the basis of the report but rather solely because he infers this from his delusional belief that Jones confessed to the killings. The standard and proper verdict in this case is that the detective does not know that Jones is the murderer.
>
> (Warfield, 2005, 411)

In this example, the detective bases his belief in Jones's guilt on the wrong evidence, namely, his delusional belief. Common sense ("the standard and proper verdict") tells us that Jones does not know. His delusional belief is not the right evidence because it has no connection to or does not otherwise support the belief that Jones is guilty. (I leave the terms 'connection' and 'supports' as primitive here given the clarity of the example.) The basing condition requires that the evidence supporting my belief that p really supports p. I may believe that the meteorologist is reliable, that she has told me that it will be sunny outside tomorrow; but if I base my belief that it will be sunny tomorrow on the basis of what a shaman told me, my belief is not justified.[4]

The intuitions informing the basing condition are most strong when we are answering specifically epistemological questions, i.e., what is a necessary condition for having a justified belief? But when a patient refuses a means of sustaining or saving life (hereafter L), in what sense is the refusal a justified *belief*? Viewed in one way, it clearly is not since a patient's refusal of L is not simply a belief. It is better classified as a *decision*; in particular, a decision to refuse L based on a belief that L is not worth it.

However, the same intuitions apply to both justified belief and reasoned decision-making. Consider a decision-making case that is analogous to Warfield's. Suppose a patient believes correctly that she has severe mitral valve prolapse and that without open-heart surgery she will likely die. Suppose that she refuses, not on the basis of the burdens of open-heart surgery, but rather on the basis of a delusional belief that her husband – who is supposedly an angelic power – will heal her. Intuitively, if the decision to refuse is based on a delusional belief, it is not a strong reason to refuse. And this is enough to highlight the importance of the basing condition as it pertains to reasoned decision-making as well. (Whether we actually respect the refusal is a more difficult question. I deliberately selected a heart surgery case because such surgery is quite burdensome objectively considered. There are good reasons for refusing the surgery, just as there are good reasons for thinking that Jones is guilty. But because the refusal is not *based on* those reasons, we view the refusal with suspicion.) Conversely, if she were relatively young with a good prognosis otherwise, but she refuses because the burdens of heart surgery and rehab are 'not worth it,' then she has rendered a competent refusal. The point is that when we focus on the *source* of the belief or the decision, we find ourselves having the same intuitions: both a belief and a decision must satisfy something like a basing condition. In regard to decisions, the decision to refuse L must be based on true beliefs about the medical facts, and the reason for refusing must be *relevant* to or *support* the judgment that 'L is not worth it.'[5] The patient must cite a burden, financial cost, or lack of benefit and issue a value judgment according to which the burden, cost, or lack of benefit 'is not *worth* it.'[6]

Another popular intuition in epistemology was discussed in Chapter 3, namely, the epistemic effects of risk. Suppose you are a juror in a capital case. The cost of being wrong about p is that you would send an innocent person to his death – you know that the judge has no scruples about capital punishment. You would not rely on, say, the testimony of one eyewitness as being sufficient for guilt. You would want a substantial amount of strong evidence.

I pause here to note the importance of these ideas to our present issue. The basing condition is relevant to assess the quality of a patient's judgment to refuse a procedure in a high-stakes context. If the 30-year-old female stated that she did not want the BKA, this may not be enough to morally justify respecting her refusal. Clinicians need more than a dislike for something – after all, no one really *wants* her ankles cut off. Viewed in one way, not wanting the BKA is a sign of reasonableness, but it is still not a reason for refusing the BKA. If the refusal is not based on a reason, it does not satisfy the basing condition. Because the cost of being wrong is so high, we need the patient to assess the procedure's burdens or costs paired with her value preferences. The high cost in being wrong *requires* clinicians to know that she has satisfied the basing condition by citing reasons, for example: 'the burden of losing my bodily integrity is, in my view, too onerous.' The risk condition captures the idea that clinicians should protect patients from their own ill-considered decisions.[7] Another reason why we need a reason is that a patient's value preference paired with an accurate understanding of the sequelae of the procedure/treatment is typically more *stable* than a desire or emotional reaction to the procedure/treatment.

Atul Gawande offers an anecdotal story to illustrate the importance of stability. The patient had undergone abdominal surgery. Several days post-op he spiked a fever, his heart rate sped up, and he became short of breath (SOB). His SOB was only mildly addressed by wearing an oxygen mask on full O2. He had pneumonia which very likely could be addressed. However, it would take a few days and the patient would need ventilator support for that time. Upon hearing this, the patient adamantly refused intubation. Over the next few moments he eventually tired of his labored breathing and passed out. At that point, the chief resident and Gawande intubated the patient. Over the next 24 hours the patient improved significantly, and was ready for extubation. Gawande describes the extubation thus:

> I cut the ties and deflated the balloon cuff holding the tube in place. Then I pulled it out, and he coughed violently a few times. "You had pneumonia," I told him, "but you're doing just fine now." I stood there silent and anxious for a moment, waiting to see what he would say. He swallowed hard, wincing from the soreness. Then he looked at me, and, in a hoarse but steady voice, he said, "Thank you."
>
> (Gawande, 2010, 97)

I assume that intubating the patient was the correct action. The patient did not offer a reason for his refusal, and likely refused out of fear or misunderstanding. His 'truest' and 'deepest' desires, to use a common metaphor, have the feature of being 'deep' because of their stability and possibly because of their proximity to the patient's self-identity and self-understanding. We want reasons because reasons implicate the person at a more fundamental and stable level.[8]

Because the stakes are high for the clinicians, and some putatively competent patients can make refusals that do not satisfy the basing condition, a more sensitive criterion for honoring a patient's refusal is required. What we need to know is not merely that the patient is competent, but also that she has rendered a *competent refusal*. What is this distinction and why is it relevant?

Competency Assessments[9]

What counts as *being* competent? Paul Appelbaum (2007) and Berg, Appelbaum, and Grisso (1996) have provided what I take to be the most comprehensive and conceptually clear account of competency (understood as giving an account of the necessary *abilities* a patient must manifest in being declared 'competent'). They identify four conditions which constitute the notion of competency: "(i) ability to communicate a choice, (ii) ability to understand relevant information, (iii) ability to appreciate the nature of the situation and its likely consequences, and (iv) ability to manipulate information rationally" (Berg, Appelbaum, & Grisso 1996, 351).

A few comments are noteworthy as Berg, Appelbaum, and Grisso offer helpful explanations of each, and I consider the latter three. The ability to understand relevant information involves comprehending the concepts that described the patient's clinical situation. Berg, Appelbaum, and Grisso do not give examples, but I suspect they would include the notions of diagnosis and prognosis, and concepts specific to the treatment option. For example, if the option involves general anesthesia, the patient needs to understand that this means complete unconsciousness. However, the ability to understand is different from *appreciating* the information, as Berg, Appelbaum, and Grisso rightly observe. The ability to appreciate information is a more advanced cognitive ability than the previous two. It requires that a competent patient must be able to evaluate or assess the gravity or seriousness of the patient's situation. It is important to note that this assessment must be *true*; there is an embedded alethic component to the appreciating condition.

That an alethic component is required can be illustrated by considering cases discussed by Berg, Appelbaum, and Grisso, such as *In re Roe*.[10] For this case, the court ruled that a man with schizophrenia was not competent to refuse his medication because he denied that he was mentally ill. In calling this a failure to appreciate the medical evidence, the appreciation criterion includes an alethic component according to which the patient must have some true beliefs about his clinical status – he must believe that he has a serious problem. But how many true beliefs or which beliefs have to be true? In answer to this question, Berg, Appelbaum, and Grisso consider a patient who believed truly both that she had a cancerous uterus and that she would die without treatment.[11] However, she preferred faith healing over hysterectomy and she believed falsely that her husband was a faith healer. The court declared, and apparently Berg,

Appelbaum, and Grisso concur, that the patient was competent since she did have the necessary true beliefs, even if her false ones were both obviously false and they were the ones upon which she based her treatment decisions. The appreciation criterion includes an alethic component, but this component is limited to true beliefs regarding one's general status and the consequences of not receiving treatment.

The fourth criterion Berg, Appelbaum, and Grisso canvas is the ability to manipulate information rationally. They note that the courts have not recognized the importance of this criterion in competency assessments and this is likely because it is the hardest one to measure objectively. Nevertheless, they offer the following informative description:

> It addresses the patient's reasoning capacity or ability to employ logical thought processes to compare the risks and benefits of treatment options. This criterion does not look at the outcome of a decision, but, like understanding and appreciation, it is concerned with the patient's decision-making process.
>
> (Berg, Appelbaum, & Grisso, 1996, 357)

One way to capture this criterion is that, if a patient demonstrates logically valid reasoning, then she has satisfied this criterion; the reasoning need not be sound (by 'validity' and 'soundness' I mean what every logic textbook means by these terms). In this regard, they state,

> As we define the rational manipulation criterion, a patient need not be able to give objectively "rational" reasons for her choice as long as she can demonstrate that the final decision follows logically from *whatever* reasons are offered. . . . Our reasoning criterion would allow a patient to rest on any premises (even a false one) as long as the conclusion drawn follows logically from those premises.
>
> (358, emphasis added)

The Argument for Stricter Conditions

Each of these conditions is sensible and clear. My argument in this section is that clinicians need to know more than that certain abilities fulfilling these conditions are present. To see why, consider a case offered by Jonsen, Seigler, and Winslade:

> Mr. Cure, a 24-year-old white graduate student, has been brought to the emergency room by a friend. Previously in good health, he is complaining of a severe headache and stiff neck. Physical examination shows a somnolent patient without focal neurologic signs but with a temperature of 39.5 C and nuchal rigidity. An examination of spinal fluid reveals cloudy fluid with a white count of 2,000; a

Gram's stain of the fluid shows many gram-positive diplococci. A diagnosis of bacterial meningitis is reached. . . . He is informed that he needs immediate hospitalization and administration of antibiotics. He refuses treatment and says he wants to go home. The physician explains the extreme dangers of going untreated and the minimal risks of treatment [intravenous antibiotics]. The young man persists in his refusal. Apart from this strange demand, he exhibits no evidence of mental derangement or altered mental status.

(2002, 14, 58)

Most of us would say that the mere desire not to have the antibiotic treatment is not enough to justify not giving it to the patient. The case illustrates that we need more than just an assessment of his reasoning abilities – for he obviously retained these – we need his reason for refusing. A simple desire not to have the antibiotic is insufficient justification for respecting the refusal. A refusal based on an irrational fear of needles, for example, does not by itself merit respect. We need reasons and these reasons must advert to the benefits, burdens, or costs of the treatment modality and whether L is worth it. And we need to know whether the refusal is *based on* those reasons that support the judgment 'L is not worth it.'

Now a reason is constituted by two features. The first is a belief about the benefits (or lack thereof), burdens, and financial costs of L. In regard to this belief, Appelbaum (2007) and Berg, Appelbaum, and Grisso (1996) are correct to note that such beliefs must be true. Second, these beliefs must be paired with an evaluative judgment about the burdens, costs, or lack of benefit, and this judgment should reflect the patient's value commitments. That evaluative judgment takes into account the probability and magnitude of the burdens, financial costs, or lack of benefit and how important or meaningful those benefits or burdens are to the patient.[12]

A case offered by LaPuma and Schiedermayer (1994, 143–145) illustrates nicely the nature and importance of this evaluative judgment. The case involved a 27-year-old female with advanced Friedrich's ataxia, cardiomyopathy, scoliosis, and respiratory depression. She was admitted due to shortness of breath and required intubation. Although her family wanted her to have a DNR order, the patient herself, through yes/no questioning, indicated that she wanted CPR in the event of a cardiac arrest. For such a patient, the likelihood of success is exceedingly low and CPR involves significant burdens – chest compressions and shocks. The patient made an evaluative judgment that the low likelihood is worth it, and that the burdens were not so bad as not to tolerate them. Evaluative judgments are of course subjective – I may not assess the value of CPR the same way – and it requires that the patient ask 'is it worth it?' Only the patient can answer that question since it is only the patient who is the *patient* of the treatment. It is important to note that the evaluative component of a reason for refusing is not an expression of a desire or an emotion; it is an *assessment* – it is what the patient *considers* worthwhile. Strictly speaking, this is not a report about how one feels, but rather what one believes. The latter implicates the person's fundamental beliefs about what counts as valuable. A feeling towards x may *indicate* that a person values x. Of course the worry is that feelings and emotional reactions are fleeting. What a clinician needs, then, is a value judgment since we are searching for that which expresses the person's enduring and fundamental self.

To illustrate the importance of issuing a value *judgment*, consider Rufus, a 70-year-old male who is recently diagnosed with myelodysplastic syndrome (MDS) (a pathology of the blood cells leading to a lack of either white or red blood cells). The patient is not a candidate for stem cell transplantation, but Azacitidine may work. The patient, however, requires red blood cell (RBC) and plasma transfusions. The patient refuses, thinking that blood from another person is gross – he does not fear it, he just thinks receiving it into one's body is gross. Contrast Rufus with Jed, who is an age- and disease-matched Jehovah's Witness who refuses blood because of his religious beliefs. Even if we rule out misunderstanding and any other psychopathology, I am still inclined to override Rufus's refusal; whereas Jed's may be respected.[13] In what sense does one offer a competent refusal and the other one not?

Jed's refusal cites a significant burden if he were to receive the blood, namely, the loss of eternal life. Even if we think that the causal belief of 'receiving another's blood causes the loss of one's salvation' is false, the value judgment cites the loss of something of significant value, i.e., eternal life. As such, Jed's refusal is a competent refusal. Rufus does not cite a significant value that would be lost upon receiving the blood. He just thinks that it is gross. If we ask him, 'what would happen if we gave you the blood?' he only responds, 'I just think that's gross.' He does not cite, for example, the probability (albeit very low) of contracting an infectious disease, the fatigue and malaise that can follow upon receiving another's blood, or a concern about saving a scarce health care resource. Because his refusal is a statement of his repugnance, it is not a value judgment strictly understood; Rufus is reporting his feelings but is not issuing a judgment that L is not meaningful, important, or worthwhile. Permutations of these cases illustrate the principal point. For example, suppose Jed continues to self-identify as Jehovah's Witness but is very unreflective about those beliefs. He mentions the resulting loss of salvation but cannot say anything further about it, and it looks like Jed doesn't understand that aspect of his religion. Even though our intuitions in this permutation might be different than the original, we are still looking for the same thing, namely, does Jed offer a competent refusal which requires basing his refusal on beliefs that he has. Does he really believe that he'll lose his salvation? And, if not, the reasons for refusing are not based on reasons that are *his*.

The 24-year-old male who refused an antibiotic did not, let us suppose, offer a reason for refusing; there was no judgment expressed regarding the burdens or costs of the IV antibiotics, much less was there an evaluation of those burdens as being too onerous or not worth it. In such a case, the clinicians have no reason to respect the patient's wish since there is not a competent refusal of the antibiotic.[14]

In general, what accounts for our ethical worries in high-stakes cases is that the patients are refusing something that could clearly contribute to their overall well-being and health. And yet, we cannot just ignore a patient's refusal when she can communicate and reason about her clinical situation. What we care most about patient autonomy, however, is that we are respecting a patient's stable self. To do that we need to know the patient's *reasons* for refusing since it is only in offering a reason that the patient's own fundamental value commitments are implicated. Respecting a patient's reasons respects the patient. Typical assessments of competency, however, focus on one's *abilities*. Since these assessments do not consider the quality of a patient's *judgment*, they risk ignoring the patient's more stable self. Consequently, in high-stakes contexts, we need to move from assessing a patient's 'competency to refuse' to assess her 'competent refusal.'

Clarifications and Application to Cases

Though my argument extends the discussion on the ethics of competency assessment, it remains consistent with what previous authors have noted. My argument is largely consistent with Appelbaum's and others' approaches since they countenance the importance of there being a process of reasoning (i.e., rational manipulation). In one important respect, my argument is stricter. Berg, Appelbaum, and Grisso require a reasoning process that must be logically valid, but the reasons can be 'whatever' (1996, 358, quoted above). I think the 'whatever' criterion is too permissive. Suppose the patient in Jonsen, Seigler, and Winslade's example cites a fear of needles as a reason to refuse the antibiotics. This looks like it satisfies the 'whatever' criterion, but clearly it is not a competent refusal on my account and should not be respected. Of course, this may be an uncharitable interpretation of what Berg, Appelbaum, and Grisso mean by 'whatever' since they do not think *any* reason is a respectful reason either; for example, they do not think that refusals based on delusions should be respected. It may be, then, that my argument is consistent with Berg, Appelbaum, and Grisso's and Appelbaum's approach but more would need to be said on their part.

Thomas May offers informative reflections on what we should take competence to mean, namely, "'competence' is used to denote the eligibility to assume responsibility for decision-making that affects one's own welfare" (May, 1998, 250). He goes so far as to say that "Competence . . . *should not focus on the patient's abilities as such,* but upon the patient's eligibility to assume decision-making responsibility" (May, 1998, 256, emphasis added). May does not tell us how to determine who is *eligible* – he is suggesting only that we should not focus on the patient's rational abilities *as such* to determine who is. May correctly observes that competent people can make bad decisions and that there are other societal values that encroach upon the exercise of one's autonomy. However, his fundamental point is that we should resist defining into the notion of competency these other societal values as, by doing so, we preempt a discussion on just which of these values in which circumstances justifiably encroach autonomy. For example, May notes that competent people make ill-advised financial decisions which ruin their lives, why should people "not be allowed to ruin their lives through similar medical decisions" (1998, 254). He then suggests that there should at least be a discussion here and intimates that there is no principled distinction between the two.

I have a few points in reply to situate my argument alongside May's. First, there is a relevant distinction between damaging one's financial standing and damaging one's health and life. Money and wealth are instrumental goods, whereas health and life are more fundamental and basic. So, indeed, we should have stringent standards on just how ill-advised a patient's high-stakes decisions are in health care. I doubt May would disagree with this. (To repeat, he only suggests that we need to discuss the issue, and defining competency so that such a discussion is preempted is wrongheaded). Second, and more importantly, my argument is simply that there is a conceptual distinction between having certain abilities and rendering a reasoned judgment. In applying the basing and moral risk conditions to high stakes contexts, we need to know both whether the patient *has* certain abilities and whether she is *exercising* them in a token instance. Nothing May says appears to challenge this idea. After all, it would be an odd argument for respecting competency to ignore whether the capacities that constitute competency are being exercised in token instances. Of note, I agree with May that one is *eligible* to take responsibility for her decision-making when she retains certain rational abilities.[15] The question I set out to answer is, 'What justifies a *health care professional's judgment* that the patient has rendered a competent refusal of L? Has the exercise of the patient's rational abilities informed her refusal?' And, to repeat, the reason we need to ask these further questions is because of the basing condition as it applies to patients, and the moral risk condition as it applies to clinicians insofar as they are tasked with acting on high-stakes refusals.

Because of my emphasis on providing a reason in high-stakes refusals, one may charge me with intellectualism or elitism. The critic may note that, even if I am correct, implementing my thesis in the practical setting would be impossible because many people do not have the medical expertise or the philosophical training to think through and justify their high-stakes refusals. Consider an actual case from my own experience: a patient suffering from early-stage vascular dementia and a medical history of diabetes-mellitus was admitted with a chief complaint of a gangrenous foot. He needed a unilateral BKA to stave off a life-threatening infection. He refused. When the ethics team arrived and we asked him for his reasons he remarked, "I came into this world with two legs, I'm goin' to leave with two legs." We took that as sufficient. Given my argument so far, did we respect a patient's *competent refusal* of L? It seems not since the reason appears to show little reflection on the values at stake.

In defending our assessment, I would say that he did offer us a reason, namely, bodily integrity. Bodily integrity was an important value to him and he believed correctly that a unilateral BKA is incompatible with the preservation of this value. In general, my requirements for a competent refusal are no more intellectualist as Appelbaum's requirements for competency. A competent refusal must include true beliefs about the disease/pathology, the benefits, burdens, and costs of the proposed treatment; and a value judgment that such burdens, costs, or lack of benefits are not worth it.

But this case, suitably revised, invites us to probe further regarding whether clinicians should respect *any* value judgment. Consider a case entertained by Michael Wreen (2004) of a man named Albert H. Albert who is

> [H]opelessly but happily senile who needs antibiotics in order to survive. Years before, when competent, Albert executed an advance directive that said that were he to become seriously mentally impaired, he should not be given any life-sustaining treatments, including antibiotics. It's now against Albert's past wishes but in keeping with his present interests—Albert's current life does have value for him—to receive antibiotics. His son pleads that he should be given the antibiotics.
>
> (Wreen, 2004, 322)[16]

At least as here described, I am inclined to side with Wreen that, all else being equal, the patient should receive antibiotics – *pace* Mappes (2006). But suppose that the patient foresaw that being happily demented was a distinct possibility and that he would enjoy life. But he refused any treatment even on this contingency, reasoning that 'anything less than full competency is not a life worth living.' Is the value judgment that '*any* degree of mental disability entails that no life-sustaining measure is worth it' a judgment that clinicians should respect?

Before answering this question, consider for comparison the following case. The patient, call her Jane, was a 34-year-old female with a past medical history of diabetes. She needed a unilateral BKA secondary to stubbing her left toe and did not know it until the toe became gangrenous. She was in good health otherwise. She refused, and in the initial report to me, the infectious disease doctor described her as a "diva" and that she has "huge issues with physical appearance." In speaking with Jane, she refused the amputation because it would make her "look bad." She also offered some comment to the effect that she would not be able to put on her new Ugg boots. I thought she was joking, but in the course of talking with her for over an hour, it became clear she was not. Here is a patient with radically shallow and puerile value commitments who was not acutely depressed and understood the medical information well. Did she offer a competent refusal on my view?

Before attempting to answer this question, one must bear in mind that the cases of Albert and Jane pose problems for *any* clinical ethics analysis. Any argument for, say, respecting the refusal versus not respecting it can only enjoy a modicum of plausibility.

Having said that, I am inclined to judge that Albert should receive the antibiotics, even in my permutation; and Jane should be discharged home with hospice care, unless or until she changes her mind (which she did). Albert should receive the antibiotics because his previous judgment that life *would* have no value to him is false since it *presently* does – insofar as he is clearly enjoying it.[17] The value judgment by Jane is not false, rather it is shallow and puerile. She is making the correct judgment that amputation is incompatible with something she values considerably – i.e., maintaining her current physical appearance. We may disagree with such a judgment, but it reflects the patient's stable and enduring self. Respecting Jane's refusal respects Jane – tragic as it is.

Conclusion

Standard competency assessments are not sensitive to what is morally required in high-stakes refusals since they only test for the presence of certain intellectual *abilities* and not whether the refusal is based on *reasons*. But, if the clinician does not have justification for believing that the patient is refusing based on reasons, the practical interest condition tells her not to act upon such a refusal. In this regard, my account takes seriously the moral gravity of such situations. What is required is that the patient offers a *competent refusal*. In order for clinicians to judge that the refusal in question may be acted upon, they need the patient to offer a reason for refusing. A reason for refusing includes a value commitment, and we should tolerate a broad range of such commitments unless they are obviously erroneous. If a patient offers a competent refusal, it should be respected. In this regard my account allows for respecting a person's considered high-stakes refusal.

In the interest of helping clinicians implement what I am suggesting here, consider the following decision-tree:

- Is the patient competent (on Appelbaum's (2007) criteria)?
- If yes: is the proposed treatment (L) objectively beneficial to the extent that it is life-saving or sustaining, and does it promise manageable or even low burdens?
- If yes: does the patient refuse L?
- If yes: does the patient understand the medical details accurately? (It may be helpful to invite the patient to discuss any fears, possible skepticism of the plan of care, and past hospital experiences.)
- If yes: does the patient cite a burden, cost, or lack of benefit *of L*?
- If yes: does the value judgment involved *support* the judgment 'L is not worth it'?
- If yes: respect the refusal.

Of course, there are a number of clinically important hurdles affecting the implementation of my argument (Howe, 2014). For instance, my argument appears to suggest that, if the clinician cannot make sense of the patient's refusal, she should determine whether the patient is issuing a competent refusal. In the context of the 30-year-old female's refusal of the BKA, matters are much more complicated. Twenty-four hours earlier, she was able-bodied, and her life plans and projects were largely made assuming that she can walk on her own two feet. Now she is being told that we are going to cut her legs off below the knee. How would you feel? Would you consent immediately with no questions, no stress, or no traumatic feelings? John Briere and Cheryl Langtree observe in their work on treating trauma that a patient's activated stress may diminish "in the presence of acceptance, validation, and nurturing. . . . The more positive and supportive the relationship . . . the greater the amount of positive emotionality available to counter condition previous negative emotional responses" (Briere & Langtree, 2011, 117; quoted in Howe, 2014, 181). My argument should not be interpreted as simply a justification for ignoring a patient's wishes. Properly situated, it should be understood as an opportunity to love our patients more deeply by, for example, validating the patient's fears and helping the patient problem-solve by canvassing information on what life might look like after the amputation, etc. Simply respecting her refusal shortcuts this important opportunity to love the patient better.

Notes

1 An important feature of high-stakes cases is that the patient stands to benefit from the procedure or treatment that is being refused and the refusal is from the first-person standpoint – i.e., they are currently alert and oriented. The more significant the benefit, the higher the stakes. And the notion of a

'benefit' should be understood in this chapter as not just preserving someone's life, but as enabling him to realize his plans and projects.

2 It is fairly well known that amputees and even bilateral BKA amputees adapt quite well. Consider Hugh Herr, Oscar Pistorius, and Aimee Mullins. See especially Mullins (2010) for a critique of the idea that amputees are 'disabled.'

3 In the actual case, the patient consented to a BKA after a clinician *listened* to her concerns instead of telling her what to do.

4 Epistemologists agree that the basing relation is a necessary condition for justification (see Pollock & Cruz, 1999, 35; and Korcz, 1997). More technically stated, a belief that p is justified for S only if S believes p on the basis of other beliefs or experience.

5 The concepts of relevance and support are key components of the basing condition, but I leave them undefined. Analytical philosophers may consider this a cop-out. Consequently, a brief comment on my philosophical method is in order. The first point is that the cases used to illustrate these notions seem clear enough – we know supportive reasons when we see them. Second, analytical philosophers (of which I consider myself) are predisposed to define key terms, and the *definiens* must be in the form of necessary and sufficient conditions. Definitions are typically in the form of, for example, 'A supports B if and only if . . . [an outline of conditions follows].' However, the stipulation of such conditions is often motivated by entertaining cases or thought experiments – cases that, if well-described, highlight our intuitions on what counts as A being a supportive reason for B. Since the generation of these conditions appeals ultimately to our intuitions (i.e., to what we 'see' with our mind's eye, or worse, to our gut reactions) the analytical method is a roundabout and complicated way of saying 'you will know it when you see it.' There is no reason to take a detour into the land of thought experiments when we rely on our intuitions all along. Consequently, I circumvent such a discussion here.

6 Below I recapitulate how Berg, Appelbaum, and Grisso (1996) address the difference between a refusal based on delusional beliefs and refusals based on "unconventional" religious beliefs. I agree largely with their analysis, though there are additional issues to consider. For instance, it is uncontroversial that refusals based on unconventional religious beliefs (for adults) may be respected, but refusals based on delusional beliefs should not be. What task remains is to explain why this is so. What properties do delusional beliefs have (or lack) that unconventional religious beliefs have (or lack) such that we may respect one but not the other? Fortunately, answering this question is not necessary for my argument. My point is limited to argue that typical competency assessments are not morally sufficient to tell us whether clinicians may respect a putatively competent patient's refusal of L in a high-stakes context.

7 Both Wreen (2004, 321) and the President's Commission for the Study of Ethical Problems in Medicine and Biomedical and Behavioral Research (1983, 121–122) endorse this commitment.

8 Terence Ackerman (2010) recapitulates examples of putatively competent patients who refuse in high-stakes scenarios due to misunderstanding, denial, acute depression, fear, or social role (see especially 80–81). In each case, the patients retained their intellectual abilities but Ackerman points out, correctly, that such refusals should not be respected.

9 Readers already familiar with Berg, Appelbaum, and Grisso (1996) and Appelbaum (2007) may proceed to the next section. I say nothing new here.

10 *In re Roe*, 583 N.E. 2d 1282, 1286 (Mass. 1992).

11 This is the case of *In re Milton* 505 N.E. 2d. 255 (Ohio, 1987) which is discussed by Berg, Appelbaum, and Grisso (1996, 357).

12 One may think that there is an omission here in that I do not mention desires. The reason for the omission is that desires *alone* are not the kinds of things that can function as normative reasons. Expressing one's desire not to have L is like the detective in Warfield's example who believes that the criminal is guilty, not on the basis of the evidence, but instead on a delusion, or, we may add, a desire that Jones is guilty because, say, the detective does not like him. Wishes/desires, superstitious beliefs, and delusions do not function as normative reasons for our moral judgments. If they were, the patient in Jonsen et al.'s example should not receive the antibiotic, period. But the whole reason why the case gives us pause is because there is no reason cited for the refusal, only an expression of his desire not to have the antibiotic. So desires are not the kinds of things which I am including in my notion of a *competent refusal*.

13 By 'override Rufus's refusal' I mean that I (as the clinician) could not morally justify respecting the refusal. Legally, restraining him and doing the transfusion anyway might very well amount to battery instead of health care delivery. One point of presenting cases like Rufus is to fix our moral intuitions on a continuum of cases where the borders between battery and health care delivery are porous. A slight permutation of this case might suggest that it is both morally and legally permissible to provide the treatment that is being refused, as in the case of a severely anorexic patient continually refusing tube feeding (see Hebert & Weingarten, 1991).

14 As to *how* the clinicians should administer the antibiotic given the refusal of an IV, one may try an oral preparation or an intramuscular injection with an anesthetic first, even if such modes may not be ideal from a strict clinical standpoint.

15 Though it is unclear whether May's understanding of eligibility entails that clinicians *must* follow the decision-making of a patient who retains rational abilities.

16 Wreen notes that the case originated with Thomas Mappes (2006, 355) and Mappes's assessment is that the past wishes take precedence.

17 Speaking of a 'false' value commitment is a delicate matter. I would only judge a value commitment false if it is *obviously* not applicable in the circumstances. Albert's present enjoyment of life renders the previous judgment that life *would* not have value for him false. Jane's judgment, however, involves *weighing* values, namely, the value of putting on Ugg boots is more important than life itself. And we may tolerate a diversity of such weighing. Albert's judgment is not a matter of weighing or ranking a seemingly unimportant value over one that is obviously more important. Rather, it is that his subjunctive judgment 'were I to decline mentally, life would have no value for me' is simply false because he has declined mentally but his life *is* of value. Of course, my answer would change if Albert were not happily senile but were instead belligerent and delirious.

11 Risky Research on Competent Adults
Justice and Autonomy

The previous two chapters addressed issues in clinical medicine. At a certain level of abstraction, the argument is the same: one should have epistemic diffidence concerning the claim that it is permissible to honor a patient's refusal of certain life-sustaining interventions. This chapter aims to extend the basic structure of my argument to research on competent adult subjects. The principal reason for allowing research that involves more than minimal risk without expected benefit is that we should respect the autonomy of competent subjects. In this chapter I argue that we have additional moral intuitions stemming from commutative justice. Specifically, I argue that commutative justice serves as an additional criterion for assessing permissible research. Integrating my specific goal in this chapter into the overall argument of this book, I aim to justify having epistemic diffidence for the claim that 'risky research on competent adults is permissible because the subjects *consent* to it.'

The purpose of research is to obtain knowledge, not to provide therapy. Because of this, research looks like a case of using people. People may disagree about whether this use is immoral in itself, but everyone seems to agree that research on human subjects is an ethically risky activity, though justifiable in many cases. The ethical risks become more obvious when discussing vulnerable populations such as children. Most of us have the intuition that pediatric subjects should enjoy greater protection from wrongdoing in research than research on competent adults. Call this the 'pediatric intuition.' I argue that this intuition conflicts with the virtue of commutative justice and specifically with what we take to justify one agent (i.e., a researcher) exposing another agent (i.e., a subject) to a risk of harm. I argue that all human subjects, including competent adult subjects, should enjoy the same protections from wrongdoing in research as pediatric subjects enjoy; therefore, the latter should not enjoy *greater* protection. A key objection to my conclusion is that the pediatric intuition is plausible because of the ethical role informed consent plays in justifying risky research on competent subjects. My argument, then, is to circumscribe the importance of informed consent and situate it alongside concerns of justice. The conclusions reached can function as a first step toward rebutting the important 'anti-paternalistic' arguments developing in research ethics (Miller & Wertheimer, 2007).

As ambitious as my argument sounds, its scope is limited enough so as to avoid obvious counterexamples. My argument has in mind studies that present more than minimal risks to competent healthy adult subjects, and, in some cases, competent sick adults. These studies both do not offer a direct benefit to the subjects and it is arguable whether they offer knowledge of vital importance.[1] Examples of such studies are airway insult studies on healthy or asthmatic adults, and studies using transbronchial biopsy on healthy adults.

Of course, the notions of 'benefit' and 'vital importance' are degreed and case-specific concepts. It is plausible to suppose that *any* knowledge of disease pathophysiology where the disease in question has no known cure and afflicts a large population may be considered vital, but not for, say, a less serious and rare disease. And obviously, the knowledge gained has to be weighed in relation to the magnitude and probability of the research risks. Consequently, I do not offer the following reflections without acknowledging the central importance of practical wisdom in reviewing the ethical quality of research. Acknowledging this does not reduce my reflections to the jejune. Rather, I offer my arguments here as *prima facie* challenges to certain types of research, challenges which can be overridden; but, at the same time, the challenge I offer is novel and, I shall argue, important.

Another limitation on my conclusion is that some randomized controlled trials (RCTs) should be judged permissible on the account I give of morally sufficient reasons. On my understanding, a morally sufficient reason for allowing harm is that, for more than minimal risk research, there must be a prospect of direct benefit *even for research on competent adults*. However, the requirement of a direct benefit is waived for studies that satisfy clinical equipoise. The reason is that, if clinical equipoise is satisfied, the researchers do not know whether or not subjects in the intervention arm will be exposed to risks of the drug with no compensating benefit or whether subjects in the placebo arm will be deprived of a beneficial new drug. My argument should be understood to focus on cases where there is *knowledge* of risk, or at least strong evidence of risk paired with weak evidence of benefit.

The present argument improves upon previous work which supports a similar conclusion (Kong, 2005) in that the present work focuses on the virtue of commutative justice, which is certainly relevant for morally assessing research. Commutative justice is the virtue that perfects the relationships between individuals. To date, criticisms of certain types of research have focused on specific trial designs, arguing that such designs evince an unreasonable risk/benefit ratio (Anderson & Kimmelman, 2010); or the language of justice has been used to justify limiting autonomy, but the notion of justice used seems utilitarian.[2] I do not think these approaches are wrongheaded, but they are incomplete. The goal of this project is to take the critique deeper. Both pediatric and adult subjects should enjoy the same level and kind of research protection, not by lowering the bar for pediatric subjects, but by raising it for competent adults. I argue for this claim by focusing on what can count as just interaction between persons where one agent harms the other.

Consistent with the argument in this book, concerns about justice impresses epistemic diffidence onto the belief that risky research on *consenting* adults is morally permissible. It may be morally permissible, but I argue that mere consent hardly suffices to justify it.

Children Actually Enjoy Greater Protection

The regulations governing human subject research were developed to ensure the ethical conduct of research both on competent adult subjects and on vulnerable[3] populations, e.g., pregnant women/fetuses, prisoners, and children.[4] These vulnerable populations enjoy further protection (i.e., subparts B, C, and D respectively) in that such subjects are or may be compromised with respect to their capacity to give informed consent.[5] Richard Behrman notes, "because of the inherent vulnerabilities arising from their immaturity, infants, children, and adolescents need additional protections beyond what is provided to competent adults when they participate in research" (Field & Behrman, 2004, xiii). The traditional reason given for these extra protections is that competent subjects can judge whether the risks are worth taking, but non-competent subjects cannot. Therefore, the justification for exposing non-competent subjects to risks focuses on whether there is a compensating benefit.[6] On the traditional account, informed consent can turn an otherwise immoral act into one that is permissible.[7] So, too, a compensating benefit can turn an otherwise immoral act (of exposing a child to significant risks) into one that is permissible.

This line of thinking is reflected in the DHHS regulations, subpart D. The regulations give us a matrix of risk/benefit categories. If the research is permissible, it must fall into one of four categories. The first category of approvable research for children (and adults) is research presenting no more than minimal risk to the child. Since the ethical protections are the same between adults and children here, discussion of it is not needed for my ultimate conclusion (which is that both adults and children should enjoy the same level of moral protection).[8] Even if serious harms were to occur in minimal risk studies, the harms would be unexpected and a commutatively just researcher (discussed below) cannot be held culpable for what is entirely improbable or atypical given current medical knowledge. The next category, however, is the chief focus of this chapter because most risky research on children is approved via this category. Research that exposes subjects to greater than minimal risks is permissible if the interventions hold out a prospect of direct benefit. The following quotation is from section 405 of 45 CFR Part 46,

> HHS will conduct or fund research in which the IRB finds that more than minimal risk to children is presented by an intervention or procedure that holds out the prospect of *direct benefit* for the individual subject, or by a monitoring procedure that is likely to contribute to the subject's well-being, only if the IRB finds that:
>
> (a) The risk is *justified by* the anticipated benefit to the subjects;
> (b) The *relation of the anticipated benefit to the risk* is *at least as favorable* to the subjects as that presented by available alternative approaches; and
> (c) Adequate provisions are made for soliciting the assent of the children and permission of their parents or guardians, as set forth in §46.408.
>
> (US Code of Federal Regulations, 2009)

Now consider the following quotation from section 111 of 45 CFR Part 46, which outlines criteria adult research must satisfy:

> (a) In order to approve research covered by this policy the IRB shall determine that all of the following requirements are satisfied:[9]
>
> (2) Risks to subjects are *reasonable* in relation to anticipated benefits, if any, to subjects, and the importance of the knowledge that may reasonably be expected to result. In evaluating risks and benefits, the IRB should consider only those risks and benefits that may result from the research (as distinguished from risks and benefits of therapies subjects would receive even if not participating in the research).
>
> (US Code of Federal Regulations, 2009)

The key concepts governing pediatric research are "direct benefit," "anticipated benefit," and a risk/benefit ratio that is "favorable" in relation to alternatives. Furthermore, the risks must be "justified by" the anticipated benefits. Concepts governing adult research do not explicitly mention "direct benefit," but section 111 includes the requirement that the risks must be "reasonable" in relation to the anticipated benefits. In the next section I address what is meant by direct benefit since that concept marks a key difference between 46.405 (children) and 46.111 (adults). My aim is to argue that the fundamental reasons supporting a direct-benefit requirement inform *all* research that is more than minimal risk.

Children Should Not Enjoy Greater Protection: Direct Benefit and Theodicy

A research project does not satisfy the contours of category 405 until it presents more than minimal risk and a prospect of direct benefit. Following closely here Nancy King (2000) and Field and Behrman (2004), I take the term 'direct' to be a causal notion and 'benefit' as referring to specific *types* of benefits, not the degree of magnitude for the benefit in question. A direct benefit is a benefit "arising from receiving the intervention being studied" (King, 2000, 333). Typically, this benefit will be related to the overall health of the subject in question. Suppose that the risks of the intervention are the toxic effects of the test drug. If the benefits are caused by the very intervention, i.e., administering the drug, they are of the same *sort* as the risks – they improve the health of the subject such as, for example, reduction in tumor size. Likewise, pain from a biopsy can be justified by improved liver function. In general, where the risks are to one's health (mental or physical) a direct benefit must be to one's health as well. This does not mean that for each risk there must be a distinct offsetting benefit; rather, cumulative risks can be offset by cumulative benefits (Weijer & Miller, 2004).

Considering 'direct benefit' as a causal notion is not only conceptually sensible –that is what we typically understand by 'direct' – it satisfies important ethical criteria as well. Those working in research ethics typically eschew the idea of 'extra' benefits compensating for risks of harm due to the research intervention. Supporting this point Friedman, Robbins, and Wendler (2010, 3) quote the Kenyan guidelines on the ethical conduct of research,

> Extraneous benefits such as payment, or adjunctive medical services, such as the possibility of receiving a hepatitis vaccine not related to the research, cannot be considered in delineating the benefits compared with the risks, otherwise simply increasing payment or adding more unrelated services could make the benefits outweigh even the riskiest research.[10]

In order to count as a *justifying* benefit, the intervention being tested must *cause* it.

We can glean from this analysis of direct benefit an underlying moral intuition according to which subjecting someone (who cannot consent) to risks of harm can be justified only if there is a (likely) compensating benefiting. What I wish to argue for now is that this intuition remains even when we negate the parenthetical 'who cannot consent.' I focus on how an agent exuding the virtue of commutative justice would behave when she causes or allows harm to another. Arguing for why commutative justice is important in the setting of strong intuitions that favor autonomy requires highlighting a different set of moral intuitions that I think we hold just as strongly. These other intuitions are displayed most clearly in discussions on the problem of evil.

A caveat before continuing: I offer these reflections on theodicy to be read in one of two ways corresponding to two different moral epistemologies. Read the first way, my aim is simply to highlight our intuitions on what counts as just treatment of another. This does not require an analogical argument. My strategy is similar to how Gettier-type counterexamples function in epistemology (Gettier, 1963). Gettier-type counterexamples are thought experiments that aim to highlight our intuitions on what counts (or does not count) as knowledge. They function solely as intuition highlighters. Similarly, the present excursion into theodicy is offered as an intuition highlighter on what counts as just treatment of another in settings where one agent causes/allows suffering on another.

A second way to read my reference to theodicy is through the lens of moral exemplar or ideal observer (IO) epistemologies. The basic approach for such epistemologies is to envision a moral exemplar and test a norm or action against what we would expect the exemplar to do. Linda Zagzebski explains,

> The reason that moral judgments can be defined by the responses of an IO is that we see when exposed to an IO that those are the judgments that we ultimately would make ourselves if we assumed the standpoint at which we are implicitly aiming. The features that make a being an IO are therefore the features that make him a judge who judges in such a way that those who experience his judgment want to assume his point of view.
>
> (Zagzebski, 2004, 353)

The moral exemplar in the theodicy case is, of course, God, or our idea of how God (as defined by classical monotheism) would behave toward others. And the key aspects of the IO I wish to draw attention to are the benevolent dispositions and motivations the IO would have towards others for whom the exemplar allows suffering. Read in this way, reflection on theodicy can paint a partial but informative picture of what the *virtue* of commutative justice looks like.

Now we can turn to my intuition highlighter. The problem of evil arises when we recognize that the existence of an omni-benevolent, omnipotent, and omniscient God is in tension with what appear to be gratuitous evils. If God is all-powerful, God *could* prevent evils, and being all-loving, God would *want* to prevent all evils – unless such evils are necessary for a greater good. Gratuitous evils are evils for which there is no greater good that could justify God in allowing them. Solutions (and replies to solutions) abound. A principal issue in this debate is whether there really are gratuitous evils and how would we know that they are gratuitous.

It is not my task to adjudicate this principal issue, but rather to note the assumptions on which both theist and atheist alike agree. Most parties agree that a morally sufficient reason for allowing suffering is that there is (i) outweighing compensation (sometimes called a greater good), (ii) to the sufferer.[11] The second restriction is pertinent for my purposes in that a *just* God would not *use* someone for the greater good of another. If the sufferer is suffering desolation or loneliness, for example, the greater good might be to bring about in the sufferer a greater sense of communion with others or with God. Furthermore, we should understand the benefit to the sufferer to be more than merely making up for one's suffering but it must also provide a reason for it. In connection with the Kenyan guidelines quoted above, financial compensation, for example, does not justify the exposure to harms caused by the test article even if it might make up for it.

The thought experiment on theodicy has us ask the question: 'what would a wholly-just being's relationship to suffering look like?' A justifying reason for allowing suffering must meet strict criteria. Weaken the criteria and the problem of evil evaporates. An exemplar of justice would not expose someone to suffering to benefit others.

Consequently, what justifies a virtuous agent in causing or allowing another to suffer must involve a compensating benefit that accrues to the sufferer and is a function of the suffering itself. An exemplar of commutative justice would not use persons for the good of others without any compensating benefit to the sufferer. If this is correct, we can understand why justifying the risks in relation to the benefits is an independent ethical criterion governing the permissibility of any research project (Emanuel, Wendler, & Grady, 2000). Even if subjects give informed consent to a study that does not meet a direct-benefit requirement, the study remains impermissible. This is important in regard to my thesis that the regulations governing pediatric research should not afford greater protection than what ought to be afforded competent adults. My point so far is that a moral exemplar would not cause or allow suffering in another without a compensating benefit to the sufferer. This is what an agent with commutative justice would do, and since commutative justice is the virtue that perfects relations between two or more persons, these reflections apply to the researcher's actions on human subjects. Risky research with no prospect of a direct benefit is *prima facie* unjust.

Objections

The previous section outlined my core argument for why adult subjects should receive moral protection equivalent to that which pediatric subjects enjoy. This section takes on several objections to this argument, chief of which is that adult subjects can consent. A second objection is that my argument would require radical changes in how research is actually practiced. A third objection considers discrete cases where my argument would appear to deliver the wrong judgment. Finally, I address a technical difference between 46.405 and 46.111 which putatively undermines my argument. I take these in turn.

Consent

My conclusion entails, roughly, that even for adult research, a prospect of direct benefit is required in the setting of risky research. The critic may note that consent turns otherwise immoral actions into moral ones: it "turns a rape into love-making, a kidnapping into a Sunday drive, a battery into a football tackle, a theft into a gift, and a trespass into a dinner party" (Hurd, 2005, 504).

I agree with Hurd and others (Dempsey, 2012) that consent does *something* to one half of an action dyad – making one action permissible and the other not. But there are other cases in the neighborhood which complicate matters. These latter cases include prostitution, dwarf throwing, voluntary slavery, and the actual and rather macabre case of Armin Meiwes. Meiwes posted an advert on an internet site devoted to cannibalism saying, "[S]eeking well-built man, 18–30 years old, for slaughter" (Finn, 2003). Bernd Juergen Brandes accepted the invitation and, after several email exchanges, Brandes visited Meiwes's home where the consensual killing took place. Initially Meiwes was convicted of manslaughter and not murder because, his defense argued, the victim consented. Germany's highest court eventually charged him with murder and sentenced Meiwes to life.[12] For some cases, then, even if the recipient of harm consents (hereafter, the inflicted), the action by the agent of the harm (the inflicter) is left without justification. I shall argue that the difference consent makes in Hurd's cases and the irrelevance of consent in the cases just enumerated is not a function of the degree of harm, but is a categorical difference.

The cases Hurd mentions have a common feature vis-à-vis consent. For each dyad (e.g., theft vs borrowing), consent is part of the definition of the action dyad.[13] Theft is taking another's property without the owner's permission; borrowing is taking another's property with the owner's permission. 'Love-making' is sexual intercourse with the other's consent; rape is sexual intercourse without the other's consent. Consent functions as an essential feature that identifies the action-types in question. But there are other action-types that can be specified without reference to consent. The Meiwes case suggests that murder is one of them; maiming, torture, enslavement, and possibly bullying are other examples. One may consent to being bullied but the act of bullying remains wrong – even when the consent is altruistic, for example, the inflicted is distracting the bully away from one's younger sibling. These reflections suggest that there are two classes of action in relation to consent. There are actions for which consent changes the action-type, as, for example, taking another's property is theft without consent and is borrowing when done with consent. And there are actions for which consent does not function to specify or define the action-type in question. Under this second category there is a further subset for which consent does not *justify* harmful actions. Hurd's cases are ones where consent does *not* perform the function of justifying the action in question, but changes the action-type because of the specifying or defining role it plays.

To bring out the distinction between consent's role in specifying action-types and its irrelevance in justifying action-types, consider first a logical point. Victor Tadros provides numerous and welcome insights on the relationship between consent of the inflicted and the inflicter's actions. But on at least one point he slips, though in an instructive and not uncommon way. He notes at one point that "It is often wrong to harm a person as a means to the greater good without that person's consent. If the person consents, however, it is permissible to harm the person as a means to the greater good" (Tadros, 2011, 30). Suppose A performs a harmful action H on S, and that H being performed on S is a means to a greater good. Tadros appears committed to making the following inference:

(P)   If S does not consent to H, then H is not permissible.

And,

(Q)   If S consents to H, then H is permissible.

Clearly, however, if we deny the antecedent in (P), we cannot derive that H is not permissible – that would involve the fallacy of denying the antecedent.

Tadros offers us an enthymeme linking (P) with (Q) according to which performing H on S (in the case of consent) "shows respect for her end-setting capacities, and hence we do not treat her as an object" (Tadros, 2011, 30). But there seem to be numerous ways in which S can be wronged in addition to being used as an object, and respect for someone's end-setting capacities would at most obviate only the wrong of treating the person merely as an object. But even this reply grants too much. S's consent does not entail that A must no longer view S as an object. S's consent has no apparent causal link with how A *sees* S; it does not entail that A must now respect her end-setting capacities. On a related point, S's consent fails to change the action-type of A's action H. H could still be an action of the type *using S as a means*; it is certainly logically possible that S consents to *being used* or to *being harmed by another*. S's consent alone neither specifies nor justifies A's action H.

A similar inference should be resisted when discussing the relevance of consent in research. Consider a research study that presents more than minimal risks to subjects without a prospect of direct benefit. Label the action-type of performing this study R~DB. One cannot infer from,

(Ped):   If R~DB is done on incompetent subjects (who cannot consent to it), then R~DB is not permissible.

To,

(Comp):   If R~DB is done on competent subjects (who do consent to it), then R~DB is permissible.

This inference, as well, is an instance of the fallacy of denying the antecedent.

But what we find plausible in this inference is instructive. The plausibility stems from conflating consent's *specifying role* in defining certain action-types, Hurd provides a nice list of examples, and consent's putative *justifying role* in justifying another agent's action. Consider again the criteria for a successful theodicy. Even if a sufferer S consents to God using her for the good of another, the action of using S still requires justification. Neither goods in the afterlife nor goods to the ultimate benefactor justify God using S. The theodicy thought experiment brings into relief the distinction between justifying an agent's act of using S and S's consent to being used; consent to H does not morally justify H itself.

One may object noting that, for example, borrowing is justified but theft is not, and the only difference between them is consent. Consent, therefore, justifies borrowing. I agree that consent may play a justifying role when it serves to specify certain action-types. The two roles need not be mutually exhaustive. But granting this does not affect my argument since research is not specified by consent. If consent is not part of the *definiens* for research activities, it cannot define otherwise immoral research actions into moral ones. Even so, it is doubtful that consent justifies an action even when consent specifies it. To justify an action requires reference to the goods to which the action is ordered. An owner's consent in borrowing does not justify that act when one borrows a weapon to be used on an innocent person. Conversely, borrowing money to support one's starving children is justified by reference to the goods at stake. What *justifies* (or fails to justify) the act of borrowing in both cases makes essential reference to the goods or evils the act is ordered to, not to consent of the owner.

But suppose what Tadros and others mean to say is not that there is an *inference* from (Ped) to (Comp), but that (Comp) is plausible on its own – consent is sufficient justification. I think our moral intuitions go in the other direction. The principle criterion on what counts as a morally sufficient reason for allowing evil is compensation to the sufferer, getting informed consent is an *additional* requirement. Stump notes, "Undeserved suffering which is uncompensated seems clearly unjust; but so does suffering compensated only by benefits to someone other than the sufferer" (Stump, 1996, 66). She then gives the example of the US military's LSD experiments on soldiers. Assuming this study was well-designed and promised to deliver knowledge worth having, we still think that it was a violation of justice. Part of an explanation for this injustice is "a consequence of the fact that the end aimed at did not directly or primarily benefit those who suffered to achieve it" (Stump, 1996, 66). It is important to note that this explanation functions as an independent reason for the injustice. Assume that the soldiers voluntarily consent to high doses of LSD, and you still have a reason for thinking that the study is unjust; the benefits, if any, do not accrue to those suffering the harms.

The idea that consent cannot provide a sufficient reason for the permissibility of a study can be shown by another (modified) example of Stump's (1986). Consider a large chemical corporation that aims to test a new technology for cleaning up toxic chemical spills. It plans to spill chemicals into a particularly poor part of India and then release their 'clean-up chemical.' Subsequently, they follow-up with residents of the area testing for toxic effects secondary to consuming the drinking water. They promise to compensate every injured resident 1,000USD (a small fortune for such residents); in return the residents indemnify the company against any future compensation. The townspeople consent to the spill considering the money as sufficient compensation. It appears that here, too, an injustice would be committed against the residents, even in the setting of consent and in spite of what they view as sufficient compensation. Uncompensated harm (the proffered 1,000USD is not directly linked to the harm accrued) stands by itself as a reason against the study. If consent procedures were adequate and ensured understanding, the study would meet *that* ethical requirement; but it would fail the requirement not to cause uncompensated suffering or harm.

Could consent function as a form of permission to do to the subject what would otherwise be impermissible? One could appeal to Neil Manson and Onora O'Neill's understanding of consent as a waiver of rights, according to which,

> Informed consent transactions are typically used to *waive* important ethical, legal and other requirements in limited ways in particular contexts. . . . In consenting we *waive* certain requirements on others not to treat us in certain ways . . . or we *set aside* certain expectations, or *license* action that would *otherwise* be ethically or legally unacceptable.

(2007, 72)

In the research context, it is often the case that researchers do things to subjects that expose them to serious risks of injury, harm, or even death. Manson and O'Neill wish to say that informed consent functions as a waiver – it is meant to license action on oneself or to say 'okay' to the researcher allowing her to do something that would be immoral *without* such consent.

I think this is a very plausible understanding of informed consent and how it is meant to function in the research context. I do not think it effectively obviates the concerns I am raising. The first point to note is that not all waivers are created equal. Manson and O'Neill recognize that the consent of a subject in the grips of suicidal ideation is not a legitimate waiver, neither is consent to torture, serious bodily harm, or being eaten! If consent motivated by suicidality destroys it as a legitimate waiver, not all acts of consent can function as legitimate waivers. To function as a legitimate waiver, the consent must be *well-motivated*; there must be *good reasons* for consenting to the research activity with its attendant risks.

Suppose there are good reasons for giving consent, such as altruism or self-sacrifice for others who are sick. Do we now have sufficient ethical justification for risky research? I think we could have such a justification, but the typical preoccupation with autonomy stops the argument at just this point where more justification is needed. Altruism may render the *subject's* action laudable, but that says little about the *researcher's* actions. Consider again the idea that suffering must be compensated by benefits accruing to the sufferer and that these benefits cannot merely *make up for* the suffering. Rather, compensating benefits must function as morally sufficient reasons for the suffering.

What these reflections mean for the actions of the researcher are as follows. Consider a high-risk study. Such risks require some form of compensation; such compensation must refer to a *reason* for exposing the subjects to such risks, and not merely to things that may 'make up for' the suffering.[14] What could count as a reason for permitting the study makes reference to its net benefit/burden ratio, namely, whether the risks 'are reasonable in relation to the anticipated benefits.' If a justifying reason for the study cannot be articulated with reference to the benefit/burden ratio, then no amount of monetary compensation or consent waiver can justify *it*. These latter would, at best, merely 'make up for' the suffering inflicted, but do not advert us to a justifying reason for the study.

How do altruistic motives fit within this reasoning? Consider the following two cases involving consent to something risky out of altruistic motives.

1   A spectator to a dangerous plane crash in the Potomac River dives into icy water to save a child.
2   A military commander consults with a subordinate about a mission because it is a particularly dangerous mission promising little by way of advancing the country's military objectives. The subordinate is eager to engage in the mission out of love for his country.

The research setting is more like 2 than 1. Case 1 is clearly a case where altruistic motivations are present in the setting of high risks, but nothing is morally problematic about it. It counts as a paradigm example of the supererogatory. Case 2, however, is more like the kind of research I am questioning in that it involves someone (the military commander) doing something dangerous to someone else (sending the soldier on a dangerous mission), and this someone else consents. Furthermore, the feature in Case 2 that the mission promises little in terms of military objectives is analogous to research that lacks a compensating benefit or does not promise knowledge of vital importance.[15] Research that involves these features is immoral on my account. Intuitions may vary, but the actions of the military commander in Case 2 seem at best morally questionable, at worse, immoral. And this is partly a function of the risks and benefits *of the mission*. The soldier's laudable motivation (assume a just war) does not itself justify *the commander* sending him on said mission. This is partly why the focus on autonomy is limited; it fails to morally assess the actions *of the researcher* when assessing research protocols.

What ethical role does a well-motivated waiver play then? It permits involvement of a subject in a study that has already been judged reasonable – a morally sufficient reason is given for the risks. 'Justifying' the risks on the basis of subjects consenting to them simply is not a *justification* for the risks. A subject's waiver *permits* doing *to him* what the (already ethically permissible) study involves doing.

The root of my skepticism that consent can function as a justifier is that consent is a mental state – e.g., I *agree* to x. Typical justifiers for moral actions, however, refer to goods (such as health and friendship) or the satisfaction of desire – though goods are more fundamental as desires can be good or evil. Mental states are not even the right kinds of things that can function as a justifier for a moral action. Mental states, such as an agent's intentions, can specify or define a moral action (Chapter 8). But mental states appear inert as a justifier for an action – especially someone else's action. At the very least, proponents of an autonomy approach need to explain the vinculum between the inflicted's mental state of consent and justification for the inflicter's action of harm.

Before leaving this section, I wish to acuminate my approach to consent even further to avoid the charge of being overly strict. Hans Jonas's famous commentary on research (Jonas, 1969, 236) notes that the only way to right the wrong of doing research on human subjects is to require, not just consent, but "devotion." The subject must will the same thing as the researcher in order to grant morally valid consent. Many commentators think that Jonas's standard of consent is too strict, and I concur. In this respect my argument does not entail overly strict criteria on consent since my argument does not address such standards at all. My argument attempts to answer a different set of questions: is the research permissible *per se*? Is the subject consenting to be treated in morally permissible ways? The previous and present sections motivate why these questions are independent of any criteria-for-valid-consent questions.

Changes in Actual Practice

So, even in the ideal scenario, where the subjects are able to give informed consent and researchers intend knowledge that is important for disease management, the justification for the study *may* still be undermined. The goal of important knowledge is not sufficient, as indicated above with the examples of the LSD experiments and the exploitation of the Indian village. The waivers the subjects give are not themselves morally sufficient reasons for performing particularly harmful activities on them even for the potential good of others.

But would not adoption of the argument so far require wholesale changes in the way research is actually done? And would not those changes involve a potential loss of effective therapies thereby placing a burden of proof on my argument that it cannot meet? The first question assumes that actual practice is the default position and changes in it require strong argument. But actual practice is obviously not morally normative and there are numerous critiques of it that are almost universally accepted. There is, for example, the widely studied 'therapeutic misconception,' which is fairly ubiquitous, especially for subjects who have relatively intractable diseases (Appelbaum et al., 1987). Subjects (especially healthy ones) are often motivated primarily by the compensation associated with the study, not altruism (Almeida et al., 2007). Waivers motivated by compensation are morally inert since greater compensation does not itself render the research risks 'reasonable in relation to the anticipated benefits.'

Consider a particularly risky study without payment.[16] If Almeida et al. (2007) are correct, very few people would enter the study.[17] That few would consent to such research is a backhanded indicator of where the research stands from a rational choice[18] perspective. Since the study's risks and benefits which the IRB must weigh preclude considering benefits in the form of payments,[19] the risk/benefit ratio *of the study* is what provides the chief ethical justification for it. But if it is inconsistent with rational choice to enter the study *sans* payment, then the study itself presents risks that are *not* 'reasonable in relation to the anticipated benefits.' Therefore, the study would fail 46.111(a) (2).

Another aspect of actual practice that is morally questionable is the ambiguity regarding 'benefit.' Audrey Chapman observes that the term benefit can refer to widely disparate effects, not all of which either justify the study or are even promised by the study:

> Potential benefit to an individual subject is usually conceptualized in the form of an improvement in health status derived from the agent being tested, but often there is disagreement as to what kinds

of milestones constitute a therapeutic benefit. For oncology patients, for example, does an improvement in the quality of life qualify or does benefit require a clinically relevant shrinkage in the size of the tumor, a remission, or an extension in life expectancy?

(2011, 3)

Actual practice does not disambiguate these different benefits, only some of which may function as justifiers in light of the risks.

Lastly, there are the likely motivations behind the research which fail to justify the study. Motivations range from curiosity to market competitiveness – e.g., a pharmaceutical company trying to develop a me-too drug (Garattini & Bertele, 2007; Gagne & Choudhry, 2011). In this regard, Kong observes the following plausible motivations behind some research,

> Research is also the pursuit of knowledge for personal curiosity, career advancement, and prestige. . . . [M]edical research is a commercial activity, the aim of which is to create new markets, maximise profits, and satisfy shareholders.
>
> (Kong, 2005, 206)

These reflections suggest that actual practice should not be considered normative and changes in it may be welcome.

If my argument is acted upon, would that mean a loss of potentially effective therapies? My short answer is no (see Light, Lexchin, & Darrow, 2013). My ultimate conclusion is that pediatric subjects should not enjoy greater moral protection from research harm than adults, not by lowering the moral bar for children, but by raising it for adults. Adults should enjoy the same protections as pediatric subjects currently enjoy, i.e., the protections outlined in subpart D. To date, few have argued[20] that the ethical principles governing subpart D are overly restrictive, thereby preventing potentially important therapies from being tested on children. I see no reason why such an objection would apply to adults if the same ethical principles are common to each.

A clarification is in order to avoid overstating my case. Some studies on adults do not offer a direct benefit, but they are well-designed and promise knowledge of vital importance. Such studies are not ruled out by my argument. Current principles governing pediatric research recognize that "knowledge of vital importance" can justify more than minimal-risk/without-direct-benefit research (see subpart D category 406). Pediatric subjects enjoy a risk cut-off: the risk cannot be more than a minor increase over minimal. But conditions outlined in 46.406 reflect the basic ethical commitment that risks must be justified by the value of knowledge promised, once direct benefit drops out as a possible justifier, there is only so much risk that we may tolerate in the context of no direct benefit. There is no reason to suppose that these ethical commitments should not apply equally to adults, much less is there reason to suppose that a prudential application of these commitments would block important medical advances. Such advances often occur in pediatric research.

Conversely, there are some adult studies that involve more than minimal risk and do not offer knowledge of vital importance (e.g., some airway toxicity studies). We know enough about the adverse effects of air pollution on the lungs (for both sick and healthy persons) that further studies are superfluous. Enough knowledge is had to inform public policy and encourage individual responsibility in relation to decreasing pollution.

A case-by-case analysis may be the only way to answer fully whether my argument entails cutting off important medical advances, but the two considerations just offered suggest that either the study in question would meet the ethical principles informing pediatric research or, if it does not, it is not an obviously permissible study and, therefore, cannot be used as a counterexample to my argument.

Case-Specific Objections – The Marshall Case and Living Donation

A few years ago, a researcher named Barry Marshall drank a solution of bacteria which formed an ulcer in five days. He then ingested an antibiotic proving that ulcers are caused by bacteria and, therefore, respond to antibiotics. He won a Nobel Prize for his discovery (Marshall, 2005).[21] The case has two features that are morally relevant to challenge my arguments above and one feature that is not, but can easily be changed. The essential features of the case involved inoculating the subject (the researcher himself) with a disease for which he was previously naïve. He then experimented with a possible treatment (i.e., antibiotics). Deliberate inoculation of a potentially serious disease on a subject is obviously a case of exposing someone to more than minimal risk. Furthermore, the benefit of resolving the disease through the experimental treatment does not compensate for the initial inoculation. Although I find myself thinking that what Marshall did to himself was permissible, my arguments above would seem to rule differently. The one easy change to the case involves supposing that, instead of using himself, Marshall enrolls another person who understands completely the science of what he is doing, is motivated to advance science, and voluntarily consents to the risks. And, just as in the actual case, the ulcers respond to antibiotics. What can be wrong with this?

I must admit that I have no reply that would be convincing to someone with strong consequentialist intuitions. Part of the reason why we think either case is permissible is due to how things actually occurred: the disease responded to treatment, it did not debilitate the subject, and the experiment delivered knowledge that was universally recognized as vitally important for medicine. We should be cautious, however, in trusting our intuitions on cases where the outcomes are grand. Max Bazerman and Ann Tenbrunsel (2011) have presented evidence that our ethical judgments succumb to an outcome bias. They presented subjects with two sets of actions. In one set, a pharmaceutical researcher does something immoral (e.g., makes up data points); the drug goes to market and benefits many. In another set, a researcher does not do anything immoral, but breaches the protocol in a minor way. The drug goes to market and has to be withdrawn due to risks and serious adverse events. Subjects judged the second researcher's actions more reprehensible than the first, but Bazerman and Tenbrunsel note correctly, in my opinion, that the actions of the first researcher are much worse than the actions of the second. Their research is directly relevant to our moral assessment of the Marshall case. We should be cautious of our intuitions on the Marshall case given Bazerman and Tenbrunsel's research that our intuitions can latch on to arguably morally irrelevant features – the good consequences that happen to follow.

I think that is precisely what is occurring when we consider the Barry Marshall case, whose success obfuscates some morally pertinent details. Suppose that your best friend is a very ambitious scientific researcher working at the dawn of cancer research. He proposes to ingest live cancer cells of a very dangerous cancer but also to ingest a radioactive isotope on the theoretical possibility that the isotope will kill the cancer cells. Would you, being his best friend, encourage him on this dangerous endeavor or would you recommend that he not do this? Viewing the Marshall case through the lens of friendship draws our moral attention to other moral goods at stake. Absent any knowledge of what cancer cells and isotopes can do *in vivo*, I would recommend that my friend engage in less risky endeavors. Clearly, my researcher friend should not administer cells and isotopes to others.[22] And the latter intuition comports well with the overall argument in this chapter.

Live kidney donation has been used as a moral analog to risky research (Miller & Joffe, 2009). Live kidney donation exposes the donor to significant risks with no compensating *medical* benefit. Not only do we consider such acts permissible, they are laudatory in most every circumstance. But, if this is so, my argument that there must be a compensating benefit to any risk (with both being of the same type) suffers from a clear counterexample.

Two points can be made in reply. First, there is a relevant disanalogy. The causal connection between risk to donor and benefit to recipient is not duplicated in the research context, and this disanalogy is morally relevant. It is not duplicated in the research context because research aims for knowledge, not therapy. It is not, therefore, intrinsically ordered to benefit others. Research that benefits others means that the experimental drug, device, or surgical procedure worked, and, therefore, benefited the subjects as well. It is hard to find in the research context a pure example of a high-risk study with no prospect of direct benefit to subjects and, at the same time, a high promise of benefit to others. Since this is the case in donation, the risk/benefit schema in donation is not duplicated in the kind of research I wish to challenge here.

Is this a morally relevant difference? Viewed from one perspective, it is obviously so. The risk/benefit schema in donation guarantees benefit to the recipient, and the risks to the donor are part of a causal chain leading to such benefits. The risks to the donor are necessary and jointly sufficient – along with graft placement – for benefiting the recipient. Part of why we think donation laudable is that there are few intervening steps between the self-sacrifice of the donor and benefit to the recipient. Imagine intervening steps that reduce the probability of benefiting the recipient – the recipient has, for example, several comorbidities that are life-threatening as well. Even if we still think that donation in such circumstances is permissible, we would certainly need additional information to make the case; it is *prima facie* impermissible. The only change in this case from the typical high-benefit case is the reduced likelihood of benefit. So, the causal connection between risk to donor and benefit to recipient is a morally relevant one; and this connection is absent in the research I wish to challenge.

Even if it can be argued that donation and risky research do not differ in morally relevant respects, it is not obvious that we should still hold that donation is permissible. Our intuitions on the permissibility of donation are not unrevisable. Carl Elliot (1995) makes a case along this line by focusing, not on the actions of the donor, but on the recipient and the one doing the extraction.

> To get at what is troubling about a person who knowingly and willingly consents to a harmful medical procedure, it is necessary to look not simply at the person making the decision to participate, but beyond him to the other people involved in and affected by the exchange.
>
> (Elliot, 1995, 93)

It is easy to admire someone's self-sacrifice for others, but at the same time we should not honor the person who takes advantage of that self-sacrifice. Elliot notes, "while we admire the person who *undergoes* harm to himself for the sake of another, we do not necessarily admire the person who *inflicts* harm on one person for the sake of another" (Elliot, 1995, 95). And these reflections apply equally to donation or research. Although morally important analogs may exist between donation and research, we should not assume organ transplantation involves permissible actions by everyone involved; and the same assessment applies to research.

Conclusion

To summarize the argument, certain kinds of research on adults involve a researcher knowingly inflicting harm on subjects. A plausible principle of just treatment of another says that, if A knowingly inflicts harm on B, A must compensate B. And A compensates B only if A has a morally sufficient reason for inflicting harm. Exploiting an analogy with theodicy, our intuitions on what counts as a morally sufficient reason for inflicting harm on someone must involve a compensating benefit to the one who is harmed. Since our moral intuitions in the theodicy case apply to *any* just agent for which the agent causes/allows suffering on another, our intuitions ground an ethical requirement governing risky research on human subjects, i.e., there must be something like a prospect of direct benefit in the setting of more than minimal risk. The principal challenge to this conclusion focuses on the ethical role of consent. I argued that consent itself cannot justify a risky study – it is a categorical error to suppose that a subject's consent can justify an action by a researcher who does not have a morally sufficient reason for causing/allowing harm in the first place. Thinking that it would justify suffers peer disagreement, and the justification canvassed above is not sufficient to offset the cost in violating commutative justice.

Notes

1 For a good description of "vital importance" see Field and Behrman (2004, 134).
2 Kong (2005, 206) notes the following, "Medical research is a social activity whose principle justification is medical progress for which the assumed beneficiary is society."
3 Vulnerable populations are ones for whom informed consent is severely compromised through developmental immaturity (fetus, children), degenerative disease (mentally disabled/Alzheimer's), or through environmental factors which may be coercive (prisoners and the economically/educationally disadvantaged).
4 A new subpart and/or Guidance document is being considered for adult subjects who do not have decision-making capacity. In this category would be advanced Alzheimer's patients, or the mentally disabled/mentally ill. See SACHRP (2008–2009).
5 There are, however, other sources of vulnerability; see Coleman (2009, 15ff.).
6 The *Belmont Report*, for example, states, "The principle of respect for persons thus divides into two separate moral requirements: the requirement to *acknowledge* autonomy and the requirement to *protect* those with diminished autonomy" (emphasis mine). Reprinted in Bankert and Amdur (2006, 482).
7 Neil C. Manson and Onora O'Neill (2007, 72ff) note that a subject's consent has the effect of waiving her rights not to be harmed or experimented upon. For a related though more radical account, see Hurd (1996).
8 There are, however, problems with the concept of 'minimal risk.' According to Wendler et al. (2005), IRBs are too strict in their interpretation of minimal risk. They point out that the statistical prevalence of injury and death from 'daily life' are fairly high and yet people tolerate such risks. But Wendler (2005) points out that daily life risks are not analogous to research-induced

risks. First, many risks of daily life cannot be controlled, but choosing to be a research subject is. Second, we tolerate risks of certain activities because of the joy or pleasure we derive from competitive activity, this includes even risky sports like football. But research that presents the risk of broken bones or torn ACLs does not always supply, on its own, a compensating benefit. Instead, Wendler (2005) settles on a "charitable participation" standard.

9 The other requirements pertain to scientific design, equitable selection of subjects, informed consent issues, and safety monitoring.

10 Friedman et al. quote from the National Council for Science and Technology (2004, n. 6).

11 See Stump (2010, 378). I should note here that the sufferer is one who suffers *undeservedly*. Self-inflicted harm, of any sort, is a species of wrongdoing and suffering caused by one's own wrongdoing is not considered a problem for theism. I should also note that I disagree with the typical framing of this issue, but my objections do not affect the point about commutative justice I wish to extract from this frame.

12 This case is discussed by many, notably Bergelson (2008) and Tadros (2011). Most commentators on this case assume that consent does not justify Meiwes's act of killing. I use this case, not to draw an analogy with what researchers do, but to explore the 'moral magic' of consent.

13 A possible complication with my analysis is her example of getting a tattoo. My reading of this is that tattoo-giving is a service and *qua giving a service* it depends on consent insofar as service-giving typically involves a request for the service. Taking a needle with ink on it to a non-requesting person is not the giving of a service but is rightly categorized by Hurd as an instance of maiming.

14 The notion of harm I am assuming here overlaps with suffering. Harm involves damage to one's health broadly construed (including psychosocial health so as to include risky behavioral research). I do not hold to an interest account of harm strictly, see Chapter 5.

15 Recall that, although my argument emphasizes the need for a compensating benefit, I would add that knowledge of vital importance can function as a justifier for causing or allowing harms on another. But adding this feature does not impugn my overall thesis because justification of risky pediatric research countenances knowledge of vital importance as a legitimate justifier as well. If both adult and pediatric research are justified in virtue of the same ethical considerations, pediatric subjects do not enjoy greater protection.

16 To tether my reflections here to a particular case, I am thinking of the TGN 1412 trial which offered subjects ~3,500USD. Now, consider the study without such a payment offer. It is apparent that no one would consent to it. See Emanuel and Miller (2007).

17 Resnik and Koski (2011) recommend having a national registry of health volunteers since quite a few of them participate in numerous trials. The worry is that some do not wait for the required 'wash out' period which may magnify the risks to their health.

18 I relegate to a footnote what is likely a key premise in my argument here only because this is not a chapter on rational choice or human action theory. Following Talbot Brewer (2009), I consider a rational action as involving, at least, an apprehension of something good or worthwhile. Intentional actions must involve reasons, and the motivational force of such reasons is explained by an apprehension of something good. In a discussion on the desire-satisfaction theory of rational action, Brewer notes in response: "One does not count as an agent simply in virtue of consistently behaving in ways that effectively bring about certain describable state of affairs [affairs seen as desirable]. . . . To be an agent is to set oneself in motion . . . on the strength of

one's sense that something counts in favor of doing so. That performing some action would bring about some state of affairs cannot intelligibly be regarded as counting in favor of performing the action unless one sees the state of affairs, or the effort to produce it, as itself good or valuable. . . . Desires can figure centrally in the rationalizing explanation of actions only if they involve a sense of the point or value of acting in the way they incline us to act, and only if they motivate us by inducing us to act on the strength of this evaluative outlook" (2009, 28). On Brewer's view, apprehending an end as good is a necessary condition for rational action. Returning to the example of entering into a study with risks grossly overriding any benefits, it is hard to appreciate any reason for entering the study focusing just on the benefits and burdens the study promises.

19 The Office of Human Research Protections (n.d.) give the following guidance, "Direct payments or other forms of **remuneration** offered to potential subjects as an incentive or reward for participation should not be considered a 'benefit' to be gained from research. . . . Although participation in research may be a personally rewarding activity or a humanitarian contribution, *these subjective benefits should not enter into the IRB's analysis of benefits and risks*" (emphasis added).

20 For a potentially representative voice see Rosenfield (2008). I say only 'potentially' since, although Rosenfield says he thinks that subpart D is a "barrier" to good clinical research, he never argues for this claim. His only protestations concern the extended review process of his own study, which was reviewed under category §46.407. No discernible challenge to the ethical standards of subpart D is presented.

21 Cited in Resnik (2012).

22 Instead of functioning as a counterexample to my argument, the Barry Marshall case might just as well illustrate that I might be permitted to do to my own body what somebody else is not permitted to do.

12 Conclusion

Suppose you and I are crystal ball gazers in which our respective crystals bequeath moral judgments. Your crystal ball churns out the judgment that it is permissible to kill X, and mine delivers the opposite judgment. Suppose further that our crystals are the only means by which we form moral judgments. We do not know that they are reliable, and we cannot use their very outputs to confirm their reliability for that would be circular. Suppose, finally, that there are significant goods that would be compromised if one is wrong that it is permissible to kill X; and only somewhat significant goods would be compromised if one is wrong that it is impermissible to kill X. Our crystal balls represent our moral perception. That we cannot confirm their reliability refers, of course, to the argument in Chapter 2, and the presence of competing outputs from our crystal balls represent the epistemic significance of peer disagreement (Chapter 3). Continuing with the analogy, it is clear that acting on what your crystal ball tells you to do is incongruent with intellectual humility regarding the reliability of your own crystal ball, and incongruent with intellectual justice vis-à-vis the outputs of my crystal ball.

Of course, this is merely an analogy, or rather a heuristic to illustrate the basic epistemological points upon which this project relies. The advance my project wishes to make is that it is ecumenical in nature. What I mean by that is that my interlocutors need not adopt the positions I defend in favor of, for example, the substance view of the person. There are two reasons for this. The first is that my argument in Chapter 4 ended by pointing out that the psychological account of the person is underdetermined as a justification for abortion rights. It was no part of that argument to adjudicate who has the better account of the person (substance view versus functional brain view). It is agreed that they are different theories; but both can accommodate the intuitions highlighted in the thought experiments typically understood to motivate the functional brain view. Since only one such account provides a reason for the permissibility of abortion, and the other arguably does not, the justification for abortion suffers underdetermination. This is an ecumenical conclusion because I am not arguing there that the functional brain view is false – I do not necessarily do so earlier in the chapter given my suspicion that McMahan and I are answering different questions (see Chapter 4, pages 68–69).

A second reason for understanding my argument as ecumenical is that my overall conclusion is that one should not *act on* judgments of permissible killing, not that one should not have those beliefs at all. I will say, however, that my arguments are strong enough for the conclusion that those with whom my interlocutors may disagree are epistemic peers – with a nod to the epistemic effects that disagreement exerts. The arguments are also strong enough to set the burden of proof. But, again, agreement is not required to grant presumptions in a dialectical exchange. A prosecuting attorney does not believe that the defendant is innocent but crafts her case considering the presumption in favor of innocence.

My project aims first to push us out of ourselves, so to speak, and look at human moral cognition and the multiple non-alethic affects to which that cognition is susceptible. Taking seriously how we typically think (Chapter 2), and that others may be just as morally attuned as we are (Chapter 3) in the setting of serious risk in being wrong on judgments of permissible killing, grounds a local skepticism on those very judgments. The basic idea in the chapters which followed are that coherence, or wide reflective equilibrium, is still tenuous epistemic comfort given the original epistemological lessons learned. Again, the conclusion reached here is ecumenical in nature. One can grant that she has a widely coherent network of beliefs in favor of a moral position, and yet acknowledge the tenuous comfort that coherence provides (Depaul, 1993).

In light of these points, my hope is that this work will be viewed with the same intellectual disposition from which it is offered, namely, an ecumenical discourse on how we should inquire on matters involving a serious moral risk in being wrong.

Bibliography

Ackerman, T. F. (2010). Why doctors should intervene. In *Bioethics: Principles, Issues, and Cases*, ed. Lewis Vaughn, pp. 79–83. New York: Oxford University Press.

Aijaz, I., McKeown-Green, J., and Webster, A. (2013). Burdens of proof and the case for unevenness. *Argumentation* 27(3): 259–282.

Aimar, S. (2018). Disposition ascriptions. *Philosophical Studies* (online, doi. org/10.1007/s11098-018-1084-9, accessed 7/18/2018).

Almeida, L., Azevedo, B., Nunes, T., Vaz-da-Silva, M., and Soares-da-Silva, P. (2007). Why healthy subjects volunteer for phase I studies and how they perceive their participation? *European Journal of Clinical Pharmacology* 63(11): 1085–1094.

Alston, W. P. (1991). *Perceiving God: the epistemology of religious experience.* Ithaca, NY: Cornell University Press.

Alston, W. P. (2005). *Beyond "justification": dimensions of epistemic evaluation.* Ithaca, NY: Cornell University Press.

Anderson, J. A. and Kimmelman, J. (2010). Extending clinical equipoise to phase 1 trials involving patients: unresolved problems. *Kennedy Institute of Ethics Journal* 20(1): 75–98.

Andrews, K., Murphy, L., Munday, R., and Littlewood, C. (1996). Misdiagnosis of the vegetative state: retrospective study in a rehabilitation unit. *British Medical Journal* 313(7048): 13–16.

Anscombe, E. (2000). *Intention.* Cambridge, MA: Harvard University Press.

Anscombe, G. E. M. (1958). Modern moral philosophy. *Philosophy*, 33(124): 1–19.

Appelbaum, P. S. (2007). Assessment of patients' competence to consent to treatment. *New England Journal of Medicine*, 357(18): 1834–1840.

Appelbaum, P. S., Lidz, C. W., and Klitzman, R. (2009). Voluntariness of consent to research: a conceptual model. *Hastings Center Report* 39(1): 30–39.

Appelbaum, P. S., Roth, L. H., Lidz, C. W., Benson, P., and Winslade, W. (1987). False hopes and best data: consent to research and the therapeutic misconception. *Hastings Center Report* 17(2): 20–24.

Aristotle (1941). *The basic works of Aristotle.* Ed. Richard McKeon. New York: Random House.

Armour, S., and Haynie, D. L. (2007). Adolescent sexual debut and later delinquency. *Journal of Youth and Adolescence* 36(2): 141–152.

Armstrong, D. M. (1980). *A theory of universals: volume 2: universals and scientific realism.* Cambridge, UK: Cambridge University Press.

Aronson, E. (1968). Dissonance theory: progress and problems. In *Theories of cognitive consistency: a sourcebook*, eds, R. P. Abelson, E. E. Aronson, W. J. McGuire, T. M. Newcomb, M. J. Rosenberg, and P. H. Tannenbaum, pp. 5–27. Chicago, IL: Rand McNally.

Arras, J. (2010). Physician-assisted suicide: a tragic view. In *Bioethics: principles, issues, and cases*, ed., L. Vaughn, pp. 565–579. New York: Oxford University Press.

Arthur, A., Rychkov, G., Shi, S., Koblar, S. A., and Gronthos, S. (2008). Adult human dental pulp stem cells differentiate toward functionally active neurons under appropriate environmental cues. *Stem Cells* 26(7): 1787–1795.

Aru, J., and Bachmann, T. (2015). Still wanted—the mechanisms of consciousness! *Frontiers in Psychology* 6: 5.

Audi, R. (2001). *The architecture of reason: the structure and substance of rationality*. New York: Oxford University Press.

Audi, R. (2013). *Moral perception*. Princeton, NJ: Princeton University Press.

Austin, C. J. and Marmodoro, A. (2017). Structural powers and the homeodynamic unity of organisms. In *Neo-Aristotelian perspectives on contemporary science*, eds, W. M. Simpson, R. C. Koons, and N. J. Teh, pp. 183–198. New York: Routledge.

Austriaco, N. P. G. (2002). On static eggs and dynamic embryos: a systems perspective. *The National Catholic Bioethics Quarterly* 2(4): 659–683.

Austriaco, N. P. G. (2004). Immediate hominization from the systems perspective. *The National Catholic Bioethics Quarterly* 4(4): 719–738.

Bach, J. R. (2003). Threats to "informed" advance directives for the severely physically challenged? *Archives of Physical Medicine Rehabilitation* 84 Supplement 2: S23–S28.

Bai, Y., Xia, X., Kang, J., Yang, Y., He, J., and Li, X. (2017). TDCS modulates cortical excitability in patients with disorders of consciousness. *NeuroImage: Clinical* 15: 702–709.

Baker, L. R. (2000). *Persons and bodies: a constitution view*. Cambridge, UK: Cambridge University Press.

Baker, L. R. (2005). When does a person begin? *Social Philosophy and Policy*, 22(2): 25–48.

Baldwin, T. (2003). From knowledge by acquaintance to knowledge by causation. In *The Cambridge Companion to Bertrand Russell*, ed., N. Griffin, pp. 420–448. New York: Cambridge University Press.

Bankert, E. A. and Amdur, R. eds (2006). *Institutional review board: management and function*, 2nd ed. Sudbury, MA: Jones and Bartlett.

Bargh, J. A. and Chartrand, T. L. (1999). The unbearable automaticity of being. *American Psychologist* 54(7): 462–479.

Baron, J. (1995). Myside bias in thinking about abortion. *Thinking and Reasoning* 1: 221–235.

Bastardi, A., Uhlmann, E. L., and Ross, L. (2011). Wishful thinking: belief, desire, and the motivated evaluation of scientific evidence. *Psychological Science* 22(6): 731–732.

Bazerman, M. H. and Tenbrunsel, A. E. (2011). Ethical breakdowns. *Harvard Business Review* 89(4): 58–65.

Beauchamp, T. L. and Childress, J. F. (2001). *Principles of biomedical ethics*, 5th ed. New York: Oxford University Press.

Beckwith, F. J. (2007). *Defending life: a moral and legal case against abortion choice*. New York: Cambridge University Press.

Berg, J. W., Appelbaum, P. S., and Grisso, T. (1996). Constructing competence: formulating standards of legal competence to make decisions. *Rutgers Law Review* 48: 345–396.

Bergelson, V. (2008). Autonomy, dignity, and consent to harm. *Rutgers Law Review* 60: 723–736.

Bergmann, M. (2004). Epistemic circularity: malignant and benign. *Philosophy and Phenomenological Research*, 69(3): 709–727.

Bertalanffy, L. V. (1952). *Problems of life*. New York: John Wiley and Sons.

Blair, R. and James, R. (1995). A cognitive developmental approach to morality: investigating the psychopath. *Cognition* 57: 1–29.

Blum, L. (1994). *Moral perception and particularity*. New York: Cambridge University Press.

Bonevac, D., Dever, J., and Sosa, D. (2011). The counterexample fallacy. *Mind*, 120(480): 1143–1158.

Boonin, D. (2003). *A defense of abortion*. New York: Cambridge University Press.

Braddock, M. (2016). Evolutionary debunking: can moral realists explain the reliability of our moral judgments? *Philosophical Psychology* 29(6): 844–857.

Braddock, M. (2017). Should we treat vegetative and minimally conscious patients as persons? *Neuroethics* (online, February 15, 2017): 1–14, doi:10.1007/s12152-017-9309-8.

Brakman, S.-V. (2008). Natural embryo loss and the moral status of the human fetus. *American Journal of Bioethics* 8(7): 22–23.

Brandt, M. J., Reyna, C., Chambers, J. R., Crawford, J. T., and Wetherell, G. (2014). The ideological-conflict hypothesis: intolerance among both liberals and conservatives. *Current Directions in Psychological Science* 23: 27–34.

Brandt, R. (2006). The rationality of suicide. In *Biomedical Ethics*, 6th ed., eds, T. Mappes and D. Degrazia, pp. 388–394. New York: McGraw-Hill.

Brandt, R. B. (1975). A moral principle about killing. In *Beneficent euthanasia*, ed., M. Kohl. Buffalo, NY: Prometheus Books.

Bratman, M. (1981). Intention and means-end reasoning. *The Philosophical Review* 90(2): 252–265.

Bratman, M. (2000). Reflection, planning, and temporally extended agency. *The Philosophical Review* 109(1): 35–61.

Breitbart, W., Rosenfeld, B., Pessin, H., Kaim, M., Funesti-Esch, J., Galietta, M., Nelson, C. J., and Brescia, R. (2000). Depression, hopelessness, and desire for hastened death in terminally ill patients with cancer. *JAMA: The Journal of the American Medical Association* 284: 2907–2911.

Brennan, W. (1995). *Dehumanizing the vulnerable: when word games take lives*. Chicago, IL: Loyola University Press.

Brewer, T. (2009). *The retrieval of ethics*. New York: Oxford University Press.

Briere, J. N. and Langtree, C. B. (2011). *Treating complex trauma in adolescents and young adults*. Los Angeles, CA: Sage Publications.

Broackes, J. (2006). Substance. *Proceedings of the Aristotelian Society* 106(1): 133–168.

Brock, D. W. (1992). Voluntary active euthanasia. *Hastings Center Report* 22(2): 10–22.

Brody, B. (1996). Withdrawal of treatment versus killing of patients. In *Intending death: the ethics of assisted suicide and euthanasia*, ed. Tom Beauchamp (pp. 90–103). Upper Saddle River, NJ: Prentice Hall.

Brown, M. T. (2007). The potential of the human embryo. *Journal of Medicine and Philosophy* 32(6): 585–618.

Bruner, J. S. and Postman, L. (1949). On the perception of incongruity: a paradigm. *Journal of Personality* 18(2): 206–223.

Bruno, M. A., Bernheim, J. L., Ledoux, D., Pellas, F., Demertzi, A., and Laureys, S. (2011). A survey on self-assessed well-being in a cohort of chronic locked-in syndrome patients: happy majority, miserable minority. *BMJ Open* 1:e000039, doi:10.1136/bmjopen-2010-000039.

Bruno, M. A., Majerus, S., Boly, M., Vanhaudenhuyse, A., Schnakers, C., Gosseries, O., Boveroux, P., Kirsch, M., Demertzi, A., Bernard, C., and Hustinx, R. (2012). Functional neuroanatomy underlying the clinical sub-categorization of minimally conscious state patients. *Journal of Neurology* 259(6): 1087–1098.

Bubela, T., Li, M. D., Hafez, M., Bieber, M., and Atkins, H. (2012). Is belief larger than fact: expectations, optimism and reality for translational stem cell research. *BMC Medicine* 10(1): 1–10.

Burke, M. B. (1996). Sortal essentialism and the potentiality principle. *Review of Metaphysics* 49(3): 491–514.

Callahan, D. (1984). Autonomy: a moral good, not a moral obsession. *Hastings Center Report* 14(5): 40–42.

Campbell, T. and McMahan, J. (2010). Animalism and the varieties of conjoined twinning. *Theoretical Medicine and Bioethics* 31(4): 285–301.

Carlin, R., Davis, D., Weiss, M., Schultz, B., and Troyer, D. (2006). Expression of early transcription factors Oct-4, Sox-2 and Nanog by porcine umbilical cord (PUC) matrix cells. *Reproductive Biology and Endocrinology* 4(1): 1–13.

Casarett, D., Pickard, A., Bailey, F. A., Ritchie, C., Furman, C., Rosenfeld, K., Shreve, S., Chen, Z., and Shea, J. A. (2008). Do palliative consultations improve patient outcomes? *Journal of the American Geriatrics Society* 56(4), 593–599.

Cavanaugh, T. A. (2006). *Double-effect reasoning: doing good and avoiding evil.* New York: Oxford University Press.

Chaiken, S. (1987). The heuristic model of persuasion. In *Social influence: the Ontario symposium*, eds, M. P. Zanna, J. M. Olson, and C. P. Herman, pp. 3–39. Hillsdale, NJ: Erlbaum.

Chapman, A. R. (2011). Addressing the ethical challenges of first-in-human trials. *Journal of Clinical Research and Bioethics* 2(4): 1–8, http://dx.doi.org/10.4172/2155-9627.1000113.

Chappell, S.-G. (2004). Persons as goods: response to Patrick Lee. *Christian Bioethics* 10(1): 69–78.

Chappell, S.-G. (2008). Moral perception. *Philosophy* 83(4): 421–437.

Chappell, S.-G. (2011). On the very idea of criteria for personhood. *The Southern Journal of Philosophy* 49(1): 1–27.

Charlotte Lozier Institute (2017). Fact sheet: adult stem cell research and transplants (November, 21). Available at: https://lozierinstitute.org/fact-sheet-adult-stem-cell-research-transplants, accessed 5/22/2018.

Chartrand, T. L. and Bargh, J. A. (2002). Nonconscious motivations: their activation, operation, and consequences. In *Self and motivation: emerging psychological perspectives*, eds, A. Tesser, D. A. Stapel, and J. V. Wood, pp. 13–41. Washington, DC: American Psychological Association.

Chen, J., Sanberg, P. R., Li, Y., Wang, L., Lu, M., Willing, A. E., Sanchez-Ramos, J., and Chopp, M. (2001). Intravenous administration of human umbilical cord blood reduces behavioral deficits after stroke in rats. *Stroke* 32(11): 2682–2688.

Chen, S. and Chaiken, S. (1999). The heuristic-systematic model in its broader context. *Dual-Process Theories in Social Psychology*, 15: 73–96.

Christensen, D. (2007). Epistemology of disagreement: the good news. *Philosophical Review* 116(2): 187–217.

Christensen, D. (2011). Disagreement, question-begging and epistemic self-criticism. *Philosophers Imprint* 11(6): 1–22.

Chudnoff, E. (2013). *Intuition*. New York: Oxford University Press.

Chudy, D., Deletis, V., Almahariq, F., Marčinković, P., Škrlin, J., and Paradžik, V. (2018). Deep brain stimulation for the early treatment of the minimally conscious state and vegetative state: experience in 14 patients. *Journal of Neurosurgery* 128(4): 1189–1198.

Coady, C. A. J. (1992). *Testimony: a philosophical study*. New York: Oxford University Press.

Coleman, C. H. (2009). Vulnerability as a regulatory category in human subject research. *Journal of Law, Medicine and Ethics* 37(1): 12–18.

Coleman, C. H., Menikoff, J. A., Goldner, J. A., and Dubler, N. N. (2005). *The ethics and regulation of research with human subjects*. Newark, NJ: LexisNexis.

Condic, M. L. (2008). *When does human life begin? A scientific perspective.* Westchester Institute White Paper 1: 1–31. Valhalla, NY: Westchester Institute for Human Development.

Condic, M. L. (2011). A biological definition of the human embryo. In *Persons, moral worth, and embryos*, ed., Stephen Napier, pp. 211–235. Dordrecht: Springer Science and Business Media.

Condic, M. L. (2013). When does human life begin: the scientific evidence and terminology revisited. *University of St. Thomas Journal of Law and Public Policy* 8: 44–81.

Condic, M. L. and Rao, M. (2010). Alternative sources of pluripotent stem cells: ethical and scientific issues revisited. *Stem Cells and Development* 19(8): 1121–1129.

Conly, S. (2013). *Against autonomy: justifying coercive paternalism*. New York: Cambridge University Press.

Contessa, G. (2013). Dispositions and interferences. *Philosophical Studies* 165: 401–419.

Cooper, J. and Fazio, R. H. (1984). A new look at dissonance theory. In *Advances in Experimental Social Psychology*, vol. 17, ed. L. Berkowitz, pp. 229–266. New York: Academic Press.

Coss, D. (2018). Interest-relative invariantism and indifference problems. *Acta Analytica* 33(2): 227–240.

Crain, B. J., Tran, S. D., and Mezey, E. (2005). Transplanted human bone marrow cells generate new brain cells. *Journal of the Neurological Sciences*, 233(1–2): 121–123.

Daniels, N. (1979). Wide reflective equilibrium and theory acceptance in ethics. *The Journal of Philosophy* 76(5): 256–282.

D'Arcy, E. (1963). *Human acts and their moral evaluation*. New York: Clarendon Press.

Darley, J. M. and Berscheid, E. (1967). Increased liking as a result of the anticipation of personal contact. *Human Relations* 20(1): 29–40.

Davis, J. K. (2009). Precedent autonomy, advance directives, and end-of-life care. *The Oxford Handbook of Bioethics*, ed., B. Steinbock, pp. 1–28. Oxford, UK: Oxford Handbooks Online, doi: 10.1093/oxfordhb/9780199562411. 003.0016.

Debes, R. (2009). Dignity's gauntlet. *Philosophical Perspectives* 23(1): 45–78.

DeGrazia, D. (2005). *Human identity and bioethics*. New York: Cambridge University Press.

DeGrazia, D. (2006). Moral status, human identity, and early embryos: a critique of the president's approach. *The Journal of Law, Medicine and Ethics* 34(1): 49–57.

Delaney, J. and Hershenov, D. B. (2009). Why consent may not be needed for organ procurement. *The American Journal of Bioethics* 9(8): 3–10.

Dempsey, M. M. (2012). Victimless conduct and the *volenti* maxim: how consent works. *Criminal Law and Philosophy*, online May 27, 2012, doi 10.1007/s11572-012-9162-0.

DePaul, M. (1993). *Balance and refinement: beyond coherence methods in ethics*. New York: Routledge.

DeRose, K. (1992). Contextualism and knowledge attributions. *Philosophy and Phenomenological Research* 52(4): 913–929.

Diamond, C. (1982). Anything but argument? *Philosophical Investigations* 5(1): 23–41.

Diamond, C. (1995). *The realistic spirit: Wittgenstein, philosophy, and the mind*. Cambridge, MA: MIT Press.

Ditto, P. H., Pizarro, D. A., and Tannenbaum, D. (2009). Motivated moral reasoning. *Psychology of Learning and Motivation* 50: 307–338.

Doble, J. E., Haig, A. J., Anderson, C., and Katz, R. (2003). Impairment, activity, participation, life satisfaction, and survival in persons with locked-in syndrome for over a decade: follow-up on a previously reported cohort. *The Journal of Head Trauma Rehabilitation* 18(5): 435–444.

Dodson, C., Toth-Fejel, T., and Stangebye, Z. (2008). For what we do, and fail to do. *American Journal of Bioethics* 8(7): 29–31.

Douglas, T. and Savulescu, J. (2009). Destroying unwanted embryos in research: talking point on morality and human embryo research. *EMBO Reports* 10(4): 307–312.

Dresser, R. and Robertson, J. A. (1989). Quality of life and non-treatment decisions for incompetent patients: a critique of the orthodox approach. *Law, Medicine and Health Care* 17/3: 234–244.

Dworkin, R. (2013). *Justice for hedgehogs*. Cambridge, MA: Harvard University Press.

Dworkin, R., Nagel, T., Nozick, R., Rawls, J., Scanlon, T. M., and Thomson, J. J. (2013). Assisted suicide: the philosophers' brief. In *Bioethics: principles, issues, and cases*, 2nd ed., ed., L. Vaughn, pp. 661–669. New York: Oxford University Press.

Eberl, J. T. (2009). Do human persons persist between death and resurrection? In *Metaphysics and God: essays in honor of Eleonore Stump*, ed., K. Timpe. Abingdon, UK: Routledge.

Eberl, J. T. (2010). Fetuses are neither violinists nor violators. *The American Journal of Bioethics* 10(12): 53–54.

Edwards, K. and Smith, E. E. (1996). A disconfirmation bias in the evaluation of arguments. *Journal of Personality and Social Psychology* 71(1): 5–24.

Elder, C. L. (2005). *Real natures and familiar objects*. Cambridge, MA: The MIT Press.

Elga, A. (2007). Reflection and disagreement. *Noûs* 41(3): 478–502.

Elga, A. (2010). How to disagree about how to disagree. In *Disagreement*, eds, T. Warfield and R. Feldman, pp. 175–186. New York: Oxford University Press.

Elliot, C. (1995). Doing harm: living organ donors, clinical research and the tenth man. *Journal of Medical Ethics* 21: 91–96.

Ellis, R. D. (2001). Implications of inattentional blindness for 'enactive' theories of consciousness. *Brain and Mind* 2: 297–322.

Ellis, R. D. (2005). *Curious emotions: roots of consciousness and personality in motivated action*. Amsterdam: John Benjamins Publishers.

Elsayem, A., Smith, M. L., Parmley, L., Palmer, J. L., Jenkins, R., Reddy, S., and Bruera, E. (2006). Impact of a palliative care service on in-hospital mortality in a comprehensive cancer center. *Journal of Palliative Medicine* 9(4): 894–902.

Eltis, D. (1987). *Economic growth and the ending of the transatlantic slave trade*. New York: Oxford University Press.

Emanuel, E. J. and Miller, F. G. (2007). Money and distorted ethical judgment about research: ethical assessment of the TeGenero TGN1412 trial. *American Journal of Bioethics* 7: 76–81.

Emanuel, E. J., Wendler, D., and Grady, C. (2000). What makes clinical research ethical? *JAMA: The Journal of the American Medical Association* 283(20): 2701–2711.

Fagerberg, D. (2010). The Christian hypothesis. In *Persons, moral worth, and embryos*, vol. 111, ed., S. Napier, pp. 100–111. Dordrecht: Springer Science and Business Media.

Fantl, J. and McGrath, M. (2009). *Knowledge in an uncertain world*. New York: Oxford University Press.

Feinberg, J. (1978). Voluntary euthanasia and the inalienable right to life. *Philosophy and Public Affairs* 7(2): 93–123.

Fergusson, D. M., Horwood, J., and Boden, J. M. (2009). Reactions to abortion and subsequent mental health. *British Journal of Psychiatry* 195: 420–426.

Festinger, L. (1962). *A theory of cognitive dissonance*, vol. 2. Stanford, CA: Stanford University Press.

Field, J. M. and Behrman, R. E., eds (2004). *Ethical conduct of clinical research involving children*. Washington DC: National Academies Press.

Finer, L. B., Frohwirth, L. F., Dauphinee, L. A., Singh, S., and Moore, A. M. (2005). Reasons US women have abortions: quantitative and qualitative perspectives. *Perspectives on Sexual and Reproductive Health* 37(3): 110–118.

Finn, P. (2003). Cannibal case grips Germany: suspect says internet correspondent volunteered to die. *Washington Post* December 4, at A26.

Finnis, J. (1973). The rights and wrongs of abortion: a reply to Judith Thomson. *Philosophy and Public Affairs* 2(2): 117–145.

Fins, J. J. (2015). *Rights come to mind: brain injury, ethics, and the struggle for consciousness*. New York: Cambridge University Press.

Fischer, J. M. and Ravizza, M. (1998). *Responsibility and control: a theory of moral responsibility*. New York: Cambridge University Press.

Foot, P. (1967). The problem of abortion and the doctrine of double effect. *Oxford Review* 5: 5–15.

Forsythe, C. D. (2013). *Abuse of discretion: the inside story of Roe v. Wade*. New York: Encounter Books.

Frances, B. (2014). *Disagreement*. Malden, MA: Polity Press.

Freeman, J. B. (2005). *Acceptable premises. An informal approach to an informal logic problem*. New York: Cambridge University Press.

Friedman, A., Robbins, E., and Wendler, D. (2010). Which benefits of research participation count as 'direct'? *Bioethics* 26(2): 60–67, doi:10.1111/j.1467-8519.2010.01825.x.

Gage, F. H. (2000). Mammalian neural stem cells. *Science* 287(5457): 1433–1438.

Gagne, J. J. and Choudhry, N. K. (2011). How many "Me-Too" drugs is too many? *JAMA: The Journal of the American Medical Association* 305(7): 711–712.

Gaita, R. (2004). *Good and evil: an absolute conception*. New York: Routledge.

Ganzini, L. and Farrenkopf, T. (1998). Mental health consultation and referral. In *The Oregon Death with Dignity Act: a guidebook for health care providers*, eds, K. Haley and M. Lee, pp. 30–32. Portland, OR: Oregon Health Sciences University.

Garattini, S. and Bertele, V. (2007). Non-inferiority trails are unethical because they disregard patient's interests. *The Lancet* 370: 1875–1877.

Garcia, J. L. A. (1997). Intentions in medical ethics. In *Human lives: critical essays on consequentialist bioethics*, eds, J. A. Laing and D. Oderberg, pp. 161–181. London: Palgrave Macmillan.

Garcia, L. L. (2008). Natural kinds, persons, and abortion. *The National Catholic Bioethics Quarterly* 8(2): 265–273.

Gawande, A. 2010. Whose body is it anyway? In *Bioethics: principles, issues, and cases*, ed., L. Vaughn, pp. 88–97. New York: Oxford University Press.

George, R. P. and Tollefsen, C. (2011). *Embryo: a defense of human life*, 2nd ed. Princeton, NJ: Witherspoon Institute.

Georgiopoulos, M., Katsakiori, P., Kefalopoulou, Z., Ellul, J., Chroni, E., and Constantoyannis, C. (2010). Vegetative state and minimally conscious state: a review of the therapeutic interventions. *Stereotactic Functional Neurosurgery* 88: 199–207.

Gerhart, K., Koziol-McLain, J., Lowenstein, S. R., and Whiteneck, G. G. (1994). Quality of life following spinal cord injury: knowledge and attitudes of emergency care providers. *Annals of Emergency Medicine* 23(4): 807–812.

Gettier, E. (1963). Is justified true belief knowledge? *Analysis* 23: 121–123.

Ghorbel, S. (2002). *Statut fonctionnel et qualité de vie chez le locked-in syndrome a domicile*. Montpellier, France: DEA Motricite Humaine et Handicap, Laboratory of Biostatistics, Epidemiology and Clinical Research, Universite Jean Monnet Saint-Etienne.

Giacino, J. T., Fins, J. J., Machado, A., and Schiff, N. D. (2012). Central thalamic deep brain stimulation to promote recovery from chronic posttraumatic minimally conscious state: challenges and opportunities. *Neuromodulation* 15: 339–349.

Giacino, J. T., Ashwal, S., Childs, N., Cranford, R., Jennett, B., Katz, D. I., Kelly, J. P., Rosenberg, J. H., Whyte, J. O. H. N., Zafonte, R. D., and

Zasler, N. D. (2002). The minimally conscious state: definition and diagnostic criteria. *Neurology* 58: 349–353.

Gianelli, D. (1993). Abortion providers share inner conflicts. *American Medical News*, July 12.

Gill-Thwaites, H. (2006). Lotteries, loopholes and luck: misdiagnosis in the vegetative state patient. *Brain Injury* 20(13–14): 1321–1328.

Gilovich, T. (1991). *How we know what isn't so: the fallibility of human reason in everyday life*. New York: Free Press.

Glannon, W. (2013). Burdens of ANH outweigh benefits in the minimally conscious state. *Journal of Medical Ethics* 39(9): 551–552.

Goering, S. (2008). 'You say you're happy, but': contested quality of life judgments in bioethics and disability studies. *Journal of Bioethical Inquiry* 5: 125–135.

Goldman, A. (2010). The refutation of medical paternalism. In *Bioethics: principles, issues, and cases*, ed., L. Vaughn, pp. 73–78. New York: Oxford University Press.

Gómez-Lobo, A. (2002). *Morality and the human goods: an introduction to natural law ethics*. Washington, DC: Georgetown University Press.

Gómez-Lobo, A. (2007). Inviolability at any age. *Kennedy Institute of Ethics Journal* 17(4): 311–320.

Gómez-Lobo, A. and Keown, J. (2015). *Bioethics and the human goods: an introduction to natural law bioethics*. Washington, DC: Georgetown University Press.

Goodin, R. (1985). *Protecting the vulnerable*. Chicago, IL: University of Chicago Press.

Graham, J., Haidt, J., Koleva, S., Motyl, M., Iyer, R., Wojcik, S. P., and Ditto, P. H. (2013). Moral foundations theory: the pragmatic validity of moral pluralism. In *Advances in experimental social psychology*, vol. 47, eds, P. Devine and A. Plant, pp. 55–130. Cambridge, MA: Academic Press.

Graham, J., Nosek, B. A., and Haidt, J. (2012). The moral stereotypes of liberals and conservatives: exaggeration of differences across the political spectrum. *PLoS ONE*, 7(12), e50092, http://doi.org/10.1371/journal.pone.0050092.

Guerrero, A. A. (2007). Don't know, don't kill: moral ignorance, culpability, and caution. *Philosophical Studies* 136(1): 59–97.

Hacker, P. M. S. (2010). *Human nature: the categorial framework*. Malden, MA: Wiley-Blackwell.

Haidt, J. (2001). The emotional dog and its rational tail: a social intuitionist approach to moral judgment. *Psychological Review* 108(4): 814–833.

Haidt, J. (2012). *The righteous mind: why good people are divided by politics and religion*. New York: Pantheon Books.

Haji, I. (2010). Psychopathy, ethical perception, and moral culpability. *Neuroethics* 3(2): 135–150.

Hamilton, N. G. and Hamilton, C. (2004). *Competing paradigms of responding to assisted-suicide requests in Oregon: case report*. Yakima, WA: Physicians for Compassionate Care Education Foundation. Available at: www.pccef.org/articles/art28.htm, accessed 7/18/2018.

Hanson, R. (2002). Why health is not special: errors in evolved bioethics intuitions. *Social Philosophy and Policy* 19(2): 153–179.

Harman, E. (2015). The irrelevance of moral uncertainty. *Oxford studies in metaethics*, vol. 10, ed., R. Shafer-Landau, pp. 53–79. New York: Oxford University Press.

Haslett, D. W. (1987). What is wrong with reflective equilibria? *The Philosophical Quarterly* 37(148): 305–311.

Hawley, K. (2005). Fission, fusion and intrinsic facts. *Philosophy and Phenomenological Research* 71(3): 602–621.

Haybron, D. M. (2008). *The pursuit of unhappiness: the elusive psychology of well-being.* New York: Oxford University Press.

Hebert, P. C. and Weingarten, M. A. (1991). The ethics of forced feeding in anorexia nervosa. *CMAJ: Canadian Medical Association Journal* 144(2): 141–144.

Hendin, H. (1999). Suicide, assisted suicide, and euthanasia. In *Harvard Guide to Suicide Assessment and Intervention*, ed., D. G. Jacobs, pp. 540–560. San Francisco, CA: Jossey-Bass Publishers.

Henley, K. (1977). The value of individuals. *Philosophy and Phenomenological Research* 37: 345–352.

Henry, D. (2005). Embryological models in ancient philosophy. *Phronesis* 50(1): 1–42.

Henry, D. (2008). Organismal natures. *Apeiron* 41(3): 47–74.

Hershenov, D. B. (2001). Abortions and distortions: an analysis of morally irrelevant factors in Thomson's violinist thought experiment. *Social Theory and Practice* 27(1): 129–148.

Hershenov, D. B. (2008a). A hylomorphic account of thought experiments concerning personal identity. *American Catholic Philosophical Quarterly* 82(3): 481–502.

Hershenov, D. B. (2008b). Misunderstanding the moral equivalence of killing and letting die. *National Catholic Bioethics Quarterly* 8(2): 239–245.

Hershenov, D. B. (2011). Soulless organisms?: hylomorphism vs. animalism. *American Catholic Philosophical Quarterly* 85(3): 465–482.

Hill, B. J. (2010). Abortion as health care. *The American Journal of Bioethics* 10(12): 48–49.

Hinckley, C. C. (2005). *Moral conflicts of organ retrieval: a case for constructive pluralism* (No. 172). Amsterdam: Rodopi Publishers.

Howe, E. G. (2014). What should care providers do when a patient "won't budge"? *The Journal of Clinical Ethics* 25(3): 179–188.

Howsepian, A. A. (2011). Fetal pains and fetal brains. In *Persons, moral worth, and embryos*, vol. 111, ed., S. Napier, pp. 187–210. Dordrecht: Springer Science and Business Media.

Huemer, M. (2011). Epistemological egoism and agent centered norms. In *Evidentialism and its discontents*, ed., Trent Dougherty, pp. 17–33. New York: Oxford University Press.

Humber, J. M. and Almeder, R. F., eds (2004). *Stem cell research.* Dordrecht: Springer Science and Business Media.

Hurd, H. M. (1996). The moral magic of consent. *Legal Theory* 2(2): 121–146.

Hurd, H. M. (2005). Blaming the victim: a response to the proposal that criminal law recognize a general defense of contributory responsibility. *Buffalo Criminal Law Review* 8: 503–522.

Ishii, T. and Eto, K. (2014). Fetal stem cell transplantation: past, present, and future. *World Journal of Stem Cells* 6(4): 404–420.

Iyengar, S. and Westwood, S. J. (2015). Fear and loathing across party lines: new evidence on group polarization. *American Journal of Political Science* 59(3): 690–707.

Jackson, E. and Keown, J. (2012). *Debating euthanasia*. Portland, OR: Hart Publishing.

Jansen, L. A. (2010). Disambiguating clinical intentions: the ethics of palliative sedation. *Journal of Medicine and Philosophy* 35(1): 19–31.

Jiang, Y., Jahagirdar, B. N., Reinhardt, R. L., Schwartz, R. E., Keene, C. D., Ortiz-Gonzalez, X. R., Reyes, M., Lenvik, T., Lund, T., Blackstad, M. and Du, J. (2002). Pluripotency of mesenchymal stem cells derived from adult marrow. *Nature* 418(6893): 41.

Johnson, A. and Detrow. K. (2016). *The walls are talking: former abortion clinic workers tell their stories*. San Francisco, CA: Ignatius Press.

Jonas, H. (1969). Philosophical reflections on experimenting with human subjects. *Daedalus* 98(2): 219–247.

Jones, D. A. (2015). Assisted suicide and euthanasia: a guide to the evidence. Available at: www.bioethics.org.uk/evidenceguide.pdf, accessed 7/18/2018.

Jonsen, A. R., Siegler, M., and Winslade, W. J. (2002). *Clinical ethics: a practical approach to ethical decisions in clinical medicine*, 5th ed. New York: McGraw-Hill.

Kaczor, C. (2011). *The ethics of abortion: women's rights, human life and the question of justice*. New York: Routledge.

Kaczor, C. (2013). *A defense of dignity: creating life, destroying life, and protecting the rights of conscience*. South Bend, IN: University of Notre Dame Press.

Kagan, S. (2018). The value of life, part II; other bad aspects of death, part I. Lecture, Open Yale Courses, Yale University. Available at: https://oyc.yale.edu/philosophy/phil-176/lecture-20, accessed 7/18/2018.

Kass, L. R. (2008). Defending human dignity. *Human Dignity and Bioethics: Essays Commissioned by the President's Council on Bioethics*, ed., Adam Schulman, pp. 297–332. Washington DC: Government Printing Office.

Kaveny, C. M. (2000). Appropriation of evil: cooperation's mirror image. *Theological Studies* 61(2): 280–313.

Kelly, T. (2008). Disagreement, dogmatism, and belief polarization. *Journal of Philosophy* 105(10): 611–633.

Kelly, T. (2013). Disagreement and the burdens of judgment. In *The epistemology of disagreement: new essays*, eds, D. Christensen and J. Lackey, pp. 31–53. New York: Oxford University Press.

Keown, J. (2006). Restoring the sanctity of life and replacing the caricature: a reply to David Price. *Legal Studies* 26(1): 109–119.

Keown, J. (2009). *Should we legalize voluntary euthanasia and physician-assisted suicide? A review of the ethical arguments and of the empirical evidence from the Netherlands and Oregon*. Washington DC: Family Research Council.

Khushf, G. (2006). Owning up to our agendas: on the role and limits of science in debates about embryos and brain death. *The Journal of Law, Medicine and Ethics* 34(1): 58–76.

Kim, SU and de Vellis, J. (2009). Stem cell-based cell therapy in neurological diseases: a review. *Journal of Neuroscience Research* 87: 2183–2200.

King, N. (2000). Defining and describing benefit appropriately in clinical trials. *Journal of Law, Medicine, and Ethics* 28: 332–343.

King, N. L. (2012). Disagreement: what's the problem? Or a good peer is hard to find. *Philosophy and Phenomenological Research* 85(2): 249–272.

Kiraly, M., Porcsalmy, B., Pataki, A., Kádár, K., Jelitai, M., Molnár, B., Hermann, P., Gera, I., Grimm, W. D., Ganss, B., Zsembery, A., and Varga, G. (2009).

Simultaneous PKC and cAMP activation induces differentiation of human dental pulp stem cells into functionally active neurons. *Neurochemistry International* 55(5): 323–332.

Kittay, E. F. (1999). *Love's labor: essays on women, equality and dependency*. New York: Routledge.

Koch, P. (2016). A theory of patient welfare. Dissertation, University of Buffalo.

Kong, W. M. (2005). Legitimate requests and indecent proposals: matters of justice in the ethical assessment of phase I trials involving competent patients. *Journal of Medical Ethics* 31: 205–208.

Korcz, K. A. (1997). Recent work on the basing relation. *American Philosophical Quarterly* 34: 171–192.

Kramer, K., Zaaijer, H. L., and Verweij, M. F. (2017). The precautionary principle and the tolerability of blood transfusion risks. *The American Journal of Bioethics* 17(3): 32–43.

Kramer, M. H. (2009). *Moral realism as a moral doctrine*, vol. 3. Hoboken, NJ: Wiley-Blackwell.

Kuczewski, M. (1997). *Fragmentation and consensus: communitarian and casuist bioethics*. Washington, DC: Georgetown University Press.

Kuhn, T. S. (1996). *The structure of scientific revolutions*, 3rd ed. Chicago, IL: Chicago University Press.

Kuhse, H. and Singer, P. (2009). *Defining the beginning and end of life: readings on personal identity and bioethics*, ed. J. P. Lizza. Baltimore, MD: Johns Hopkins University Press.

Kunda, Z. (1987). Motivation and inference: self-serving generation and evaluation of evidence. *Journal of Personality and Social Psychology* 53: 636–647.

Kunda, Z. (1990). Motivated reasoning. *Psychological Bulletin* 108(3): 480–498.

Kunda, Z. (1999). *Social cognition*. Cambridge, MA: MIT Press.

Kwak, K. A., Lee, S. P., Yang, J. Y., and Park, Y. S. (2018). Current perspectives regarding stem cell-based therapy for Alzheimer's Disease. *Stem Cells International* 1 Mar: 6392986, doi: 10.1155/2018/6392986.

Lacewing, M. (2015). Emotion, perception, and the self in moral epistemology. *Dialectica* 69(3): 335–355.

Lachs, J. (2010). When abstract moralizing runs amok. In *Bioethics: principles, issues, and cases*, ed., L. Vaughn, pp. 561–565. New York: Oxford University Press.

Lackey, J. (2010). A justificationist view of disagreement's epistemic significance. In *Social Epistemology*, eds, A. Haddock, A. Millar, and D. Pritchard, pp. 298–325. New York: Oxford University Press.

LaFleur, W. R., Bohme, G., and Shimazono, S., eds (2008). *Dark medicine: rationalizing unethical medical research*. Bloomington, IN: Indiana University Press.

LaPuma, J. and Schiedermayer, D. (1994). *Ethics consultation: a practical guide*. London: Jones and Bartlett Publishers.

Laughlin, M. J., Barker, J., Bambach, B., Koc, O. N., Rizzieri, D. A., Wagner, J. E., Gerson, S. L., Lazarus, H. M., Cairo, M., Stevens, C. E. and Rubinstein, P. (2001). Hematopoietic engraftment and survival in adult recipients of umbilical-cord blood from unrelated donors. *New England Journal of Medicine* 344(24): 1815–1822.

Laureys, S., Perrin, F., Schnakers, C., Boly, M., and Majerus, S. (2005a). Residual cognitive function in comatose, vegetative and minimally conscious states. *Current Opinion in Neurology* 18: 726–733.

Laureys, S., Pellas, F., van Eeckhout, P., Ghorbel, S., Schnakers, C., Perrin, F., Berre, J., Faymonville, M. E., Pantke, K. H., Damas, F., and Lamy, M. (2005b). The locked-in syndrome: what is it like to be conscious but paralyzed and voiceless? In *Progress in brain research, vol. 150: the boundaries of consciousness: neurobiology and neuropathology*, ed., S. Laurey, pp. 495–511. Amsterdam: Elsevier.

Lear, J. (1988). *Aristotle: the desire to understand*. New York: Cambridge University Press.

Lee, P. (2004). A Christian philosopher's view of recent directions in the abortion debate. *Christian Bioethics* 10: 7–31.

Lee, P. (2010). *Abortion and unborn human life*. Washington, DC: CUA Press.

Lee, P. and George, R. P. (2008). The nature and basis of human dignity. *Ratio Juris*, 21(2): 173–193.

Leibniz, G. W. (1996). *New essays concerning human understanding*. Trans. P. Remnant and J. Bennett. New York: Cambridge University Press.

Lemos, R. M. (1995). *The nature of value*. Gainesville, FL: University of Florida Press.

Leon-Carrion, J., van Eeckhout, P., and Dominguez-Morales Mdel, R. (2002). The locked-in syndrome: a syndrome looking for a therapy. *Brain Injury* 16: 555–569.

Liao, M. (2006). The embryo rescue case. *Theoretical Medicine and Bioethics* 27(2): 141–147.

Light, D. W., Lexchin, J., and Darrow, J. J. (2013). Institutional corruption of pharmaceuticals and the myth of safe and effective drugs. *Journal of Law Medicine and Ethics* 41(3): 590–600.

Little, M. O. (1995). Seeing and caring: the role of affect in feminist moral epistemology. *Hypatia* 10(3): 117–137.

Littlejohn, C. (2013). Disagreement and defeat: Clayton Littlejohn. In *Disagreement and skepticism*, ed., D. E. Machuca, pp. 178–201. New York: Routledge.

Lockhart, T. (2000). *Moral uncertainty and its consequences*. New York: Oxford University Press.

Longino, H. (1979). Evidence and hypothesis: an analysis of evidential relations. *Philosophy of Science* 46(1): 35–56.

Lord, C. G., Ross, L., and Lepper, M. R. (1979). Biased assimilation and attitude polarization: the effects of prior theories on subsequently considered evidence. *Journal of Personality and Social Psychology* 37(11): 2098–2109.

Loux, M. J. (1998). *Metaphysics: a contemporary introduction*. New York: Routledge.

Lowe, E. J. (1991). Substance and selfhood. *Philosophy* 66(255): 81–99.

Lu, T. M. (2018). Review of: Kate Greasley and Christopher Kaczor, *Abortion rights: for and against*, Cambridge University Press. *Notre Dame Philosophical Reviews*. Available at: https://ndpr.nd.edu/news/abortion-rights-for-and-against, accessed 7/16/2018.

Lulé, D., Zickler, C., Hacker, S., Bruno, M. A., Demertzi, A., Pellas, F., Laureys, S. and Kübler, A. (2009). Life can be worth living in locked-in syndrome. *Progress in Brain Research* 177: 339–351.

Lulé, D., Pauli, S., Altintas, E., Singer, U., Merk, T., Uttner, I., Birbaumer, N. and Ludolph, A. C. (2012). Emotional adjustment in amyotrophic lateral sclerosis (ALS). *Journal of Neurology* 259(2): 334–341.

Mack, A. and Rock, I. (2000). *Inattentional blindness*. Cambridge, MA: MIT Press.

MacNair, R. M. (2009). *Achieving peace in the abortion war*. New York: iUniverse Inc.

Manfredi, P. L., Morrison, R. S., Morris, J., Goldhirsch, S. L., Carter, J. M., and Meier, D. E. (2000). Palliative care consultations: how do they impact the care of hospitalized patients? *Journal of Pain and Symptom Management* 20: 166–173.

Manninen, B. A. (2010). Rethinking Roe v. Wade: defending the abortion right in the face of contemporary opposition. *The American Journal of Bioethics* 10(12): 33–46.

Manson, N. C. and O'Neill, O. (2007). *Rethinking informed consent in bioethics*. New York: Cambridge University Press.

Mappes, T. A. (2006). Some reflections on advanced directives. In *Biomedical Ethics*, 6th ed., eds, T. A. Mappes and D. DeGrazia, pp. 350–357. New York: McGraw-Hill.

Marino, T. A. (2008). Natural embryo loss—A missed opportunity. *The American Journal of Bioethics* 8(7): 25–27.

Marquis, D. (2010). Manninen's defense of abortion rights is unsuccessful. *The American Journal of Bioethics* 10(12): 56–57.

Marshall, B. J. (2005). Nobel Prize in physiology and medicine: autobiography. Nobel Foundation. Available at: http://nobelprize.org/nobel_prizes/medicine/laureates/2005/marshall-autobio.html, accessed 5/7/2012.

Martinez-Morales, P. L., Revilla, A., Ocana, I., Gonzalez, C., Sainz, P., McGuire, D., and Liste, I. (2013). Progress in stem cell therapy for major human neurological disorders. *Stem Cell Reviews and Reports* 9(5): 685–699.

Masek, L. (2009). Intentions, motives and the doctrine of double effect. *The Philosophical Quarterly*, 60(240): 567–585.

May, T. (1998). Assessing competency without judging merit. *Journal of Clinical Ethics* 9(3): 247–257.

McDowell, J. (1997). Virtues and reasons. In *Virtue ethics*, vol. 10, eds, R. Crisp and M. Slote, pp. 141–162. New York: Oxford University Press.

McLachlan, H. V. (1977). Must we accept either the conservative or the liberal view on abortion? *Analysis* 37(4): 197–204.

McMahan, J. (2002). *The ethics of killing: problems at the margins of life*. New York: Oxford University Press.

McMahan, J. (2007). Killing embryos for stem cell research. *Metaphilosophy* 38(2/3): 170–189.

Meilaender, G. (1984). On removing food and water: against the stream. *The Hastings Center Report* 14(6): 11–13.

Meilaender, G. (1998). *Terra es animate*: on having a life. In *On moral medicine: theological perspectives in medical ethics*, eds, A. Verhey and S. Lammers, pp. 390–400. Grand Rapids, MI: Wm. Eerdman's Publishing.

Miller, F. and Joffe, S. (2009). Limits to research risks. *Journal of Medical Ethics* 35(7): 445–449.

Miller, G. F. and Wertheimer, A. (2007). Facing up to paternalism in research ethics. *Hastings Center Report* 37(3): 24–34.

Mills, E. (2008). The egg and I: conception, identity, and abortion. *Philosophical Review* 117(3): 323–348.

Mitford, J. (1974). *Kind and usual punishment: the prison business*, vol. 1. New York: Vintage Books.

Mitscherlich, A. and Mitscherlich, M. (1975). *The inability to mourn: principles of collective behavior*. New York: Grove Press.

Moller, D. (2011). Abortion and moral risk. *Philosophy* 86(3): 425–443.

Monti, M. M., Vanhaudenhuyse, A., Coleman, M. R., Boly, M., Pickard, J. D., Tshibanda, L., Owen, A. M., and Laureys, S. (2010). Willful modulation of brain activity in disorders of consciousness. *New England Journal of Medicine* 362(7): 579–589.

Moon, M. (2011). The effects of divorce on children: married and divorced parents' perspectives. *Journal of Divorce and Remarriage* 52: 344–349.

Morrison, S. (2010). *Palliative care 2020: the future of palliative care*. Available at: www.youtube.com/watch?v=yar-iXPug0A, accessed, 5/17/2018.

Mosteller, T. (2005). Aristotle and headless clones. *Theoretical Medicine and Bioethics* 26(4): 339–350.

Mullins, A. (2010). The opportunity of adversity. *TED Talks*. Available at: www.ted.com/talks/aimee_mullins_the_opportunity_of_adversity.html, accessed 1/17/14.

Murphy, M. C. (1999). The simple desire-fulfillment theory. *Noûs* 33(2): 247–272.

Murrell, W., Féron, F., Wetzig, A., Cameron, N., Splatt, K., Bellette, B., Bianco, J., Perry, C., Lee, G., and Mackay-Sim, A. (2005). Multipotent stem cells from adult olfactory mucosa. *Developmental Dynamics: An Official Publication of the American Association of Anatomists* 233(2): 496–515.

Myles-Worsley, M., Johnston, W. A., and Simons, M. A. (1988). The influence of expertise on X-ray image processing. *Journal of Experimental Psychology: Learning, Memory, and Cognition* 14(3): 553–557.

Nachev, P. and Hacker, P. M. S. (2010). Covert cognition in the persistent vegetative state. *Progress in Neurobiology* 91(1): 68–76.

Nakase-Richardson, R., Whyte, J., Giacino, J. T., Pavawalla, S., Barnett, S. D., Yablon, S. A., Sherer, M., Kalmar, K., Hammond, F. M., Greenwald, B., and Horn, L. J. (2012). Longitudinal outcome of patients with disordered consciousness in the NIDRR TBI Model Systems Programs. *Journal of Neurotrauma* 29(1): 59–65.

Napier, S. (2008). *Virtue epistemology: motivation and knowledge*. New York: Bloomsbury.

Napier, S. (2009). A regulatory argument against human embryonic stem cell research. *Journal of Medicine and Philosophy* 34(5): 496–508.

Napier, S. (2010). Vulnerable embryos: a critical analysis of twinning, rescue, and natural-loss arguments. *American Catholic Philosophical Quarterly* 84(4): 781–810.

Napier, S. (2015). The justification of killing and psychological accounts of the person. *American Catholic Philosophical Quarterly* 89(4): 651–680.

Napier, S. (2016). Thought experiments, the reliability of intuitions, and human embryonic stem cell research. *International Philosophical Quarterly* 56(1): 77–99.

National Bioethics Advisory Commission (NBAC) (1999). *Ethical issues in human stem cell research*, vol. 1. Rockville, MD: National Bioethics Advisory Commission. Available at: https://bioethicsarchive.georgetown.edu/nbac/stemcell.pdf, accessed, 7/18/2018.

National Commission for the Protection of Human Subjects of Biomedical and Behavioral Research (NCPHSBBR) (1975). *Report and recommendations:*

research on the fetus. DHEW Pub. No. (OS) 76–127. Washington, DC: US Department of Health, Education, and Welfare.

National Commission for the Protection of Human Subjects of Biomedical and Behavioral Research (NCPHSBBR) (1976). *Report and recommendations: research involving prisoners.* DHEW Publication No. (OS) 76–131. Washington, DC: US Department of Health, Education, and Welfare.

National Council for Science and Technology (2004). *Guidelines for ethical conduct of biomedical research involving human subjects in Kenya.* Nairobi: National Council for Science and Technology.

Nettleman, M., Ingersoll, K. S., and Ceperich, S. D. (2006). Characteristics of adult women who abstain from sexual intercourse. *BMJ Sexual and Reproductive Health* 32(1): 23–24.

NIH Stem Cell Information Home Page (2016). In *Stem cell information* [website], [cited April 5, 2018]. Bethesda, MD: National Institutes of Health, US Department of Health and Human Services, Available at: www//stemcells.nih.gov/info/basics/1.htm.

Noë, A. (2004). *Action in perception.* Cambridge, MA: MIT Press.

Noonan, H. W. (1985). The closest continuer theory of identity. *Inquiry* 28(1–4): 195–229.

Norton, S. A., Hogan, L. A., Holloway, R. G., Temkin-Greener, H., Buckley, M. J., and Quill, T. E. (2007). Proactive palliative care in the medical intensive care unit: effects on length of stay for selected high-risk patients. *Critical care medicine* 35(6): 1530–1535.

Not Dead Yet (2018). *Not Dead Yet disability activists oppose assisted suicide as a deadly form of discrimination.* Not Dead Yet [website]. Available at: http://notdeadyet.org/assisted-suicide-talking-points, accessed 7/18/2018.

Nozick, R. (1981). *Philosophical explanations.* Cambridge, MA: Harvard University Press.

Nussbaum, M. C. (1990). *Love's knowledge: essays on philosophy and literature.* New York: Oxford University Press.

Oderberg, D. S. (1997a). Modal properties, moral status, and identity. *Philosophy and Public Affairs,* 26(3): 259–276.

Oderberg, D. S. (1997b). Voluntary euthanasia and justice. In *Human lives: critical essays in consequentialist bioethics,* eds, J. Laing and D. Oderberg, pp. 225–240. London: Palgrave Macmillan.

Oderberg, D. S. (2008a). *Real essentialism.* New York: Routledge.

Oderberg, D. S. (2008b). The metaphysical status of the embryo: some arguments revisited. *Journal of Applied Philosophy* 25(4): 263–276.

Oderberg, D. (unpublished). The origination of a human being: rejoinder to Persson. Available at: https://drive.google.com/file/d/0B7SKlRTfkUiecmdYN2lRQm8zdFE/view, accessed, 7/18/2018.

Office of Human Research Protections (n.d.). *Institutional review board guidebook: chapter III basic IRB review.* Rockville, MD: Office of Human Research Protections. Available at: www.hhs.gov/ohrp/irb/irb_chapter3.htm, accessed 9/21/2011.

Okita, K., Matsumura, Y., Sato, Y., Okada, A., Morizane, A., Okamoto, S., . . . and Shibata, T. (2011). A more efficient method to generate integration-free human iPS cells. *Nature Methods* 8(5): 409–412.

Okita, K., Nagata, N., and Yamanaka, S. (2011). Immunogenicity of induced pluripotent stem cells. *Circulation Research* 109(7): 720–721.

Olson, E. T. (1997). *The human animal: personal identity without psychology.* New York: Oxford University Press.

Olson, E. T. (2002). Thinking animals and the reference of 'I'. *Philosophical Topics* 30(1): 189–207.

Olson, E. T. (2007). *What are we? A study in personal ontology.* New York: Oxford University Press.

Olson, E. T. (2017). Personal identity [definition], *The Stanford encyclopedia of philosophy* (Summer 2017 Edition), ed., Edward N. Zalta. Available at: https://plato.stanford.edu/archives/sum2017/entries/identity-personal.

Ord, T. (2008). The scourge: moral implications of natural embryo loss. *American Journal of Bioethics* 8(7): 12–19.

Oregon Health Division (2004). *Sixth annual report on Oregon's Death with Dignity Act.* Portland, OR: Oregon Health Division. Available at: www.ohd.hr.state.or.us/chs/pas/ar-index.cfm.

Owen, A. (2013). Detecting consciousness: a unique role for neuroimaging. *Annual Review of Psychology* 64: 109–133.

Panicola, M. R., Belde, D., Slosar, J., and Repenshek, M. (2011). *Health care ethics: theological foundations, contemporary issues and controversial cases,* 2nd ed. Winona, MN: Anselm Academic.

Parfit, D. (1971). Personal identity. *The Philosophical Review* 80(1): 3–27.

Park, H. and Kitayama, S. (2011). Perceiving through culture: the socialized attention hypothesis. In *The science of social vision,* vol. 7, eds, R. B. Adams Jr, R. B. Adams, N. Ambady, S. Shimojo, and K. Nakayama, 75–89. New York: Oxford University Press.

Pashlar, H. (1999). *The psychology of attention.* Cambridge, MA: MIT Press.

Patel A. N., Henry, T. D., Quyyumi, A. A., Schaer, G. L., Anderson, R. D., Toma, C., East, C., Remmers, A. E., Goodrich, J., Desai, A. S., and Recker, D. (2016). Ixmyelocel-T for patients with ischaemic heart failure: a prospective randomised double-blind trial. *Lancet* 387: 2412–2421, doi: 10.1016/S0140-6736(16)30137-4.

Pellegrino, E. (1996). The place of intention in the moral assessment of assisted suicide and active euthanasia. In *Intending death: the ethics of assisted suicide and euthanasia,* ed., T. Beauchamp, pp. 163–183. Upper Saddle River, NJ: Prentice Hall.

Pellegrino, E. and Thomasma, D. (1988). *For the patient's good: restoration of beneficence in health care.* New York: Oxford University Press.

Penrod, J. D., Deb, P., Luhrs, C., Dellenbaugh, C., Zhu, C. W., Hochman, T., Maciejewski, M. L., Granieri, E., and Morrison, R. S. (2006). Cost and utilization outcomes of patients receiving hospital-based palliative care consultation. *Journal of Palliative Medicine* 9(4): 855–860.

Perkins, D. N., Farady, M., and Bushey, B. (1991). Everyday reasoning and the roots of intelligence. In *Informal reasoning and education,* eds, J. F. Voss, D. N. Perkins, and J. W. Segal, pp. 83–105. Hillsdale, NJ: Erlbaum.

Persson, I. (2009). The origination of a human being: a reply to Oderberg. *Journal of Applied Philosophy* 26(4): 371–378.

Pilsner, J. (2006). *The specification of human actions in St Thomas Aquinas.* New York: Oxford University Press.

Pizarro, D. (2000). Nothing more than feelings? The role of emotions in moral judgment. *Journal for the Theory of Social Behavior* 30(4): 355–375.

Plantinga, A. (1974). *The nature of necessity.* New York: Oxford University Press.

Plantinga, A. (2006). Against materialism. *Faith and Philosophy* 23(1): 3–32.

Plantinga, A. (2007). Materialism and Christian belief. In *Persons: human and divine*, eds, P. Van Inwagen and D. Zimmerman, 99–141. New York: Oxford University Press.

Polanyi, M. (1962). *Personal knowledge*, rev. ed. London: Routledge and Kegan Paul.

Pollock, J. and Cruz, J. (1999). *Contemporary theories of knowledge*, 2nd ed. Savage, MD: Rowman and Littlefield.

Potack, J. Z. and Chokhavatia, S. (2008). Complications of and controversies associated with percutaneous endoscopic gastrostomy: report of a case and literature review. *Medscape Journal of Medicine* 10(6): 142.

President's Commission for the Study of Ethical Problems in Medicine and Biomedical and Behavioral Research (1983). *Deciding to forego life-sustaining treatment*. Washington, DC: U.S. Government Printing Office.

President's Council on Bioethics (2005). White paper: alternative sources of human pluripotent stem cells. Washington, DC: President's Council of Bioethics [online]. Available at: www.bioethics.gov/reports/white_paper/index.html.

Prusak, B. G. (2013). *Parental obligations and bioethics: the duties of a creator*. New York: Routledge.

Pruss, A. (2013). Aristotelian forms and laws of nature. *Analysis and Existence* 24: 115–132.

Pruss, A. (2017). Being a bad person and doing wrong [blog post]. Available at: http://alexanderpruss.blogspot.com/2017/12/being-bad-person-and-doing-wrong.html, accessed 3/15/2018.

Rachels, J. (1986). *The end of life: euthanasia and morality*. New York: Oxford University Press.

Rao, M., Ahrlund-Richter, L., and Kaufman, D. S. (2012). Concise review: cord blood banking, transplantation and induced pluripotent stem cell: success and opportunities. *Stem Cells* 30(1): 55–60.

Rawls, J. (1971). *A theory of justice*. Cambridge, MA: Harvard University Press.

Reardon, D. C. (2018). The abortion and mental health controversy: a comprehensive literature review of common ground agreements, disagreements, actionable recommendations, and research opportunities. *SAGE open medicine* 6, https://doi.org/10.1177/2050312118807624.

Reed, B. (2006). Epistemic circularity squared? Skepticism about common sense. *Philosophy and Phenomenological Research* 73(1): 186–197.

Reed, B. (2012). Resisting encroachment. *Philosophy and Phenomenological Research* 85(2): 465–472.

Rensink, R. A., O'Reagan, J. K., and Clark, J. J. (1997). To see or not to see: the need for attention to perceive changes in scenes. *Psychological Science* 8: 368–373.

Rescher, N. (2006). *Presumption and the practices of tentative cognition*. New York: Cambridge University Press.

Resnik, D. B. (2012). Limits on risks for healthy volunteers in biomedical research. *Theoretical Medicine and Bioethics* 33(2): 137–149.

Resnik, D. B. and Koski, G. (2011). A national registry for healthy volunteers in phase 1 clinical trials. *JAMA: The Journal of the American Medical Association* 305(12): 1236–1237.

Rhonheimer, M. (2009). *The perspective of morality: philosophical foundations of Thomistic virtue ethics*. Trans. G. Malsbary. Washington DC: CUA Press.

Richardson, R. C. (2000). The organism in development. *Philosophy of Science* 67: S312–S321.

Roberts, R. C. and Wood, W. J. (2008). *Intellectual virtues: an essay in regulative epistemology*. New York: Oxford University Press.

Roe, K. M. (1989). Private troubles and public issues: providing abortion amid competing definitions. *Social Science and Medicine* 29(10): 1191–1198.

Roeser, S. (2011). *Moral emotions and intuitions*. New York: Palgrave Macmillan.

Rosen, M. (2018). *Dignity: its history and meaning*. Cambridge: Harvard University Press.

Rosenfield, R. L. (2008). Improving balance in regulatory oversight of research in children and adolescents: a clinical investigator's perspective. *Annals of the New York Academy of Medicine* 1135: 287–295.

Royal College of Psychiatrists (2006). *Statement from the Royal College of Psychiatrists on physician-assisted suicide*. London: Royal College of Psychiatrists. Available at: www.rcpsych.ac.uk/pdf/CPC%2004.05.11%20 Enc%2010.pdf, accessed 5/11/2018.

Rudner, R. (1953). Scientist qua scientist makes value judgments. *Philosophy of Science* 20(1): 1–6.

Russell, B. (1989). The persistent problem of evil. *Faith and Philosophy* 6(2): 121–139.

Rutiku, R., Aru, J., and Bachmann, T. (2016). General markers of conscious visual perception and their timing. *Frontiers in Human Neuroscience* 10:23, doi: 10.3389/fnhum.2016.00023.

Sandel, M. J. (2005). The ethical implications of human cloning. *Perspectives in Biology and Medicine* 48: 241–246.

Savulescu, J. and Schuklenk, U. (2017). Doctors have no right to refuse medical assistance in dying, abortion or contraception. *Bioethics* 31(3): 162–170.

Sayre, K. (1998). *Belief and knowledge: mapping the cognitive landscape*. New York: Rowman & Littlefield Publishers.

Scaltsas, T. (1994a). *Substances and universals in Aristotle's Metaphysics*. Ithaca, NY: Cornell University Press.

Scaltsas, T. (1994b). Substantial holism. In *Unity, identity, and explanation in Aristotle's metaphysics*, eds, T. Scaltsas, D. Charles, and M. L. Gill, pp. 107–128. New York: Oxford University Press.

Schiff, N. D., Rodriguez-Moreno, D., Kamal, A., Kim, K. H. S., Giacino, J. T., Plum, F. and Hirsch, J. (2005). fMRI reveals large-scale network activation in minimally conscious patients. *Neurology* 64: 514–523.

Schumacher, E. F. (1977). *A guide for the perplexed*. New York: Harper Perennial.

Schwarz, S. D. and Tacelli, R. K. (1989). Abortion and some philosophers: a critical examination. *Public Affairs Quarterly* 3(2): 81–98.

Secretary Advisory Committee on Human Research Protections (SACHRP) (2008–2009). Meetings 03-09 and 10-08. Available at: www.hhs.gov/ohrp/ sachrp/mtgings/mtg03-09/present.html and www.hhs.gov/ohrp/sachrp/mtgings/ mtg10-08/present.html respectively, accessed 9/12/2011.

Sehgal, A., Galbraith, A., Chesney, M., Schoenfeld, P., Charles, G., and Lo, B. (1992). How strictly do dialysis patients want their advance directives followed? *JAMA: The Journal of the American Medical Association* 267: 59–63.

Shafer-Landau, R. (2005). *Moral realism: a defence.* New York: Oxford University Press.

Shaw, J. (2006). Intention in ethics. *Canadian Journal of Philosophy* 36(2): 187–223.

Shaw, J. (2015). Death and other harms: intention and the problem of closeness. *American Catholic Philosophical Quarterly* 89(3): 421–439.

Sherman, N. (1991). *The fabric of character: Aristotle's theory of virtue.* New York: Oxford University Press.

Shoemaker, S. (1963). *Self-knowledge and self-identity.* Ithaca, NY: Cornell University Press.

Shoemaker, S. (1984). Personal identity. A materialist's account. In *Personal identity,* eds, S. Shoemaker and R. Swinburne, pp. 67–132. New York: Oxford University Press.

Singer, P. (1979). *Practical ethics.* New York: Cambridge University Press.

Sinnott-Armstrong, W. (2006). *Moral skepticisms.* New York: Oxford University Press.

Sinnott-Armstrong, W. (2008). How to apply generalities: reply to Tohurst and Shafer-Landau. In *Moral psychology: the cognitive science of morality: intuition and diversity,* vol. 2, ed., W. Sinnott Armstrong, pp. 97–106. Cambridge, MA: The MIT Press.

Sloan, D. and Hartz, P. (1992). *Abortion: doctor's perspective, a woman's dilemma.* New York: Donald I Fine.

Smith, B. and Brogaard, B. (2003). Sixteen days. *The Journal of Medicine and Philosophy* 28(1): 45–78.

Snowdon, P. F. (2014). *Persons, animals, ourselves.* New York: Oxford University Press.

Staley, K. W. (2004). *The evidence for the top quark: objectivity and bias in collaborative experimentation.* New York: Cambridge University Press.

Stanford, K. (2017). Underdetermination of scientific theory. *The Stanford Encyclopedia of Philosophy* (Winter edition), ed., Edward N. Zalta. Available at: https://plato.stanford.edu/archives/win2017/entries/scientific-underdetermination.

Stanley, J. (2005). *Knowledge and practical interests.* New York: Oxford University Press.

Stanovich, K., West, R., and Toplak, M. (2013). Myside bias, rational thinking, and intelligence. *Current Direction in Psychological Science* 22(4): 259–264.

Starkey, C. (2006). On the category of moral perception. *Social Theory and Practice* 32(1): 75–96.

Steele, C. M. and Liu, T. J. (1983). Dissonance process as self-affirmation. *Journal of Personality and Social Psychology* 45: 5–19.

Steinbock, B. (2005). Alternative sources of stem cells. *Hastings Center Report* 35(4): 24–26.

Steinbock, B. (2009). Moral status, moral value, and human embryos: implications for stem cell research. In *The Oxford Handbook of Bioethics,* ed., B. Steinbock, pp. 416–440. Oxford, UK: Oxford University Press.

Stith, R. (2014). Construction vs. development: polarizing models of human gestation. *Kennedy Institute of Ethics Journal* 24(4): 345–384.

Stretton, D. (2004). Essential properties and the right to life: a response to Lee. *Bioethics* 18(3): 264–282.

Stretton, D. (2008). Critical notice—defending life: a moral and legal case against abortion choice by Francis J Beckwith. *Journal of Medical Ethics* 34(11): 793–797.

Stump, E. (1986). Providence and the problem of evil. In *Christian Philosophy*, ed., T. Flint, pp. 51–91. Notre Dame, IN: Notre Dame University Press.

Stump, E. (1996). Aquinas on the sufferings of Job. In *The evidential argument from evil*, ed., D. Howard-Snyder, pp. 49–68. Bloomington, IN: Indiana University Press.

Stump, E. (2010). *Wandering in darkness: narrative and the problem of suffering.* New York: Oxford University Press.

Sulmasy, D. P. (2008). Dignity and bioethics: history, theory, and selected applications. In *Human dignity and bioethics: essays commissioned by the President's Council on Bioethics*, ed., A. Schulman, pp. 469–504. Washington, DC: Government Printing Office.

Sun, N., Panetta, N. J., Gupta, D. M., Wilson, K. D., Lee, A., Jia, F., Hu, S., Cherry, A. M., Robbins, R. C., Longaker, M. T., and Wu, J. C. (2009). Feeder-free derivation of induced pluripotent stem cells from adult human adipose stem cells. *Proceedings of the National Academy of Sciences* 106(37): 15720–15725.

Tadros, V. (2011). Consent to harm. *Current Legal Problems* 64: 23–49.

Tang, Y., Yasuhara, T., Hara, K., Matsukawa, N., Maki, M., Yu, G., Xu, L., Hess, D. C., and Borlongan, C. V. (2007). Transplantation of bone marrow-derived stem cells: a promising therapy for stroke. *Cell Transplantation* 16(2): 159–169.

Taylor, J. S. (2016). Autonomy, competence, and end of life. In *Ethics at the end of life: new issues and arguments*, ed., J. K. Davis, pp. 101–115. New York: Routledge.

Temel, J. S., Greer, J. A., Muzikansky, A., Gallagher, E. R., Admane, S., Jackson, V. A., Dahlin, C. M., Blinderman, C. D., Jacobsen, J., Pirl, W. F., and Billings, J. A. (2010). Early palliative care for patients with metastatic non-small-cell lung cancer. *New England Journal of Medicine* 363(8): 733–742.

Thibaut, A., Di Perri, C., Chatelle, C., Bruno, M.-A., Bahri, M. A., Wannez, S., Piarulli, A., Bernard, C., Martial, C., Heine, L., and Hustinx, R. (2015). Clinical response to tDCS depends on residual brain metabolism and grey matter integrity in patients with minimally conscious state. *Brain Stimulation: Basic, Translational, and Clinical Research in Neuromodulation* 8(6): 1116–1123.

Thomson, J. J. (1971). A defense of abortion. *Philosophy and Public Affairs* 1(1): 47–66.

Thomson, J. J. (1995). Abortion. *Boston Review* (online), pp. 11–15 (print). Available at: http://bostonreview.net/archives/BR20.3/thomson.html, accessed 7/18/2018.

Thune, M. (2010). 'Partial defeaters' and the epistemology of disagreement. *The Philosophical Quarterly* 60(239): 355–372.

Tollefsen, C. (2006). Is a purely first-person account of human action defensible? *Ethical Theory and Moral Practice* 9(4): 441–460.

Tollefsen, C. (2010). Fetal interests, fetal persons, and human goods. In *Persons, moral worth, and embryos*, ed., S. Napier, pp. 163–184. Dordrecht: Springer Science and Business Media.

Tollefsen, C. (2011). Some questions for philosophical embryology. *American Catholic Philosophical Quarterly* 85(3): 447–464.

Toner, P. (2011). Hylemorphic animalism. *Philosophical Studies* 155(1): 65–81.

Tooley, M. (1972). Abortion and infanticide. *Philosophy and Public Affairs* 2(1): 37–65.

Trotter, G. (2010). Abortion, secular dogma, and the sacrament of sex: another failed attempt to impose moral idiosyncrasies through the ruse of argument. *The American Journal of Bioethics* 10(12): 51–52.

Unger, P. K. (1996). *Living high and letting die: our illusion of innocence*. New York: Oxford University Press.

US Code of Federal Regulations (2009). *Protection of human subjects*, 45 CFR 46. Bethesda, MD: Office of Human Subjects Research Protections. Available at: http://ohsr.od.nih.gov/guidelines/45cfr46.html, accessed 9/21/2011.

Varelius, J. (2013). Minimally conscious state, human dignity, and the significance of species: a reply to Kaczor. *Neuroethics* 6(1): 85–95.

Vetlesen, A. J. (1994). *Perception, empathy, and judgment: an inquiry into the preconditions of moral performance*. State College, PA: Penn State Press.

Vlastos, G. (1973). The individual as object of love in Plato. In *Platonic studies*, G. Vlastos. Princeton, NJ: Princeton University Press.

Vogelstein, E. (2017). Deciding for the incompetent. In *Ethics at the end of life: new issues and arguments*, ed., J. K. Davis, pp. 108–125. New York: Routledge.

Voss, H. U., Uluç, A. M., Dyke, J. P., Watts, R., Kobylarz, E. J., McCandliss, B. D., Heier, L. A., Beattie, B. J., Hamacher, K. A., Vallabhajosula, S., and Goldsmith, S. J. (2006). Possible axonal regrowth in late recovery from the minimally conscious state. *The Journal of Clinical Investigation* 116(7): 2005–2011.

Vuilleumier, P. (2005). How brains beware: neural mechanisms of emotional attention. *Trends in Cognitive Sciences* 9: 585–594.

Warfield, T. A. (2005). Knowledge from falsehood. *Philosophical Perspectives* 19(1): 405–416.

Warren, L., Manos, P. D., Ahfeldt, T., Loh, Y.-H., Li, H., Lau, F., Ebina, W., Mandal, P. K., Smith, Z. D., Meissner, A., and Daley, G. Q. (2010). Highly efficient reprogramming to pluripotency and directed differentiation of human cells with synthetic modified mRNA. *Cell Stem Cell* 7(5): 618–630.

Warren, M. A. (1973). On the moral and legal status of abortion. *The Monist* 57(1): 43–61.

Warren, M. A. (1992). *Moral status: obligations to persons and other living things*. New York: Clarendon Press.

Watt, H. (2000). *Life and death in healthcare ethics: a short introduction*. New York: Routledge.

Watt, H. (2006). Becoming pregnant or becoming a mother? Embryo transfer with and without a prior maternal relationship. In *Human embryo adoption: biotechnology, marriage, and the right to life*, eds, T. Berg and E. Furton, pp. 55–67. Philadelphia, PA; Thornwood, NY: The National Catholic Bioethics Center and The Westchester Institute for Ethics and the Human Person.

Weijer, C. and Miller, P. B. (2004). When are research risks reasonable in relation to anticipated benefits? *Nature Medicine* 10(6): 570–573.

Weil, S. (1968). The love of God and affliction. In *Science, necessity and the love of God*, S. Weil. New York: Oxford University Press.

Wendler, D. (2005). Protecting subjects who cannot give consent: toward a better standard for "minimal" risks. *Hastings Center Report* 35(5): 37–43.

Wendler, D. (2011). What we worry about when we worry about the ethics of clinical research. *Theoretical Medicine and Bioethics* 32: 161–180.

Wendler, D., Belsky, L., Thompson, K. M., and Emmanuel, E. (2005). Quantifying the federal minimal risk standard: implications for pediatric research without a prospect of direct benefit. *JAMA: The Journal of the American Medical Association* 294(7): 826–832.

White, D., Katz, M. H. MD, Luce, J. M. MD, and Lo. B. (2009). Who should receive life support during a public health emergency? Using ethical principles to improve allocation decisions. *Annals of Internal Medicine* 150: 132–138.

Whyte, J., Katz, D., Long, D., DiPasquale, M. C., Polansky, M., Kalmar, K., Giacino, J., Childs, N., Mercer, W., Novak, P., and Maurer, P. (2005). Predictors of outcome in prolonged posttraumatic disorders of consciousness and assessment of medication effects: a multicenter study. *Archives of Physical Medicine Rehabilitation* 86: 453–462.

Wiggins, D. (1974). Essentialism, continuity, and identity. *Synthese* 28(3–4): 321–359.

Wiggins, D. (2001). *Sameness and substance renewed.* New York: Cambridge University Press.

Willke, J. C. (1984). *Abortion and slavery: history repeats.* Cincinnati, OH: Hayes.

Wreen, M. (1988). The definition of euthanasia. *Philosophy and Phenomenological Research* 48(4): 637–653.

Wreen, M. J. (2004). Hypothetical autonomy and actual autonomy: some problem cases involving advance directives. *The Journal of Clinical Ethics* 15(4): 319–333.

Xiao, J., Nan, Z., Motooka, Y., and Low, W. C. (2005). Transplantation of a novel cell line population of umbilical cord blood stem cells ameliorates neurological deficits associated with ischemic brain injury. *Stem Cells and Development* 14(6): 722–733.

Young, R. (2018). Voluntary euthanasia [definition]. In *The Stanford encyclopedia of philosophy* (Summer edition), ed., Edward N. Zalta. Available at: https://plato.stanford.edu/archives/sum2018/entries/euthanasia-voluntary.

Zagzebski, L. T. (1996). *Virtues of the mind: an inquiry into the nature of virtue and the ethical foundations of knowledge.* Cambridge, UK: Cambridge University Press.

Zagzebski, L. (2001). The uniqueness of persons. *Journal of Religious Ethics* 29(3): 401–423.

Zagzebski, L. (2004). *Divine motivation theory.* New York: Cambridge University Press.

Zagzebski, L. T. (2012). *Epistemic authority: a theory of trust, authority and autonomy in belief.* New York: Oxford University Press.

Zhao, T., Zhang, Z. N., Rong, Z., and Xu, Y. (2011). Immunogenicity of induced pluripotent stem cells. *Nature* 474(7350): 212–215.

Ziegner, U. H., Ochs, H. D., Schanen, C., Feig, S. A., Seyama, K., Futatani, T., Gross, T., Wakim, M., Roberts, R. L., Rawlings, D. J., and Dovat, S. (2001). Unrelated umbilical cord stem cell transplantation for X-linked immunodeficiencies. *Journal of Pediatrics* 138(4): 570–573.

Zuniga, G. (2004). An ontology of dignity. *Metaphysica* 5(2): 115–131.

Index

Printed in the United States
by Baker & Taylor Publisher Services